| Wallace Library | DUE DATE (stamped in blue)<br>RETURN DATE (stamped in black) |
|---|---|
|  |  |
|  |  |
|  |  |
|  |  |
|  |  |
|  |  |
|  |  |
|  |  |
|  |  |

# HEARING CARE FOR CHILDREN

### Editors

### Frederick N. Martin

*The University of Texas, Austin*

### John Greer Clark

*HearCare, Inc., Cincinnati, Ohio*

**ALLYN AND BACON**

*Boston • London • Toronto • Sydney • Tokyo • Singapore*

**Series Editor:** Kris Farnsworth
**Editorial Assistant:** Christine Svitila
**Editorial-Production Administrator:** Joe Sweeney
**Editorial-Production Service:** Walsh Associates
**Composition Buyer:** Linda Cox
**Manufacturing Buyer:** Aloka Rathnam
**Cover Administrator:** Suzanne Harbison

**Library of Congress Cataloging-in-Publication Data**
Hearing care for children / edited by Frederick N. Martin and John
   Greer Clark.
      p.     cm.
   Includes bibliographical references and index.
   ISBN 0-13-124702-6
   1. Hearing disorders in children.   I. Martin, Frederick N.
II. Clark, John Greer.
   [DNLM:   1. Hearing Disorders—in infancy & childhood.   WV 271
   H4344   1995]
RF291.5.C45H314   1995
618.92′0978—dc20
DNLM/DLC
for Library of Congress                                    95-36484
                                                           CIP

Printed in the United States of America
10  9  8  7  6  5  4  3  2  1       00  99  98  97  96  95

# CONTENTS

# PART V
# INTERVENTION/EDUCATION FOR CHILDREN
# WITH HEARING LOSS    285

## 15  EARLY INTERVENTION    287
**Donald M. Goldberg**

## 16  EDUCATIONAL MANAGEMENT OF CHILDREN WITH
## HEARING LOSS    303
**Carolyn Edwards**

## 17  EDUCATIONAL AUDIOLOGY    316
**James C. Blair**

# PREFACE

Working with children and their families has perhaps more far-reaching effects than any other challenge audiologists undertake. The effects of sensory deprivation can be minimized only through early identification and detection, and yet generalizations in approach and procedure of management are difficult. Each child's situation is unique because of unpredictable combinations of personality traits and hearing abilities, and the equally unpredictable dynamics within each family. One fact, however, is not unpredictable. The child's ultimate use of audition to develop spoken language depends, to a large extent, on the quality of intervention we make available.

The care we provide our pediatric patients will necessarily have a determining impact on their future development, and on their potential for rehabilitation and education. As audiologists, we cannot overestimate the importance of our responsibility to their lives. Nor is our responsibility limited to the children alone. Inevitably, our efforts will have a significant effect on the future of those most closely involved with them and on their emotions. The child's immediate and extended families often discover their own lives completely restructured as they strive to cope with situations never before encountered, particularly constantly re-emerging emotional conflicts and day-to-day mechanics of meeting both communication and rehabilitative demands.

Success in (re)habilitation of children with hearing disorders requires insight from of a number of individuals, and effective interactions among them. Audiologists, otolaryngologists, pediatricians, speech-language pathologists, educators of the deaf and hearing impaired, classroom teachers, and educational support personnel must work together toward a common goal. Whether this collaboration is formal or informal, the audiologist's interaction with members of this team of professionals is crucial to successful (re)habilitation.

The diagnostic process follows a recognizable pattern. Upon suspicion of a hearing loss following neonatal or early childhood screening or in response to expressed parental concern, the child and parents will undergo a series of tests and interviews. The underlying etiologies of pediatric hearing loss may be elusive and may affect more than just the hearing mechanism. The pediatrician will consult with an otolaryngologist and professionals in genetic counseling while diagnosis is sought and any associated anomalies are identified. It is within this diagnostic process that the expertise of audiologists will first be drawn upon. Within this process audiologists are often the first professionals to provide the parents with confirmation of the existence of a permanent, handicapping condition.

Following the diagnosis of hearing impairment, professionals often talk of parent management, and/or management of the child with hearing loss. We would be wise to remember that it is actually the (re)habilitation process itself that we are attempting to manage. Debate may arise over who heads the management team, and the audiologist must be sensitive to this. Educators may argue that they are in a more regular contact with the child and parents and therefore should be considered to be in the best position to head the team. Physicians may argue that the hearing loss will require medical supervision and that this should place them as the team managers. Audiologists will frequently state that as they are usually the professionals who are in frequent or at least periodic contact with each other member of the team, they should head the (re)habilitative endeavors.

The professional egotism underlying such debates becomes readily apparent when we consider that it is the parents who accompany their children to the audiologist, the physician, and the speech-language pathologist and who hold forth the endurance that will provide the needed support throughout the child's life. It is for these reasons that one of the most important players on the hearing loss management team, and the team's inevitable head, should always be the child's parents. It becomes one of the audiologist's primary roles to facilitate the parents' efforts in meeting the challenges ahead.

Within this text we have included an overview of the medical pathologies of childhood hearing loss and a background discussion of the effects of hearing loss. However, we have striven to provide an emphasis on the actual practice of pediatric audiology. Toward this end, we have included more in-depth coverage of the psychological impact of childhood hearing loss and the audiologist's counseling responsibilities for those most closely affected; the audiologist's role in the identification and assessment of hearing loss in children; methods employed to enhance the reception of auditory signals; and the audiologist's need to understand and interact within the remediation of children with impaired hearing. We view this as a different and more (re)habilitative orientation to the topic of hearing loss in children: an approach we believe will prepare future audiologists to tackle the many challenges presented by the children they see.

The content level of this book assumes no prior knowledge on the reader's part beyond that obtained in an introductory audiology course. While primarily written for audiologists, it is hoped that the information presented may be of value to all professionals whose work impacts the lives of children with hearing loss and their caregivers. It is further hoped that this text will help promote an increased understanding of the contributions of various professionals on the hearing loss management team, thereby increasing professional dialogue and interaction on behalf of the children we serve.

*The child with no problems is easy to teach,*
*But needs and deserves all our care.*
*But the child who is challenged has further to reach,*
*And should get a more bountiful share.*

*We dedicate this book to the parents and children we have had the pleasure to know.*
*Our lives have been enriched by all they have shared with us.*

*FNM/JGC*

# CHAPTER CONTRIBUTORS

Ellyn Altman, Ph.D, P.C.
Clinical Psychologist, Great Neck, New York
and Adelphi University Postdoctoral Institute for
    the Advanced Studies of Psychotherapy and
    Psychoanalysis

Kathleen S. Arnos, Ph.D.
Genetic Services Center
Gallaudet University Research Institute

James C. Blair, Ph.D.
Department of Communicative Disorders and
    Deaf Education
Utah State University

Craig A. Champlin, Ph.D.
Communication Sciences and Disorders
The University of Texas at Austin

Patricia A. Chase, M.S.
Division of Hearing and Speech Services
School of Medicine
Vanderbilt University

John Greer Clark, Ph.D.
HearCare, Inc.
Cincinnati, Ohio

Lisa Devlin, M.S.
Department of Audiology and Speech-Language
    Pathology
Gallaudet University

Allan O. Diefendorf, Ph.D.
Department of Otolaryngology
Indiana University School of Medicine

Carolyn Edwards, M.Cl.Sc., M.B.A.
Auditory Management Services
Toronto, Ontario

Donald M. Goldberg, Ph.D.
Helen Beebe Speech and Hearing Center
Easton, Pennsylvania

James W. Hall, III, Ph.D.
Division of Hearing and Speech Sciences
and Department of Otolaryngology
    School of Medicine
    Vanderbilt University

Daniel P. Harris, Ph.D.
Healthcare Rehabilitation Center
Austin, Texas

Jamie Israel, M.S.
Genetic Services Center
Gallaudet University Research Institute

Michael Jaindl, M.D.
Private Practice
Kingsville, Texas

Danielle M.R. Kelsay, M.A.
Department of Otolaryngology
The University of Iowa Hospitals and Clinics

Frederick N. Martin, Ph.D.
Communication Sciences and Disorders
The University of Texas at Austin

Robert J. Nozza, Ph.D.
Department of Communication Sciences and
    Disorders
College of Education
The University of Georgia

Mark Ross, Ph.D.
Professor Emeritus
University of Connecticut

Linda M. Thibodeau, Ph.D.
Communication Sciences and Disorders
The University of Texas at Austin

Richard S. Tyler, Ph.D.
Department of Otolaryngology
The University of Iowa Hospitals and Clinics

Jay A. Werkhaven, M.D.
Department of Otolaryngology
School of Medicine
Vanderbilt University

Mary Pat Wilson, M.S.
Department of Audiology and Speech-Language
    Pathology
Gallaudet University

# ABOUT THE EDITORS

Frederick N. Martin, Ph.D., City University of New York, is the Lille Hage Jamail Centennial Professor in Communication Sciences and Disorders. His publications include 9 single-authored books, 4 edited books, 15 book chapters, over 100 journal articles, numerous conference and convention papers and several monographs. Martin has won the Teaching Excellence Award of the College of Communication, the Graduate Teaching Award, and the Advisor's Award of the Ex-Students' Association of The University of Texas, in addition to being the second-prize winner of the Beltone Award for Outstanding Teaching in Audiology. His research interests revolve around pediatric diagnosis and patient and parent counseling.

John Greer Clark, Ph.D., has been in independent private practice since 1982. His primary interests in audiologic rehabilitation are in hearing instrumentation and patient-family counseling. He is the recipient of the Honors of the Ohio Speech and Hearing Association and the Prominent Alumni and Distinguished Alumnus Awards from the Communication Sciences and Disorders Department at the University of Cincinnati. Dr. Clark is a member of the Board of Directors of the American Academy of Audiology and the Ohio Academy of Audiology. He has served as an associate editor of *HEARSAY* and as editorial consultant for *Ear & Hearing* and *Language, Speech, and Hearing Services in the Schools*. His more than 40 publications include two edited textbooks, and two single-authored books.

# PART ONE

# CAUSES AND EFFECTS OF CHILDHOOD HEARING LOSS

# CHAPTER 1

## HEARING LOSS AND ITS EFFECTS

*ALLAN O. DIEFENDORF*

## INTRODUCTION

Children with hearing loss are just as unique as children with normal hearing. Each child's individual "blueprint," including familial and environmental factors, provides the foundation for developmental achievement and outcome. Children with hearing loss, however, may not have immediate access to language and thus may differ from their normal hearing peers in their language development and in their facility with communication. Because language and communication serve as the foundation for normal child development, delays in the acquisition of these skills impact other aspects of child development such as literacy, academic achievement, and social development.

A widely held belief in the professional community is that children with hearing loss represent a homogeneous group with similar limitations. The use of such terms as the *deaf child* or the *hard-of-hearing child* subtly implies that youngsters, once categorized by degree of hearing loss, are more alike than different. Yet to assume that any group of children with hearing loss is a homogenous sample with similar limitations and needs will lead to a substantial number of youngsters erroneously profiled. However, any discussion of the effects of hearing loss on this heterogeneous group of children must be based on the assumption that there are some central issues affecting children with hearing loss that can be discussed for the group as a whole in spite of the diversity it represents.

The purpose of this chapter is to provide an overview of the effects of hearing loss on children and their developmental outcome. This chapter will take an introductory posture so that the complex topic of the effects of hearing loss on children will be appreciated, and an interest in pursuing various issues in detail will hopefully have been enhanced.

## FACTORS AFFECTING CHILDREN WITH HEARING LOSS

All children with hearing loss have at least one characteristic in common: They do not hear normally. Beyond that basic fact, however, children with hearing loss represent a heterogeneous population, varying on a number of factors. As a result, every child brings a unique combination of characteristics to the developmental equation. In turn, habilitative and educational needs in all cases are complex, extensive, and long term. The importance of ascertaining some of these factors is that more appropriate initial planning and intervention can be undertaken.

The age of onset of a hearing loss exerts a strong influence on the effects that it will have on a child's communicative skills and developmental outcome. From a developmental point of view, the effects of a sensory deficit will depend on the stage of development that exists at the time the deficit occurs. A child who has a congenital hearing loss is at greater risk for delays in oral language development than is the child who acquires a hearing loss after some period of normal auditory experience. The degree of hearing loss is another factor that interacts with age-of-onset of hearing loss and affects the child's communicative skill and developmental achievement. Stated simply, the greater the hearing loss, the greater the reduction in loudness for some (or all) of the component frequencies of speech. This results in a decrease in the number of acoustic cues that are available to the listener. Children with fluctuating conductive hearing loss caused by persistent otitis media, children with mild and moderate bilateral sensorineural hearing loss, and children with unilateral hearing loss usually go undetected longer than children who sustain more severe degrees of hearing loss. Most parents regard hearing loss as "all or none," and the notion of a partial impairment is unfamiliar to them. Yet each of these hearing impairments has a complex, and varied set of symptoms that accompany them (Table 1.1). The location within the auditory system of the condition causing hearing loss is another factor influencing the overall impact of hearing loss. Generally, the more peripheral the lesion site, the greater the possibility for successful auditory perception.

Other handicapping conditions (Table 1.2) can coexist with hearing loss and serve to exaggerate the effects of the hearing impairment on developmental processes. Some problems such as mental retardation, physical disabilities, or reduced visual acuity may be relatively easy to diagnose. In contrast, deficits in visual processing, visual-motor coordination, or memory, which also have been found to occur in children with hearing loss, are more difficult to identify. The advantage of identifying at the outset the array of handicapping conditions is that more appropriate initial planning and intervention can be undertaken. The audiologist must investigate the factors involved in each individual case by use of interviews, case histories, assessments by other professionals, and close observation. Provision of appropriate services depends on a thorough knowledge of the individual to be served and his or her family system.

## DISABILITY VERSUS CULTURAL MODELS: DEVELOPING A BALANCED PERSPECTIVE

Regardless of the language system (English or American Sign Language) or communication form (oral or manual) used in the home, children will be seriously compromised in the development of communication skills without early detection of hearing loss and the provision of learning environments that fit the unique needs of the child and family. When achieved, parental and educational practices with deaf or hard-of-hearing individuals from infancy to early adulthood should have as their primary goal the establishment of an easy and fluent system of communication. This system should be internalized as a language foundation on which the secondary language systems of reading and writing can then be developed. This philosophy allows each family unit to implement a model of learning (Figure 1.1) that is desirable and appropriate for their individual circumstances. While I believe in the value of both the disability and cultural models of learning, they are not without controversy. Yet if clinicians maintain a family-centered philosophy (parents and professionals engaged in a *collaborative process* to determine what is best for both the child and the family), then families decide what model is consistent with their attitudes, values, and beliefs, and the controversy need not be so polarizing.

Ogden (1984) maintains that the critical factor in creating a healthy home environment for a child with hearing loss is good communication. This recommendation carries the strong implication that a language system be quickly established. Research bears out the crucial importance of establishing a communicative attitude that requires parent-child reciprocity, or taking turns (Kretschmer and Kretschmer, 1979). Simply stated, for attachment to continue as a helpful bonding force in the process of parenting a child with hearing loss, parents must not only guide and direct the child, they must also allow for guidance and direction *from* the child. This kind of reciprocal give-and-take leads naturally to mutual expectations based on shared information and knowledge and on early learning of the rules for social communication (Hunt, 1979).

### Hearing Loss as a Disability

Some families (with hearing parents) will view their child with hearing loss with strong emotional

**TABLE 1.1**   Symptoms Associated with Conductive Hearing Loss; Unilateral Hearing Loss; Mild, Bilateral Sensorineural Hearing Loss, and Moderate-to-severe Bilateral Sensorineural Hearing Loss

|  | AUDIOLOGICAL | COMMUNICATIVE | EDUCATIONAL |
|---|---|---|---|
| **CONDUCTIVE HEARING LOSS** | • Hearing loss 30db (range 10–50 db)<br>• Poor auditory reception<br>• Degraded and inconsistent speech signal<br>• Difficulty understanding under adverse listening conditions<br>• Impaired speech discrimination<br>• HL overlays developmental requirement for greater stimulus intensity before infants can respond to and discriminate between speech<br>• Inability to organize auditory information consistently | • Difficulty forming linguistic categories (plurals, tense)<br>• Difficulty in differentiating word boundaries phoneme boundaries<br>• Receptive language delay<br>• Expressive language delay<br>• Cognitive delay | • Lower achievement test scores<br>• Lower verbal IQ<br>• Poorer reading and spelling performance<br>• Higher frequency of enrollment in special support classes in school<br>• Lower measures of social maturity |
| **UNILATERAL HEARING LOSS** | • Hearing loss moderate-to-profound<br>• Impaired auditory localization<br>• Difficulty understanding speech in presence of competing noise<br>• Loss of binaural advantage: binaural summation binaural release from masking | • Tasks involving language concepts may be depressed | • Lags in academic achievement reading spelling arithmetic<br>• Verbally based learning difficulties<br>• High rate of grade repetition<br>• Self-described embarrassment annoyance confusion helplessness<br>• Less independence in the classroom |
| **MILD BILATERAL SENSORINEURAL HEARING LOSS** | • Hearing loss 15–40 dB<br>• Speech recognition depressed<br>• Auditory discrimination depressed<br>• Amplification considered FM systems classroom amplification | • Potential problems in articulation<br>• Problems in auditory attention<br>• Problems in auditory memory<br>• Problems in auditory comprehension<br>• Possible delays in expressive oral language<br>• Impact on syntax and semantics<br>• Impact on vocabulary development | • Lowered academic achievement arithmetic problem-solving math concepts vocabulary reading comprehension<br>• Educational delays progress systematically with age |
| **MODERATE-TO-SEVERE BILATERAL SENSORINEURAL HEARING LOSS** | • Hearing loss between 41 dB–90 dB<br>• Noise and reverberation significantly affect listening and understanding<br>• Audiologic management essentials amplification recommendations monitor hearing for: • otitis media • sudden changes in hearing • progressive hearing loss Member of Educational Planning Team | • Deficits in speech perception<br>• Deficits in speech production (mild-to-moderate articulation problems)<br>• Language deficits from slight to significant syntax morphology semantics pragmatics<br>• Vocabulary deficits | • Slight to significant deficits in literacy (reading and writing)<br>• Deficits in academic achievement<br>• High rate of academic failure<br>• Immaturity<br>• Feelings of isolation and exclusion<br>• Special education supports needed |

**TABLE 1.2**  Additional Handicapping Condition(s) That Can Coexist with Hearing Loss

---

### PHYSICAL CONDITION

Brain damage or injury

Epilepsy (convulsive disorder)

Cerebral palsy

Cardiovascular defects

Orthopedic and gait abnormalities (restricted use of extremities as a result of permanent injury or paralysis)

Legal blindness

Uncorrected or uncorrectable visual problem (blindness in one eye, muscular imbalance or paralysis)

Other health impairment (asthma, thyroid, diabetes, kidney defects, other immunologic, endocrine, and metabolic disorders)

---

### COGNITIVE INTELLECTUAL CONDITION

Mental retardation

Specific learning disability (visual/auditory perceptual problems; perceptual/motor function difficulty; attention deficits; lack of control of impulse; lack of control of motor function)

Emotional/behavioral problem (behaviors include passive/withdrawn; aggressive/abusive; rapid mood changes/sudden outbursts; chronic, unfounded physical complaints and symptoms)

---

Adapted from Karchmer, M. A. (1985). A demographic perspective. In C. Cherow (ed.), *Hearing Impaired Children and Youth with Developmental Disabilities*. Washington, DC: Gallaudet College Press.

reactions very similar to the reactions of individuals who have lost a loved one through death. While it is true that the parents of these children in reality have not "lost" their child, nevertheless they have lost the hopes, dreams, and aspirations that they held for the child when they viewed the child as normal. These families may view hearing loss as a disability and approach intervention and

learning environments from this perspective. Oral English as the language and form is advocated, and different communication methodologies (aural-oral, cued speech, total communication) may be employed to achieve this goal.

The view of hearing loss as a disability maintains that deaf and hard-of-hearing people should be protected by legislative action. As such, deaf and hard-of-hearing people have joined other groups in lobbying for laws to protect people with disabilities from discrimination and to assist persons with disabilities in becoming fully participating members of society. The Rehabilitation Act of 1973, the Individuals with Disabilities Education Act, the Americans with Disabilities Act, the Fair Housing Act Amendments of 1988, the Air Carriers Access Act, the Television Decoder Circuitry Act, as well as numerous other state and federal laws have all been enacted over the past twenty years and are intended to assist and protect individuals with the disability of hearing loss.

## Hearing Loss as a Culture

Potential parents who are deaf or severely hard-of-hearing will, at one time or another, confront their innermost feelings about the hearing of the child to come. While many claim the most important thing is to have a healthy child (apparently viewing hearing ability as secondary), the parents' real feelings are manifested to varying degrees at the time of diagnosis. In general, parents who are deaf or severely hard-of-hearing often express a desire for deaf children for the sake of easy assimilation into the family. American Sign Language as the native language is advocated, and English as a second language is recognized.

These families view hearing loss from a cultural perspective, with a realization that deafness is not synonymous with disability unless thwarted by barriers caused by a lack of information and reasonable accommodations in the environment. This model recognizes people who are deaf as a minority with its own language and culture; deafness is not a disability, in the sense that nothing is "broken" that needs to be fixed.

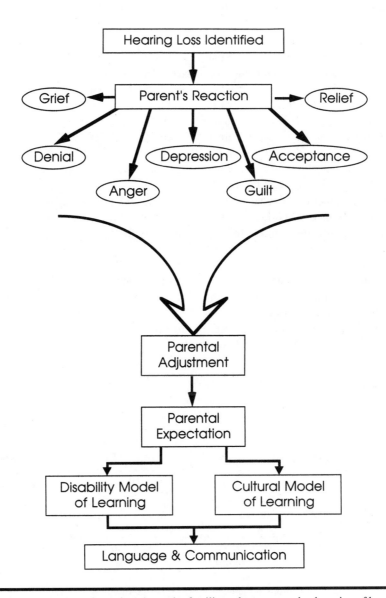

**FIGURE 1.1**   Models of learning chosen by families subsequent to the detection of hearing loss. Both approaches emphasize language and communication.

Either model is appropriate, depending on the characteristics of the family. As seen from Table 1.3, an outcome that does not fit either model, but must be acknowledged, is children with normal hearing born to deaf or severely hard-of-hearing parents. Eighty to 90 percent of children born to congenitally or prelingually deaf individuals have normal hearing (Schein and Delk, 1974). This can create a family dynamic in which the normal-hearing child can become a reminder to the parents of their own limitations in communication. When assigned the role of the parent's communication link or interpreter with the external world, the child with normal hearing becomes a way to compensate for these limitations. Deaf parents who are insensitive to the developing child's needs will have difficulty allowing the normal-hearing child to be a child. If the child is viewed as a normal-hearing extension of deaf parents, strains will occur in the parent–child relationship (Altschuler, 1963; Schlesinger and Meadow, 1972). These children can become either overly responsible or may look for escape through rebellion or poor compliance with parental requests.

There are, however, many deaf parents who understand the basic principles of child development. These parents have the capacity to empathize with the experiences of the children with normal hearing, valuing them as children regardless of their hearing ability. Such parents are sensitive about relying on the child with normal hearing who is willing and able to serve as interpreter or telephone conduit; they make sure the child is not overburdened. While audiologists may only deal with this family dynamic from a distance, is is important to recognize the dynamics of this constellation in counseling parents after normal hearing has been ascertained by the audiologist. Parents with hearing loss should be made aware of the possibility of speech and language problems resulting from oral language deprivation in order to accept referrals for professional help when necessary.

## DEFINITION OF TERMS

Up to this point different terms have been used in this chapter without proper definitions. Because much confusion in interpreting educational and research data in the field results from incomplete descriptions of the individuals involved, and from generalizations of findings to dissimilar populations, definition of terms is essential.

The degree of hearing loss is almost always important when discussing the effects of hearing loss on child development. The terms *deaf* and

TABLE 1.3    Interactions That Can Occur by Family Constellation and Model of Learning

|  |  | CHILDREN | | |
|---|---|---|---|---|
|  |  | Normal Hearing | Hearing Loss to Profound Level | Profound Hearing Loss to No Measurable Hearing |
| PARENTS | Normal Hearing | Native language Culture of the home | Disability model | Disability model (likely) Cultural model (possible) |
|  | Deaf | Native language/English (or both) Culture of the home | Cultural model (likely) Disability model (possible) | Cultural Model |

*hard-of-hearing* also refer to degree of loss, but these two classifications that are often used by professionals have many shades of meaning. It is becoming increasingly difficult to use these labels in a way that will enable those with varied viewpoints and perspectives to construe a common meaning. The current definitions have been adopted from the approach of Boothroyd (1982) in which definition of these terms is based on the ability of the individual to use audition to understand speech, if necessary, with amplification.

The term *deaf* describes an individual whose hearing loss is so profound that the auditory channel cannot be used as the primary one to perceive and monitor speech or to acquire language. This does not negate the possible value of amplification for children who are deaf: It does, however, imply that for them sound is a secondary and supplemental channel to vision or touch. It is an apparent contradiction of terms to talk about exploiting residual hearing in a person who is deaf. The improper application of the descriptive label deaf can lead to an educational placement and, therefore, achievement and behavioral expectations consistent with the connotations of the label rather than of the potential of the child. The term *hard-of-hearing* is used to describe an individual who uses hearing as the primary mode for speech perception, speech monitoring, and language acquisition. Information perceived through the visual modality (i.e., through speech reading or a manually coded system) may supplement information that is perceived through audition.

Although the amount of residual hearing is an important indicator for separating the hard-of-hearing from the deaf, it is not the only one. The age at which the hearing loss is detected, the family outlook on hearing impairment, and the effectiveness of early habilitative measures are just several of the all important influences on the child's ultimate status. The recognition of an individual's needs and unique status must transcend any categorical attempt of definition or description. Categories such as hard-of-hearing and deaf are guidelines, not specific prescriptions for ser-

vices or proscriptions of exclusion from certain other services.

The term *hearing impairment* is a generic term indicating a hearing loss that may range in severity from mild to profound; it includes the subsets of deaf and hard-of-hearing, although some individuals with a cultural perspective have suggested that the term *impairment* carries a negative connotation when describing individuals with hearing loss. It is not possible to draw firm boundaries between "deaf" and "hard-of-hearing" on the basis of severity of loss shown on an audiogram. However, the following classification system, based on the average of pure-tone hearing threshold levels of 500, 1000, and 2,000 Hz, is a general guide to degree of severity of hearing losses (Clark, 1981).

| | |
|---|---|
| *00–15 dB* | *Normal* |
| *16–25 dB* | *Slight or minimal hearing loss* |
| *26–40 dB* | *Mild hearing loss* |
| *41–55 dB* | *Moderate hearing loss* |
| *56–70 dB* | *Moderately severe hearing loss* |
| *71–90 dB* | *Severe hearing loss* |
| *>90 dB* | *Profound hearing loss* |

Knauf (1978) made the following observation, however, about the degree of hearing loss:

> *The hearing threshold level is perhaps the primary variable for estimating the impact of a child's hearing impairment and it frequently is the first measure available. It is not surprising then that judgments and classifications of the hearing impaired are sometimes based only on this criterion. While classifications based on hearing level are valuable in estimating the impact of a certain hearing level on an average child and in the early counseling of parents, there are many exceptions. Some unusual children with profound losses of 90 dB perform better in language and academic skills compared to other children with average intelligence and moderately severe losses of 70 dB. Similar individual variations will be found along the entire continuum of hearing levels. (p. 550)*

It is not possible to predict language or educational performance of children with hearing impairment on the basis of degree of hearing loss alone, whether the measure used is a pure-tone average or one of speech recognition threshold and/or word recognition. Thus, the audiometric classification system defines the severity of hearing loss, not the behavioral impact on communication function and developmental outcome.

Within a broad range of behavior and development there are certain outcomes that are somewhat typical of children who are hard-of-hearing and children who are deaf. This chapter will focus on children who are hard-of-hearing and their families to describe the effects of hearing loss. The problems these children exhibit in speech perception, speech and language production, academic achievement and social behavior are related to the degree of hearing loss. *Hearing* is the key; it is the major cause of the disability and the major avenue through which the disability can best be minimized or overcome. *Deafness,* on the other hand, is an entirely separate issue from hearing and that separation is recognized and respected in this chapter.

## EFFECT OF HEARING LOSS ON PARENT–CHILD INTERACTIONS

As discussed in Chapter 9, families are impacted emotionally by the confirmation of hearing loss in their child. While grief is an understandable reaction to loss, the parents' reaction to the loss may have significant influence on rehabilitation outcomes. The parents play a key role in a hearing-impaired child's intervention program, especially during the infant and preschool years. The presence of a severe or profound hearing loss can disrupt aspects of adult–child interactions. Research findings in the normal developmental literature show that adults speak to infants in special ways; this is because infants react to the conversational attempts of adults, and adults interact with infants as if they were conversational partners long before children are language users (Sachs, 1985).

Moses and Van Hecke-Wulatin (1981) have described the problems that mothers experience in attempting to interact playfully and positively with their hearing-impaired infants, suggesting that the mother may often have difficulty viewing her relationship with the child as being a reciprocal one. Results of past investigations (Goss, 1970; Kenworthy, 1986; Kricos, 1982) suggest that there is need to teach parents of young hearing-impaired children to identify and respond to their children's nonverbal communication attempts. Assuming that adult–child interchanges serve some prelinguistic function, it is easy to see how severe delays in language development can begin during early childhood for those with hearing impairment.

## SPEECH AND LANGUAGE SKILLS OF CHILDREN WITH HEARING LOSS

The effect of hearing loss on the development of speech and language skills is both varied and complex. All things being equal, the more severe the hearing loss and the earlier the onset, the greater the effects on developmental processes.

### Speech Perception

One function of the peripheral auditory system is to convert the auditory speech signal into a neural code for input to the central nervous system. When this function is disrupted by hearing loss, some or all of the information in the speech signal may be coded inaccurately or not at all. The problems of speech perception by persons with hearing loss cannot be treated only in terms of audibility. There is also a loss of frequency resolution, and possibly of temporal resolution, which interferes with the discriminability of phonemes and speech features. Thus, hearing loss introduces much more complex signal distortions than simple filtering and attenuation.

It is convenient to classify consonant phonemes according to their characteristic subphonemic features. Although many different and more elaborate sets of subphonemic features have been devised, it is possible to describe all consonants in terms of the three-feature set consisting of manner, voicing, and place. The manner feature describes the specific articulatory gesture used to produce the consonant. The voicing feature classifies consonants according to the presence or absence of the laryngeal tone as a sound source. The place feature relates to the point in the vocal tract at which the consonant is produced. Listeners with moderate and severe hearing losses are able to perceive consonant voicing and manner of articulation distinctions (e.g., /ba/ versus /pa/; /ba/ versus /ma/; or /ba/ versus /za/), but they have a great deal of difficulty in distinguishing place of articulation (e.g., /ba/ versus /da/ versus /ga/). Erber (1972) found that children with severe hearing losses not only had trouble distinguishing place of articulation, they also often confused consonants with differing manners of articulation (e.g., /ba/ versus /va/). The children with severe hearing loss in Erber's study were able to distinguish nasal versus nonnasal consonants (e.g., /ma/ versus /ba/), although their labeling of /m/ and /n/ was not always correct.

The spectrum of any vowel will contain energy at the fundamental frequency of the speaker's voice and its harmonics. Yet each vowel will be distinguished by certain peaks in the spectrum that result from the placement of the articulators and the size and shape of the vocal tract as it forms that particular vowel. These peaks of energy are called *formants,* and vowels can be defined in terms of the formant frequencies associated with them. All vowels of English can be distinguished from each other on the basis of the lowest frequency formants. The lowest frequency formant (F1) corresponds roughly to the degree of tongue constriction employed during vowel production; those vowels that are produced with a relatively narrow constriction (high vowels) are characterized by a relatively low-frequency F1. Vowels produced with the tongue lower in the mouth have a higher frequency F1. The second formant (F2) corresponds to the front-back place of major vocal tract constriction; the frequency of F2 is high for front vowels and then decreased as the place of constriction moves to the back of the oral cavity.

Vowel confusions occur much less frequently than consonant confusions. However, children with moderate to severe hearing losses can have difficulty distinguishing one vowel from another. Confusions may involve vowels with high-frequency second formants (e.g., /i/ (bee) versus /I/ (big)) or they may involve confusions between front and back vowels that have similar first frequency formants (e.g., /i/ (tea) versus /u/ (two)).

The effect of hearing loss on phoneme perception is almost entirely predictable on the basis of the frequency location of acoustic cues in the speech signal. Vowels are the most intense phonemes, and energy in the first formant region accounts for much of the energy in the long-term speech spectrum. It is therefore not surprising that vowels are perceived more accurately than consonants, because vowel energy would likely remain audible even if some consonant energy were rendered inaudible by hearing loss. Errors on front vowels may occur most often because front vowels have higher frequency second formants. Because the amplitude of vowel formants decreases as their frequency increases, the F2 energy in front vowels is also lower in amplitude than is F2 energy in back vowels. Children with hearing loss are likely to have abnormal auditory thresholds at high frequencies. This characteristic of hearing loss, combined with the acoustic structure of front vowels, results in a reduction in the audibility of F2 energy in front vowels. The lower frequency, higher intensity first formant remains audible and becomes the only information on which the child can base vowel judgments. Moreover, vowels that share F1 frequency characteristics may also be confused with each other.

The consonant errors reported also make sense in terms of the frequencies associated with speech information. Children with hearing loss at high frequencies have little difficulty perceiving low-frequency voicing information. The low-frequency nasal murmur, which is a powerful cue for nasal manner information, is also usable. This is reflected in the low incidence of phoneme errors involving nasality. Other types of manner information, however, extend to higher frequencies and are thus more likely to be perceived inaccurately. The most disruptive effects of high-frequency hearing loss could be expected to be exerted on speech information confined to the high frequencies. Place information fits this description well. However, most children with severe hearing losses are able to perceive place of articulation through lipreading. Thus, with combined auditory and visual cues, information perceived through the two sensory channels complement one another: That is, manner and voicing are perceived through intact low-frequency hearing and place of articulation for consonants, and lip shape cues for vowels are perceived through lipreading.

It is important to point out that large individual differences exist in speech perception abilities among individuals who have a similar degree and configuration of hearing loss. Thus, the information relating degree of hearing loss and speech perception abilities should be used only as a framework for understanding the problem and for planning an approach for selecting assessment procedures and planning an intervention program.

## Speech Production

At the same time that phonemes are being decoded and stored in memory, other aspects of speech are being learned. These include voice inflections, rhythm of connected speech, stress patterns associated with different types of utterances, and other nonphonemic components of natural speech. The degree to which this acoustic information is available to a child directly influences the nature of the speech that will later be produced. The use of even limited residual hearing may make the difference between intelligible and unintelligible speech.

The intelligibility of speech by children who are deaf is often extremely poor. The severity and uniqueness of these speech problems sets deaf speakers apart from their peers. There are four anatomic systems that must be coordinated for adequate speech: respiration, phonation, reso-

nation, and articulation. Research has shown that speakers with hearing loss may have poor respiratory control, abnormal laryngeal function, and poor articulatory timing. Forner and Hixson (1977) and Whitehead (1983) reported that normal-hearing and intelligible deaf adults typically initiate speech between 700 and 800 cc above the functional reserve capacity. However, semi-intelligible speakers with hearing loss consistently speak at lung volumes well below functional reserve capacity. Hearing-impaired individuals frequently experience difficulty controlling laryngeal function for speech, which results in abnormal vocal qualities and irregular suprasegmental patterns. Monsen, Engebretson, and Vemula (1979) found that some individuals who are deaf have difficulty maintaining an appropriate tension balance between the vocal folds. Moreover, Gilbert and Campbell (1980) found that children, adolescents, and adults with hearing loss exhibited higher fundamental frequencies than individuals with normal hearing. Voicing errors are prevalent in the speech of hearing-impaired individuals, and it has been suggested that speakers who are deaf frequently fail to produce correct voice onset time.

There is also a lack of coordination across these systems. The reason for this lack of coordination lies in the hearing loss. To learn these complex, coordinated motor movements, a speaker must hear speech and practice reproducing it. Thus, the speech produced by children with hearing loss is directly related to the severity of the hearing loss and the degree to which an auditory–verbal feedback loop can be established.

Children with severe to profound hearing losses misarticulate both vowels and consonants, making their articulation patterns unique. These children misarticulate vowels almost as frequently as consonants (Markides, 1970). They produce vowels that cannot easily be distinguished from each other because their formant structures are poorly defined. Children with severe to profound hearing losses apparently attempt to produce different vowels by making only minimal changes in the position and movements of the articulators, a limitation that may affect vowel formant transitions. In addition to the lack of differentiation among vowels, children with severe to profound hearing loss may also prolong them to durations that are three to five times as long as those produced by normal-hearing speakers, although there is considerable variability within and between these speakers (Monsen, 1974, 1979).

Children with severe to profound hearing loss produce fewer consonants and develop them later than children with normal hearing. The research in this area has shown remarkable consistency in error patterns across different groups of children. Further, the largest difference between children is in the frequency of errors with type of error varying to a much smaller extent. The following errors are consistently reported: (1) front, voiced consonants are produced more often than other less visible sounds; consonants produced in the middle of the mouth are omitted most often, followed by consonants produced in the back of the mouth, (2) omission of consonants occurs in the word-final position most often with relatively infrequent occurrence in the word-medial and word-initial position, (3) asynchronous errors involving voicing are frequent with the voiced cognate substituted for the voiceless cognate for stop consonants, (4) consonants are frequently omitted from blends, (5) coordination of phonation with consonant production is often faulty, resulting in inappropriate voicing of voiceless consonants and vice versa, and (6) consonant production is often accompanied by hypernasality and/or audible nasal emission of air.

Abnormal patterns of speech rhythm may constitute the most deviant aspect of speech for these children. Their speech rate is often slower than that of speakers with normal hearing because the duration of consonants and vowels is longer. Other factors that contribute to slow speech rate are the insertion of frequent pauses and slow articulatory transitions. Frequent pauses may be related to poor breath control. Finally, stress patterns are inappropriate when a speaker does not distinguish

stressed and unstressed syllables by varying duration (Ling, 1976; Osberger and McGarr, 1982).

Children who are hard-of-hearing (mild to moderate hearing loss) exhibit misarticulations similar to those of children with normal hearing who have developmental disorders of articulation. They appear to develop and use speech sounds in the same order of difficulty as that experienced by children with normal hearing. However, the sounds most commonly misarticulated are fricative consonants (e.g., /s/, /z/, /ʃ/, and /θ/), affricates (e.g., /tʃ/, /dʒ/), and the initial liquid /r/. Deviations in speech in this group also include omission of final consonants, infrequent production of voiced fricatives, and rare use of voiced, back, lingual consonants such as /g/, /j/, and /ŋ/. Unless the hearing loss is severe, articulation of vowels develops normally. Moreover, voice quality and resonance are rarely affected by moderate hearing loss, and speech prosody is usually normal (Elfenbein, Hardin, and Davis 1985).

## EFFECTS ON PRIMARY AND SECONDARY LANGUAGE

Communication with others in some form is essential to every aspect of human life. Because communication is based on the use of codes or symbol systems (i.e., language), language knowledge and use serve as the basis for most human behavior and interaction. Development of self-concept and relating to others are dependent on communicative interaction within the environment. Educational achievement is totally language based. Vocational achievement depends on the educational level attained and the development of the ability to work and communicate with others. It is nearly impossible to overstate the importance of language skills to the development of individuals and thus to the development of children with hearing loss.

Children with hearing loss run the risk of failing to learn language at the normal time or rate because the learning of languages is primarily an auditory event. Its common code is composed of sounds that vary in small but important ways and of combinations of sounds into units of varying size (syllables, words, and phrases). These units are grouped into patterns associated with differing ways of expressing meaning (various sentence structures). Overlaid on the sound and sound combinations that form the basis of a spoken language are the prosodic features that provide subtle clues to shades of meaning, to the emotional state of the speaker, and to the importance of the message to be delivered. Current theories of language acquisition suggest that children with hearing loss acquire language rules and knowledge in the following three related areas to be competent communicators: form (syntax), content (semantics), and function (pragmatics).

## Form

All the information required for controlling the form of spoken messages is collected by learning finite sets of language elements. This is the case at the phonological level at which the list of phonemes and functional intonation and rhythm patterns is finite. Moreover, the use of grammar and syntax also depends on restricted sets of elements. To deal with the grammar of English, a child has to learn a small set of bound morphemes (e.g., -ing, un-, -ed), several sets of form words (e.g., pronouns, prepositions, conjunctions, articles), and a restricted number of laws concerning word order. Thereafter, the child will be learning new words (vocabulary) for the rest of his or her life, and these will afford the means of greatly extending the content of what the child says. However, the child will not learn any new prepositions or pronouns or develop any new grammatical system for use in his native language. The use of a natural language depends on the possession of a relatively small body of information that makes possible the expression of an infinite variety of contents. Were it not for this feature, a language would scarcely be learned and would certainly not be acquired in the comparatively short time in which children master their native language.

Syntax is that aspect of language that must be mastered in order to arrange words into a meaningful utterance. Thus, syntax deals with grammar, or the set of rules relating sounds of language to meaning. Syntax allows for an infinite variation within a system that uses a finite number of sounds and words; its serves as the tool to translate inner thought into the acoustical phenomena that make up spoken communication. The relations among lexical items as they are combined into messages of varying lengths and structures largely determine message meaning. Morphology represents the system of rules by which the smallest meaningful units of language (morphemes) are combined to form words and to express variations in meaning. The production of grammatical sentences depends in part on the correct usage of morphological rules.

Morphemes fall into two classes, free and bound. Free morphemes are lexical items, such as car or jump; bound morphemes are those language units that cannot stand alone, such as -s and -ing, but which change the meaning of words to which they are attached (e.g., cars, jumping). Bound morphemes are usually unstressed units of language; most of them have poor audibility and visibility. Thus, it can be hypothesized that their relative obscurity may make their learning by youngsters with hearing loss quite difficult. The observation that these children often omit the endings of words in their speech is probably related to their reduced ability to perceive and produce certain bound morphemes.

Hearing impairment affects the acquisition of grammatical rules for use in comprehension and expression of spoken language. The overall impression is that most of the common grammatical forms are used accurately by children who are hard-of-hearing. However, in addition to word endings such as plural and tense markers, adjectival markers are omitted frequently. Additionally, use of modal or auxiliary verbs is sometimes affected along with omission of prepositions, infinitives, and determiners. Complex sentence structures (passive verb construction, relative clauses) may not be comprehended or produced (Wilcox and Tobin, 1974; Davis and Blasdell, 1975). For example, sentences containing relative clauses represent one common way in which two or more English sentences can be combined to form a complex utterance. Relative clauses may occur in different positions within a sentence, and they may relate to subject or object components of the sentence. Interpretation of these sentences requires the comprehension of both sentences underlying the surface structure and the recognition of which noun is common to both sentences and referent for the relative pronoun. Very different interpretations of the sentence can result (e.g., the sentence "The boy who owned the dog ran down the street." is interpreted as "The boy owned the dog.") from an inappropriate choice of subject-verb-object relationships to represent the most complete meaning of the complex sentence presented. Quigley, Smith, and Wilbur (1974), report that complex sentences, including those containing relative clauses, appear in the second primer of a typical reading series used in regular classrooms. Thus, failure to comprehend complex spoken sentences is likely to be related to difficulty in comprehension of the same sentences in written form.

## Content

The semantic element of language is concerned with the meanings of words or what words symbolize. Knowledge of the lexical components of language by children with hearing loss has been investigated in several ways. Administration of vocabulary or concept tests, analysis of elicited language samples, and use of experimental tasks have all been employed. The descriptions of word usage that result from all of these procedures are remarkably consistent. Children with hearing loss appear to differ from their normal-hearing peers in the rate and degree to which they learn the meaning of words. Not only are overall vocabulary skills influenced by hearing impairment, certain other aspects of vocabulary knowledge are also affected.

Children with hearing loss do not learn as much incidental vocabulary as do children with normal hearing. In addition, the most common meaning of a word is usually learned first and well, with other meanings of that word being learned poorly or not at all. Moreover, the word knowledge of these youngsters differs with respect to their command of literal word meanings and the breadth of their lexicon. One major reason for the limited vocabulary skills appears to be their dependence on direct teaching of the meaning of the words that they learn, a situation in marked contrast to that of the child with normal hearing who acquires the majority of word meanings vicariously. Teachers by necessity must provide word definitions through overt demonstrations or "acting out" the concept at hand, thus making a word's meaning quite concrete. Further, there is a tendency on the part of teachers to stick to the easily demonstrated, less figurative definitions of words based on the assumption that the child who is hard-of-hearing would not be capable of dealing with other levels of definition. Thus, the vocabulary of children with hearing loss may be unduly influenced by teaching curriculum and strategies rather than by natural language experience.

Words take on varied meanings in context, and children with hearing loss have a particular difficulty in determining new meanings in this situation (Moeller, McConkey, and Osberger, 1983). Further, they often have difficulty understanding nonliteral language, such as puns, metaphors, and some aspects of humor. Slang use of common words may be confusing to children with hearing loss, making it more difficult for them to follow casual conversation. Even when slang or unusual meanings of words are understood, the ease with which they are incorporated into daily usage varies and may lag significantly behind that of other children.

The degree of vocabulary deficit appears to be related to the degree of hearing loss. Use of certain language forms (i.e., nouns, verbs, adjectives, conjunctions, prepositions) varies according to the severity of the hearing loss. While general vocabulary knowledge increases with age, the gap between children with normal hearing and children with hearing loss in word usage widens as the children grow older.

## Function

There has been a shift of focus in the language acquisition literature from a semantic–syntactic analysis of language to a more pragmatically based approach. Pragmatics is the use of language in social contexts. Clinical reports and the limited data available indicate that this is an area in which children with hearing loss demonstrate significant difficulty. Curtis, Prutting, and Lowell (1979) attempted to characterize the early pragmatic-semantic communicative development of twelve children with hearing loss acquiring spoken English as a first language. Their results showed that these youngsters used a range of pragmatic intentions, but they did so primarily through nonverbal means (i.e., gestures). The pragmatic functions used most often were labeling and naming, acknowledgement, and demand, which are some of the earliest used by children with normal hearing. Skarakis and Prutting (1977) studied semantic-pragmatic competence in preschool youngsters with hearing loss who were enrolled in an oral program. Results indicated that specific semantic functions appeared to be acquired more slowly than did pragmatic intentions. Both semantic and pragmatic skills developed, but were delayed. This and other studies indicate individual differences in the effect of hearing impairment on communicative function.

Some research has focused on a discourse analysis of spoken communicative interactions and revealed a number of difficulties that children with hearing loss demonstrate (Moeller et al. 1983). Because of problems in question comprehension, youngsters with hearing loss may fail to follow the rules for taking turns and topic-negotiation. The child's syntax problems may be a source of difficulty in following topic shifts in a conversation. Moreover, if the child has formulation and sequencing problems, these difficulties will be apparent in discourse situations. Many children with hearing loss have not learned appropriate clarification and repair strategies to use when they do not understand what has been said to them. Often, there will be a complete breakdown in communication because the child has not learned to ask for repetition of something that was misunderstood. In summary, children with hearing loss must be taught directly the rules that govern conversations, just as they are taught semantic relationships and the rules of word order and morphological usage.

## Reading

Deficits in communication function interfere seriously with the educational process during the early years and in all the school years that follow. A barrier to the child's progress that is second in importance only to oral language is a failure to learn to read. Practically all of the information not presented to the child in the form of oral language will reach him in printed form.

As a general rule children with severe hearing loss do not exhibit sufficient knowledge of language to ensure a basis for the normal development of reading skills. Several linguistic factors suspected of affecting literacy have been reported, including knowledge of vocabulary, syntax, and figurative language.

For children with hearing loss the task of learning to read is a dual one. They are expected to learn language and reading simultaneously. The fact that children with hearing loss are often taught reading readiness skills in preschool attests to their importance. Unfortunately, certain aspects of language are poorly taught through reading. Some lexical items, particularly nouns and verbs, may be successfully taught in written form because they can be represented fairly easily. Other grammatical items are difficult to teach. Included in this category are auxiliaries, and prepositions such as "of" and "for," both of which have a variety of meanings not easily explained. Another area suspected of affecting English literacy, particularly reading development, is figurative language. Knowledge of the multiple meanings of words is important in learning to read but poorly taught in written form.

Reading levels fall far below the norms for children with normal hearing. Different estimates of reading achievement have been reported. Generally, reading skills slowly increase between the ages of 8 and 14 years, and there is a leveling off of achievement in the early teens. Trybus and Karchmer (1977) reported data developed from Stanford Achievement Test scores of children with hearing loss. The median reading score for students age 20 and above was grade 4.5. The highest reading achievement was obtained by 18-year-olds, but only 10 percent of them scored at or above the eighth grade level.

The development of good reading skills depends on the development of good language skills. The two cannot be separated and under optimal conditions should be sequentially learned. The importance of language cannot be overstated. The eventual level of reading achievement is dictated by the level of language.

## CHILDREN WITH HEARING LOSS IN SCHOOLS

The underlying cause of poor academic achievement is the language deficit incurred as a result of the hearing loss. As a rule, any degree of hearing impairment can put a child at risk for reduced academic achievement (see Table 1.1). As discussed in Chapter 17, there is an inverse relationship between hearing loss and academic achievement.

Taken together, children with hearing loss may demonstrate reduced performance in those academic subjects that are language-based and/or dependent on the ability to learn new information through reading. Even mathematics performance is affected, although to a lesser extent than are other subjects (Davis, Shepard, Stelmachowicz, and Gorga, 1981; Wood, Wood, and Howarth

1983; and Davis, Elfenbein, Schum, and Bentler, 1986). These data, while pointing out general trends in educational characteristics, underscore the heterogeneous makeup of children with hearing loss and the need for audiologists to recognize the individual challenges related to the developmental and educational needs of children to be served as discussed in Chapters 16 and 17.

When children report their experiences in schools, they rarely mention academic problems. Rather, they talk about difficulty in making friends or being unpopular with other children (Davis et al., 1986). Since they are frequently the only students with hearing loss in the schools, it is not unusual for them to feel totally isolated, not fitting into either the deaf or the hearing world. Davis (1988) has hypothesized that much of the social isolation experienced by these children comes about because they are so much like children with normal hearing without being enough like them. Davis states:

> They misunderstand, they are inconsistent in their responses, they sound different when they speak, and they make "dumb mistakes" in class. They are just unusual enough to call attention to themselves, but not different enough to elicit concern, pity, or empathy. Because most school children value being just like their peers, they are unlikely to be completely comfortable with children who are different in small but significant ways. (p. 410)

Because of their difficulty in the pragmatic use of language (asking for clarification, difficulty in discourse situations), children with hearing loss often do not follow conversations and are occasionally not aware that they are being spoken to. Without facility with spoken language, these children depend on the goodwill of adults, both teachers and parents, to interpret, rephrase, and verbally mediate when necessary. As such, opportunities to interact with their peers occurs less frequently. The end result is one of social isolation and the reduced self-esteem that occurs when a child feels rejected by those children with whom daily interactions are necessary.

There is nothing inherent in hearing impairment that causes social adjustment problems in children with hearing loss. It is the reaction of the family, peers, other adults, and poor communication development that contribute to the reported self-esteem and social adjustment difficulties. Social immaturity begins to be apparent during the preschool years in the form of impulsivity, egocentricity, rigidity, and physical aggressiveness. This immaturity becomes more apparent with increasing age as greater communicative demands are made on the children. Further discussion of the challenges of adolescence for children with hearing loss may be found in Chapter 10.

## SUMMARY

In summary, we must remain cognizant of the role of audition in primary and secondary language development and of the fact that most children with hearing loss possess adequate residual hearing to exploit the auditory channel for language learning. The goal for all children with hearing loss must be early detection followed immediately by appropriate intervention. The development of language is the foundation for all other aspects of human behavior, growth, and development. Without language, subsequent effects are seen in the secondary aspects of language (literacy), academic achievement, and social development. Through early detection and appropriate intervention we must work with children and their families to enable them to achieve their optimum personal development.

## REFERENCES

Altshuler, K. Z. (1963). Personality traits and depressive symptoms in the deaf. In J. Wortis (ed.), *Recent Advances in Biological Psychiatry.* New York: Plenum Press.

Boothroyd, A. (1982). *Hearing-Impairments in Young Children.* Englewood Cliffs: Prentice-Hall.

Clark, J. G. (1981). Uses and abuses of hearing loss classification. *ASHA 23,* 493–500.

Curtis, S., Prutting, C. A., and Lowell, E. L. (1979). Pragmatic semantic development in young children with impaired hearing. *Journal of Speech and Hearing Research, 22,* 534–552.

Davis, J. M. (1988). Management of the school age child: A psychosocial perspective. In F. H. Bess (ed.), *Hearing Impairment in Children* (pp. 401–416). Parkton, MD: York Press.

Davis, J., and Blasdell, R. (1975). Perceptual strategies employed by normal hearing and hearing-impaired children in the comprehension of sentences containing relative clauses. *Journal of Speech and Hearing Research, 18,* 281–295.

Davis, J. M., Elfenbein, J., Schum, D., and Bentler, R. A. (1986). Effects of mild and moderate hearing impairment on language, educational, and psychosocial behavior of children. *Journal of Speech and Hearing Disorders, 51,* 53–62.

Davis, J., Shepard, N., Stelmachowicz, P., and Gorga, M. (1981). Characteristics of hearing-impaired children in the public schools: Part II. Psychoeducational Data. *Journal of Speech and Hearing Disorders, 46,* 130–137.

Elfenbein, J., Hardin, J., and Davis, J. (1985). *Oral Communication Skills of Hard of Hearing Children.* Paper presented at the American Speech-Language-Hearing Association Annual Convention, Washington, DC.

Erber, N. P. (1972). Auditory, visual, and auditory-visual recognition of consonants by children with normal and impaired hearing. *Journal of Speech and Hearing Research, 15,* 364–371.

Forner, T. T., and Hixon, T. J. (1977). Respiratory kinematics in profoundly hearing-impaired speakers. *Journal of Speech and Hearing Research, 20,* 373–408.

Gilbert, H. R., and Campbell, M. I. (1980). Speaking fundamental frequency in three groups of hearing-impaired individuals. *Journal Communication Disorders, 13,* 195–205.

Goss, R. (1970). Language used by mothers of deaf children and mothers of hearing children. *American Annals of the Deaf, 115,* 93–96.

Hunt, J. M. (1979). Psychological development: Early experience. *Annual Review of Psychology, 20,* 103–143.

Kenworthy, O. T. (1986). Caregiver-child interaction and language acquisition of hearing-impaired children. *Topic in Language Disorders, 6,* 1–11.

Knauf, V. H. (1978). Language and speech training. In J. Katz (ed.), *Handbook of Clinical Audiology* (pp. 549–564). Baltimore: Williams and Wilkins.

Kretschmer, R., and Kretschmer, L. (1979). The acquisition of linguistic and communicative competence: Parent-child interactions. *Volta Review, 81,* 306–322.

Kricos, P. B. (1982). Response of mothers to the nonverbal communication of their hearing-impaired preschoolers. *Journal of the Academy of Rehabilitative Audiology, 15,* 51–69.

Ling, D. (1976). *Speech and the Hearing-Impaired Child: Theory and Practice.* Washington, DC: A. G. Bell Association for the Deaf.

Markides, A. (1970). The speech of deaf and partially hearing children with special reference to factors affecting intelligibility. *British Journal of Disorders, 5,* 126–140.

Moeller, M. P., McConkey, A. J., and Osberger, M. J. (1983). Evaluation of the communicative skills of hearing-impaired children. *Audiology, 8,* 113–128.

Monsen, R. B. (1974). Durational aspects of vowel production in the speech of deaf children. *Journal of Speech and Hearing Research, 17,* 386–398.

Monsen, R. B. (1979). Acoustic qualities of phonation in young hearing-impaired children. *Journal of Speech and Hearing Research, 22,* 270–288.

Monsen, R., Engebretsen, M., and Vemula, R. (1979). Some effects of deafness on the generation of voice. *Journal Acoustical Society of America, 66,* 1680–1690.

Moses, K. L., and Van Heck-Walutin, M. (1981). The socioemotional impact of infant deafness: A counseling model. In G. T. Mencher, and S. E. Gerber, (eds.). *Early Management of Hearing Loss.* New York, Grune & Stratton.

Ogden, P. W. (1984). Parenting in the mainstream. *Volta Review, 86,* 29–39.

Osberger, M. J., and McGarr, N. S. (1982). Speech production characteristics of the hearing-impaired. In N. J. Lass (ed.), *Speech and Language Advances in Basic Research and Practice,* Vol. 8. New York: Academic Press.

Quigley, S. P., Smith, N. L., and Wilbur, R. B. (1974). Comprehension of relativized sentences by deaf students. *Journal of Speech and Hearing Research, 17,* 325–341.

Sachs, J. (1985). Prelinguistic development. In G. B. Gleason (ed.), *The Development of Language* (pp. 37–160). Columbus: CE Merrill.

Schein, J. D., and Delk, M. T. (1974). *The Deaf Population of the United States.* Silver Springs, MD: National Association of the Deaf.

Schlesinger, H., and Meadow, K. (1972). *Sound and Sign: Childhood Deafness and Mental Health.* Berkeley: University of California Press.

Skarakis, E. A., and Prutting, C. A. (1977). Early communication: Semantic functions and communicative intentions in the communication of the preschool child with impaired hearing. *American Annals of the Deaf, 122,* 382–391.

Trybus, R. J., and Karchmer, M. A. (1977). School achievement scores of hearing-impaired children: National data on achievement status and growth patterns. *American Annals of the Deaf, 115,* 527–536.

Whitehead, R. L. (1983). Some respiratory and aerodynamic patterns in the speech of the hearing-impaired. In I. E. Hochberg, H. Levitt, and M. J. Osberger (eds.), *Speech of the Hearing-Impaired: Research, Training, and Personnel Preparation.* Baltimore: University Park Press.

Wilcox, J., and Tobin, H. (1974). Linguistic performance of hard-of-hearing and normal-hearing children. *Journal of Speech and Hearing Research, 17,* 286–293.

Wood, D., Wood, H., and Howarth, P. (1983). Mathematical abilities of deaf school-leavers, *British Journal of Developmental Psychology, 1,* 67–73.

# CHAPTER 2

# GENETIC ASPECTS OF HEARING LOSS IN CHILDHOOD

*KATHLEEN S. ARNOS, JAMIE ISRAEL, LISA DEVLIN, AND MARY PAT WILSON*

## INTRODUCTION

The causes of hearing loss in childhood can be divided into two major categories: (1) genetic or hereditary and (2) environmental or acquired. Genetic hearing loss refers to that which is inherited through the family in a specific pattern. Within both etiologic categories, the hearing loss can be congenital (is present at the time of birth) or can occur at any time after birth (later onset). In fact, some types of hereditary hearing loss do not produce symptoms until the third or fourth decade of life. Recent discoveries have led to the proposal of a third category of hearing loss caused by an interaction of genetic and environmental factors (Hu et al., 1991).

The relationship between genetics and hearing loss has been recognized since the early nineteenth century (Reardon, 1992; Ruben, 1991). It was not until the last few decades, however, that considerable progress was made in the clinical characterization of various types of hereditary hearing loss as well as in the understanding of the biochemical effects and molecular nature of the hundreds of genes involved in the structure and function of the hearing apparatus. Practical applications of this new knowledge for individuals with hearing loss and their family members are beginning to occur, and many more benefits to families will be realized in the next few decades. During the past decade considerable improvements have been made in the accessibility of genetic counseling and evaluation for individuals with hearing loss and for their families (Arnos, Cunningham, Israel, and Marazita, 1992).

An understanding of basic genetics and a familiarity with hereditary types of hearing loss is critical to the clinical audiologist practicing in both pediatric and adult settings. A large proportion of those children with hearing loss encountered by the audiologist are likely to have hereditary types of hearing loss, although this etiology is often not obvious. Through genetic counseling, families can learn more about the etiology of the hearing loss and the implications for reproduction. As advances in the field of genetics occur, there will be increased availability of new genetic technologies for assisting with diagnosis and management. Audiologists will be essential in ensuring that families get the maximum benefit from these new technologies. Because audiologists are often the first professional contact the family has when the diagnosis of hearing loss is made, they can make a referral for a genetics evaluation and see that it is followed through by the family. In this and other ways, audiologists can be an important part of an interdisciplinary team for diagnosing and working with children with hereditary types of hearing loss. The goal of this chapter is to introduce audiologists to the basic concepts of genetics, the range of hereditary types of hearing loss, the impact of new technology in genetics, the process of genetic evaluation and counseling and strategies for referral.

## EPIDEMIOLOGIC AND DEMOGRAPHIC CHARACTERISTICS OF HEREDITARY HEARING LOSS

Genetic factors are known to be involved in a significant proportion of hearing loss that occurs at birth or shortly thereafter. A recent school-based survey of children with moderate to profound, congenital or early-onset (within the first few years of life) sensorineural hearing loss showed that over 60 percent of the hearing loss was due to genetic causes (Marazita et al., 1993). Recent studies have also suggested that genetic factors play an important role in later-onset hearing loss (Sill et al., 1994), although this has not yet been accurately estimated.

At least 200 types of hereditary hearing loss have been described (Konigsmark and Gorlin, 1976; McKusick, 1992). Approximately two-thirds of these types involve isolated hearing loss; there are no other associated features. The other one-third of hereditary types of hearing loss occur as part of a genetic syndrome. A syndrome is a group of medical or physical characteristics that have the same cause. Dozens of syndromes have been described in which hearing loss can occur together with external ear malformations, heart defects, ocular diseases, kidney malformations and diseases, as well as with other physical traits or medical findings. For example, Usher syndrome, which has been estimated to occur in 3 to 6 percent of children in schools for the deaf, is characterized by sensorineural hearing loss and an eye disorder called retinitis pigmentosa. Usher syndrome is inherited as an autosomal recessive condition. The eye disorder first causes difficulty with night vision in early childhood and later results in a progressive tunnel vision. Recent research has documented that several different genetic types of Usher syndrome exist. Jervell and Lange-Nielsen syndrome is another recessively inherited condition in which profound congenital sensorineural deafness occurs together with a heart problem, causing fainting spells in childhood that may result in sudden death if the heart condition is not treated.

Table 2.1 shows the commonly used classification system for hereditary types of hearing loss, which takes into account isolated hereditary hearing loss (category 1) as well as syndromic types (categories 2 through 7) or types in which a specific metabolic or biochemical defect has been identified (category 8). While audiologists need

**TABLE 2.1**  Konigsmark and Gorlin's Classification of Genetic Deafness

1. No associated abnormalities
2. External ear abnormalities
3. Eye disease
4. Musculoskeletal disease
5. Integumentary system disease
6. Renal disease
7. Nervous system disease
8. Metabolic and other abnormalities

Adapted from Konigsmark, B. W. and Gorlin, R. J. (1976).

not be familiar with all of the features of these different types of hereditary hearing loss, an appreciation of the range of additional characteristics that can be associated with hearing loss and the complexity of the inheritance patterns can assist these professionals in making appropriate referrals and in providing families with encouragement to follow through with the referrals. Appendix 4 at the end of the text lists several different hereditary types of hearing loss and their medical, audiological, and genetic characteristics. An excellent reference for speech and hearing professionals who want additional information is Jung (1989).

Several attempts have been made to further define types of hereditary hearing loss by their audiologic characteristics, however, reliable correlations between audiograms and genetic types of hearing loss have not been made (Reardon, 1992). Genetic types of hearing loss are most commonly sensorineural, but conductive or mixed hearing loss can also be hereditary. The audiometric configuration can also vary between individuals who have the same type of genetic hearing loss whether they are from the same or different families. In some genetic types of hearing loss, particularly those inherited in a dominant mode, the severity of the hearing loss can range from mild to profound, with differences in severity commonly occurring among members of the same family. In some cases, persons who have genes for hearing loss may report "normal hearing," but demon-strate mild or subtle auditory changes upon audi-tory testing. Audiometric information, together with family and medical history and the results of a physical examination, help the clinical geneticist make a specific diagnosis as to the cause of the hearing loss. Therefore, to postulate about or di-agnose a hereditary cause of hearing loss based on audiometric characteristics alone may result in in-accurate or incomplete information being provid-ed to a family.

## MODES OF INHERITANCE

### Chromosomal Inheritance

Every nucleated cell in the human body, other than the sex cells, contains a copy of the genetic material called DNA (deoxyribonucleic acid). This biochemical material, which is inherited from the parents, is organized within the nucleus of the dividing cell into structures called chromo-somes. There are forty-six chromosomes, twenty-three pairs, in the nucleus of each cell. Figure 2.1 shows a photograph of the chromosomal comple-ment (called a karyotype) of a healthy person. Each chromosome pair varies in size and has other more subtle identifying characteristics that allow them to be distinguished from one another. One of each pair of chromosomes is inherited from the fa-ther, while the other is inherited from the mother. One pair of chromosomes is called the sex chro-mosomes. Females have two X chromosomes, while males have an X and a Y chromosome.

Each of the chromosomes is composed of thousands of genes—the biochemical instructions responsible for directing the body's growth and development. Genes are much too small to be seen microscopically. The ear is an incredibly complex organ; literally hundreds of genes are in-volved in determining the structure and function of the ear. One change in a single gene in the path-way controlling the development or functioning of the hearing organ can result in hearing loss. This single gene change can also affect the struc-ture and development of other organs of the body,

leading to syndromes with a variety of physical manifestations. Although a person who has a ge-netic type of hearing loss possesses this gene from conception, the actual expression of the gene may vary in individuals, so that the onset of the hearing loss may occur at birth or later in life. The time at which a gene for hearing loss is "turned on" may depend on the type of gene, and in some instances is influenced by other genes or the environment. This explains why some types of genetic hearing loss are congenital, while others do not occur until later adulthood. The hundreds of genes that deter-mine the structure and function of the ear are not isolated to a single chromosome, but are spread across all the chromosomes. Although the specific chromosomal location and resulting biochemical function for most of these genes remain unknown, recent technology in genetics has allowed the identification and characterization of an increas-ing number of these genes.

### Mendelian Inheritance

Chromosomes come in pairs, therefore the genes that control particular traits or functions also come in pairs, one from each of the parents. Every time parents have a child, one of each pair of their chromosomes is contributed to that child, through the egg cell from the woman and the sperm cell from the man. Since the parent will contribute one of each of their pairs of chromosomes, they will also give one of each pair of genes on those chro-mosomes. A gene at a specific chromosomal loca-tion can exist in several slightly different molecular forms called *alleles*. For some traits, different alleles have slight changes but are con-sidered normal variations, for example, ABO blood type. For other traits, an altered allele may cause changes in physical, medical, or develop-mental features. Related to hearing loss, a person who has one copy of an altered gene (allele) for hearing loss and one allele for normal hearing is called a *heterozygote*. In contrast, a person who has two identical alleles for a trait is called a *ho-mozygote*. When only one copy of a gene is re-quired for a particular trait to be expressed (e.g.,

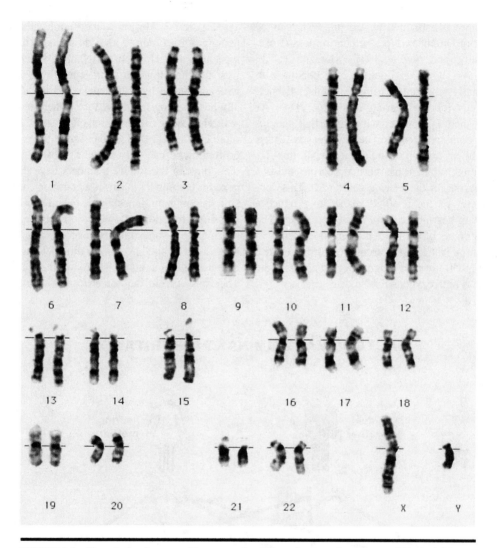

**FIGURE 2.1**    Karyotype of a normal human male. (Microphotograph courtesy of Kenneth Rosenbaum, M.D., Department of Medical Genetics, Children's National Medical Center, Washington, D.C.)

the person is a heterozygote), the trait is called *dominant*. When two copies of the allele are required (the person is a homozygote), the trait is called *recessive*. Hearing loss can be inherited in either of these ways. Occasionally, recessive genes for hearing loss are located on the X chromosome and the trait is inherited as X-linked recessive. These modes of inheritance were first identified in the late 1800s in a plant species by

Gregor Mendel, thus the term *mendelian* or single gene inheritance.

### Dominant Inheritance

A trait such as hearing loss is dominant when only a single copy of the gene for hearing loss is required (the person is a heterozygote for the deaf allele). The dominant gene is usually, but not always, inherited from one of the parents. Dominant inheritance is estimated to account for 15 to 20 percent of hereditary types of hearing loss (Rose, Conneally, and Nance, 1977; Marazita et al., 1993). As shown in Figure 2.2, a person with dominantly inherited hearing loss is usually heterozygous for the hearing loss gene (Dd). As shown, there is a 50 percent chance that persons with a dominant gene for hearing loss will pass that gene on to each of their children. In this figure, the other parent has normal hearing and is a homozygote for the hearing genes (dd). This couple, therefore, has a 50/50 chance to produce a child with hearing loss with each pregnancy. The hearing status of the first child has no bearing on the hearing status of the second child; the chance is still 50/50 for each pregnancy when one of the parents is heterozygous for the deaf gene.

Figure 2.3 illustrates the family history or pedigree of a family with a dominantly inherited type of hearing loss. In this family, hearing loss was inherited through four generations. A child with a dominant type of genetic hearing loss usually has a strong family history of hearing loss in several successive generations. However, in some families the hearing loss can range from mild to profound and can vary in the age of onset, even though all of the family members have the same gene for hearing loss. This is a common characteristic of dominant genes and is called variable expression. In addition, with dominant types of hearing loss, some members of the family may have the gene and have a very mild hearing loss or no hearing loss at all (called reduced penetrance). Therefore, careful audiometric documentation is

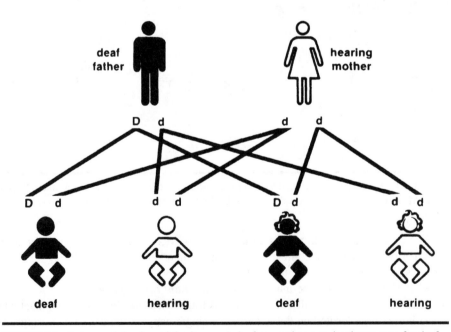

## AUTOSOMAL DOMINANT INHERITANCE

**FIGURE 2.2** Autosomal dominant inheritance. A deaf person has one dominant gene for deafness (D) and a corresponding gene for hearing (d). Each child has a 50/50 chance to inherit the deafness gene (D) from the parent who has this gene.

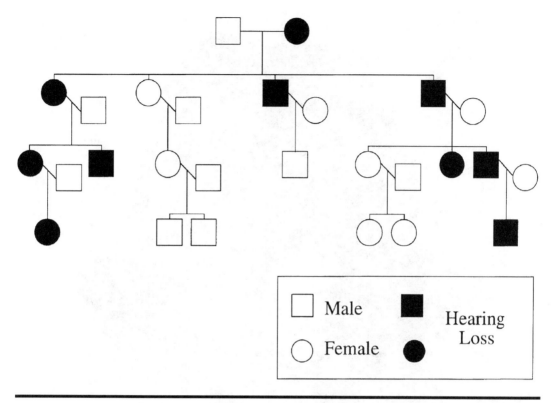

**FIGURE 2.3**    Pedigree (family tree) illustrating autosomal dominant inheritance of deafness through four generations.

required in families where this is suspected to be the case so that accurate information can be given to the family. Variable expression and reduced penetrance are exhibited in both isolated and syndromic types of hearing loss that are dominantly inherited. In syndromic types, the associated physical and medical characteristics can vary from person to person within the family.

It is also possible for a person to have a dominant gene for hearing loss for the first time in a hearing family. This is called a new mutation (gene change); this new mutation can occur during any of the cell divisions that take place in the formation of egg and sperm cells. New mutations occur frequently in sperm cells, since each sperm (twenty-three chromosomes) is the product of hundreds of divisions, depending on the age of the

father. On this basis, it would be expected that the frequency of paternal new mutations would be increased as the father ages and that certain types of mutations are more often of paternal origin. Several known dominant genetic conditions have resulted from new mutations and have been associated with advanced paternal age (Thompson, McInnes, and Willard, 1991). One such example related to hearing loss is a dominant genetic condition called Treacher-Collins syndrome (conductive hearing loss, malformations of the external ears, downward sloping eyes, depressed cheekbones, coloboma (notch or cleft of the lower eyelid), and other features (Figure 2.4). It has been estimated that approximately 60 percent of individuals with Treacher-Collins syndrome are the result of a new mutation, and many fathers in

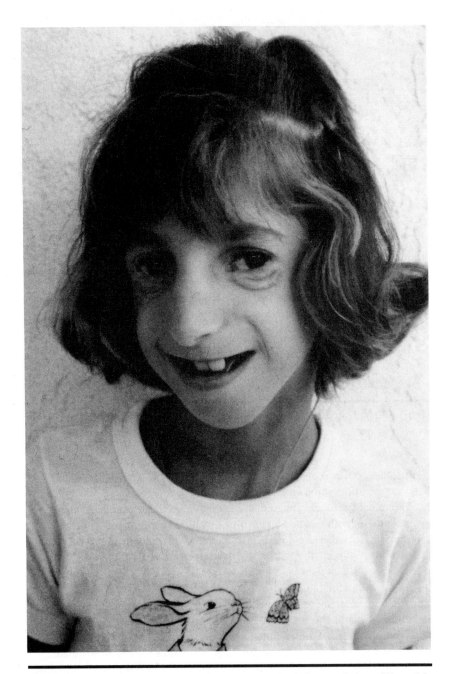

**FIGURE 2.4**    Child with Treacher-Collins syndrome. (Used by permission of Karen M. Jenson, M.E.D., Department of Communicative Sciences and Disorders, California State University Fresno.)

these cases tend to be older (Gorlin, Cohen, and Levin, 1990).

### Recessive Inheritance

In recessive inheritance, a person must receive two copies of the gene, one from each parent, in order for the trait to be expressed (the person is a homozygote). In this type of inheritance, heterozygotes do not express the trait but are called carriers. Recessive inheritance is estimated to account for approximately 80 percent of genetic hearing loss (Rose et al., 1977; Marazita et al.,

1993). As shown in Figure 2.5, in recessive inheritance, the chance that two hearing heterozygotes (Rr) will have a homozygous (deaf) child (rr) is one in four, or 25 percent with each pregnancy. The chance is the same for all pregnancies of the couple. Figure 2.6 illustrates the family history of a family in which recessive hearing loss occurred in two siblings. Since most types of recessive hearing loss are nonsyndromic and blood tests to identify genes for hearing loss are generally not available, it is often difficult to diagnose recessively inherited hearing loss when the parents

## AUTOSOMAL RECESSIVE INHERITANCE

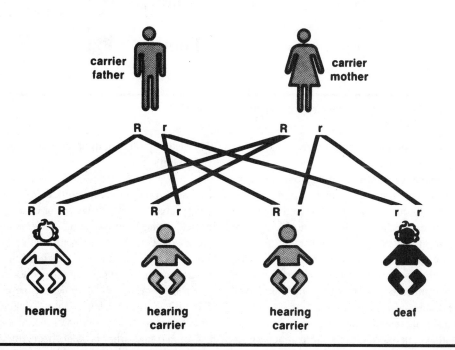

**FIGURE 2.5** Autosomal recessive inheritance. Deaf individuals must have a double dose of the gene for deafness (r), one inherited from each of the parents. The parents are hearing carriers (Rr) and have a 1/4 chance to produce a deaf child with each pregnancy.

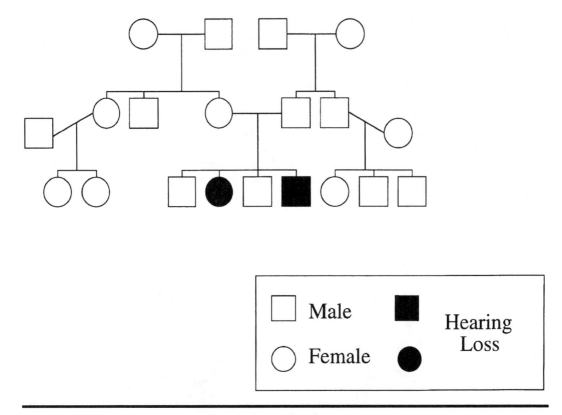

**FIGURE 2.6**    Pedigree illustrating recessive inheritance of deafness.

have only one child with hearing loss and all other family members have normal hearing.

Recessive genes for hearing loss are very common. Population studies have estimated that approximately one in eight persons in the general population carries a recessive gene for hearing loss (Rose et al., 1977). Although many hearing people are carriers for recessive types of hearing loss, the parents must have the exact same type of gene (they must match exactly) to have a chance to have a child with hearing loss. The chance for this to occur increases if the parents are related to one another. The more closely the parents are related, the more likely it is that they both inherited the same recessive gene from their common ancestor. Mating between blood relatives or "consanguinity" is important to identify in the diagnostic process, even when the parents may be only distantly related, in order to document recessive inheritance.

### X-Linked Recessive Inheritance

A very small number of genes for hearing loss are located on the X chromosome. A female who has a recessive gene for hearing loss on one of her X chromosomes (Xx) most often is hearing, but each of her sons has a 50 percent chance to inherit the X chromosome with this gene and be deaf (xY) (Figure 2.7). Each of her daughters has a 50 percent chance to be a carrier (Xx). All of the daughters of a male who is deaf from an X-linked recessive gene (whose mate is homozygous for the hearing gene) will be hearing carriers, while all the sons will be hearing but not carry the gene for hearing loss, since they inherit the Y chromosome from their father. Female carriers may

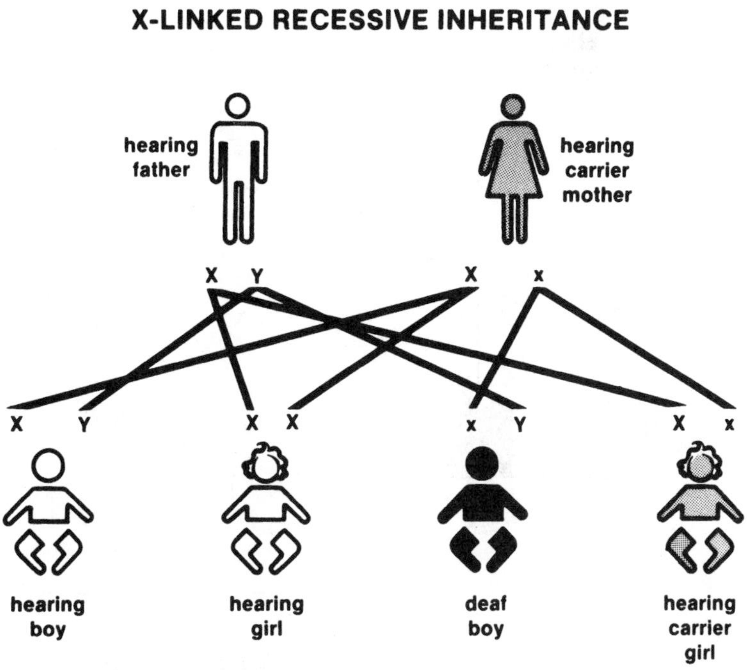

## X-LINKED RECESSIVE INHERITANCE

**FIGURE 2.7**   X-linked recessive inheritance. The sons of a woman who is a carrier of the X-linked gene for deafness have a 50/50 chance to be deaf. The daughters have a 50/50 chance to be hearing carriers.

sometimes exhibit very mild hearing loss or subtle audiologic changes. Figure 2.8 illustrates a family in which X-linked inheritance of hearing loss has occurred. In this family, hearing loss occurs only in males who are related to each other through hearing female carriers.

## Complex (Multifactorial) and Nontraditional Inheritance

Some conditions are caused by the interaction of a gene or genes with one or more environmental factors. This type of inheritance is called multifactorial. Multifactorial conditions can occur in a single person in a family or can appear to "cluster" in random family members. Examples of multifactorial conditions include heart disease, cancer, cleft lip/palate, and neural tube defects (such as spina bifida). In general, a couple with one child with a multifactorial condition have approximately a 2 to

5 percent chance for this condition to reoccur in future children. In some multifactorial conditions, other factors, such as the sex of the child or parent, may influence the chance of recurrence.

Future studies will investigate possible gene–environment interactions for such disorders as Meniere disease, presbycusis, and otitis media. Recently, it has been discovered that some individuals who have aminoglycoside (such as streptomycin) induced hearing loss possess a specific gene that makes them more susceptible to the ototoxic effects of these drugs. It is this combined interaction of a single gene and an environmental event that causes the hearing loss. A recent study (Prezant et al., 1993) identified a mutation in the mitochondrial DNA that caused hearing loss in members of some families who received small, short-duration doses of aminoglycoside antibiotics. The mitochondria, which contain a single cir-

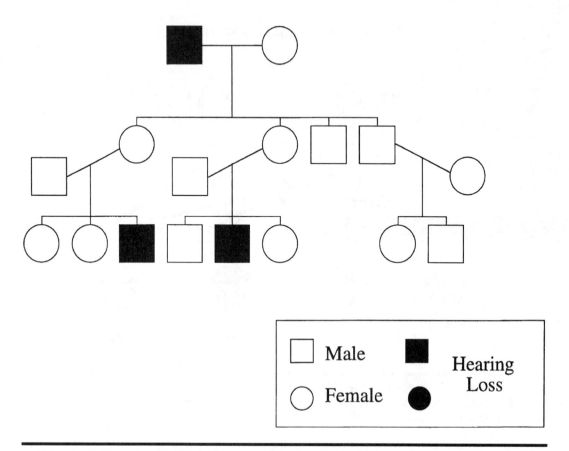

**FIGURE 2.8**    Pedigree illustrating X-linked recessive inheritance of deafness.

cular piece of DNA, are small cellular structures that are responsible for energy production for cellular activities. Mitochondria are always inherited maternally; they are passed from mother to child through the egg cell, but are not passed from father to child in the much smaller sperm cell. Mitochondrial genes are also known to be responsible for some other forms of hearing loss (i.e., nonsyndromic deafness, deafness and diabetes, and Wolfram syndrome) as well as for neuromuscular and ocular disorders (Ballinger et al., 1992; Rotig et al., 1993; Wallace, 1987).

Several types of nontraditional inheritance are also known to occur in certain genetic conditions. These include genetic imprinting, uniparental disomy, mosaicism, and anticipation. Genetic imprinting describes a phenomena in which differences in the severity or symptoms of some diseases were found to depend upon whether the gene(s) or chromosome rearrangement were inherited from the mother or the father (Hall, 1990). Uniparental disomy describes a phenomenon in which both chromosomes of a pair are inherited from one parent. For example, cases of cystic fibrosis (CF) have been described in which both copies of the CF gene and the chromosome upon which the gene resides, were inherited from one parent, instead of both of the parents (Spence et al., 1988). Mosaicism is another form of nontraditional inheritance in which only a certain proportion of the cells of a person contain a particular gene or chromosome change. In the phenomenon known as genetic anticipation, symptoms of a disorder seem to worsen as the gene is inherited through successive generations. Recent developments in molecular biology have provided an explanation for this finding at the DNA level in several genetic conditions (Sutherland and Richards, 1994). Located within a specific gene, there are repeated sequences of DNA (called trinucleotide repeats) that are unstable. Changes in the length of a segment of DNA may occur throughout a family, usually increasing in size in successive generations and contributing to the severity and age of onset of the clinical symptoms. Recent research has shown that the sex of the transmitting parent may in some cases influence the size of the unstable DNA sequence and contribute to the clinical features in the child (Ashizawa et al., 1994).

Although examples of nontraditional inheritance of hearing loss are not common, future research is likely to reveal new types of hearing loss inherited in such ways, with important implications for families. For example, genetic anticipation may occur in some families in which a child with early-onset severe to profound deafness is found to have relatives with later-onset mild to moderate hearing loss. This possibility reinforces the importance of accurately recording information about the family history of hearing loss, even when some instances of hearing loss in the family are mild and of late onset.

## GENETIC EVALUATION AND COUNSELING

Most children who are seen by the audiologist for the diagnosis of hearing loss would benefit from a genetic evaluation by qualified genetics professionals. Genetic evaluation and counseling can assist the family in getting accurate information about the cause of the hearing loss, other medical implications, the chance of recurrence in future children or other family members, and reproductive options. In addition, through genetic counseling, families can receive updated information about new technologies in genetics and learn

about any ongoing research studies that may be of benefit to them. Genetic counseling is a process of education, communication, and information-sharing. The goal of genetic counseling is to provide information and assist families in making choices. An effective genetic counselor is also able to recognize the emotional state of the family and work with them on issues related to grieving, adjustment, acceptance of the diagnosis, and making choices that are right for them.

Genetic evaluation and counseling may be appropriate for families and individuals at various times in their lives and for different reasons. The audiologist, as one of the primary care providers for a child with hearing loss, can assist the family with exploring the reasons genetic counseling might be beneficial for them and the time that is most appropriate for them to seek these services. A common family situation presented to the audiologist is hearing parents who have just received the diagnosis of hearing loss in their child. For some families, immediate referral for genetic counseling might be appropriate to help them adjust to the diagnosis and to explore the reproductive implications. For other families, the presence of other medical complications may indicate the need for immediate referral to explore the possibility that these complications may be associated with the hearing loss and to obtain appropriate information for treatment and management. Other parents, who are not planning any additional children and who may be completely overwhelmed with the educational and medical implications of newly diagnosed hearing loss in their child, may not be ready for genetic counseling for several months or years. The audiologist who sees the family on a regular basis can be responsible for informing the family about the benefits of genetic counseling and can explore whether a referral is appropriate for them at any particular point in time based on, for example, emotional adjustment, additional medical complications, and reproductive concerns.

Referring audiologists should familiarize themselves with the range of genetic services available locally, including a genetic counselor whom they can contact to discuss issues such as fees, services available, appropriateness of a referral, and follow-up. Through meetings or informal presentations, audiologists and genetic professionals can establish guidelines together for referral and follow-up. Most genetic centers encourage telephone calls from audiologists who have questions about a potential referral. Genetics professionals can often provide pamphlets, brochures and fact sheets describing genetic services that the audiologist can share with families. The audiologist who is familiar with the information and referral network developed with local genetics clinics can feel comfortable helping families who are resistant to a referral because they may not understand the purpose or benefits of genetic counseling or may feel threatened with the perceived possibility of being "blamed" for the occurrence of hearing loss in a child.

In general, a referral for genetic counseling should be made for any individual or family in whom hearing loss has occurred, but particularly for those families who have questions about the cause of hearing loss and implications for future children as well as for those children with a possible syndromic type of hearing loss. A child with hearing loss who has hearing parents, no family history of hearing loss, a negative medical history, and a normal physical examination is very likely to have a recessive genetic cause of hearing loss, although a specific diagnosis is often not possible in these children. Although parents in this situation may question why genetic counseling is important for them, genetic counseling can provide many benefits to these families. Such an evaluation can exclude syndromic causes of hearing loss, alleviate guilt feelings, and correct misunderstandings by providing the family with detailed explanations of the possible causes of the hearing loss and the possibility for recurrence in future children. Although many parents in this situation may be frustrated by the fact that an exact etiology cannot be determined for their child's hearing loss, they may feel reassured by the knowledge that other medical complications have been excluded. Additionally, it may be important for the genetics team to discuss specific events that occurred (or did not occur) that are found to be unrelated to the cause of hearing loss in their child. This may be helpful in providing reassurance and in alleviating guilt feelings.

Adults with hearing loss can also gain substantial benefits from genetic counseling (Arnos et al., 1992). As individuals with hearing loss approach reproductive age, it is natural for them to wonder about the cause of their own deafness and the possibility of having deaf or hearing children. Approximately 90 percent of profoundly deaf individuals marry another deaf person (Schein, 1989). Many deaf adults consider themselves to be culturally deaf; deafness is viewed not as a disability, but as a cultural difference (Padden and Humphries, 1988). Culturally deaf individuals share a common sign language and values and experiences, are often educated together in residential school settings, and socialize within their cultural group throughout their lives. Many of these deaf couples would prefer to have deaf children and are very motivated to learn about the cause of their own deafness (Jordan, 1991; Arnos, Israel, and Cunningham 1991). In addition, medical complications associated with some syndromic types of deafness do not have their onset until the late teenage years or adulthood, which then warrants genetic evaluation and follow-up.

Another group of individuals who can benefit from genetic evaluation and counseling are individuals with progressive types of hearing loss and adults who develop later-onset hearing loss. These persons often have concerns about whether the hearing loss will continue to progress, if there are other associated medical findings, and the implications for their children and grandchildren. The geneticist, in conjunction with audiology and otolaryngology specialists, may be able to determine the exact diagnosis and appropriate management for the individual. Recently, researchers at the University of Costa Rica and the University of California identified a gene for one type of dominantly inherited progressive hearing loss on chromosome number 5 in a large family from Costa Rica (Leon, Raventos, Lynch, Morrow, and King, 1992). Affected family members develop a low-frequency hearing loss beginning in childhood that progresses to profound bilateral deafness at all frequencies in adulthood. Research progress on this type and other types of progressive and adult-onset hearing loss will continue over the next several years.

Some audiologists may find a checklist format for identifying families with a positive family history and possible syndromic types of hearing loss helpful in the referral process. Table 2.2 includes a suggested format that can be altered by the audiologist together with the geneticists to whom they refer to best meet the needs of their clients.

## The Genetic Counseling Process

Once a referral is made, the genetic counseling process begins with assessing the needs of the individual or family and their purpose for seeking a genetic evaluation. Information that is collected for all families includes complete medical and audiologic history on the person who has hearing loss as well as family history including health and audiologic information on close family members. In addition, a physical examination of one or several family members is performed by a clinical (M. D.) geneticist.

The genetics evaluation may be performed by a team of professionals, including a clinical geneticist (M. D.), a Ph.D. geneticist, a genetic counselor (M. S.), social workers, and nurses. Geneticists have different areas of specialization, including pediatric or adult genetics, reproductive genetics, and subspecialities such as neurology or ophthalmology. In some large hospitals, specialty clinics (i.e., oral-facial, metabolic, neurofibromatosis, etc.) may exist in which geneticists as well as professionals from other disciplines all provide coordinated medical care and management for the client. Audiologists, speech-language pathologists, and otolaryngologists are often part of these teams or serve as consultants.

### Family History

An accurate family history is important to the diagnostic process and can sometimes provide the only clue as to the cause and mode of inheritance of the hearing loss. Prior to the clinic visit or at the beginning of the visit, a member of the genetics team will ask specific, detailed questions about the health and hearing status of siblings, parents, grandparents, and other close family members. Ethnicity and any possible occurrence of consanguinity (blood relationship between parents) in the family will also be explored. Information collected by face-to-face or phone interviews of family members may be supplemented by special questionnaires sent to the family prior to the visit. Questionnaires such as these have been developed for families with hearing loss (Arnos et al., 1992; Bieber, 1981). Even in those cases in which the collection of the family history is not possible, for example, because of adoption or loss of contact with family members, the other components of the genetic evaluation as specified below are often helpful in making the diagnosis.

### Medical History

The family is asked detailed questions about the medical and pregnancy history for the family member with hearing loss and for other relatives. When necessary, medical records concerning birth complications, past hospitalizations, otolaryngologic or other specialty medical examinations, and developmental evaluations are collected. This information is often helpful in making an accurate diagnosis or in excluding previously reported causes of hearing loss. When indicated by the family history, similar medical records may also be collected on other family members.

### Audiologic History

Audiograms are an important component of the genetic evaluation and diagnosis of a child with hearing loss. It is often helpful for the audiologist to provide interpretation or comments on special or unusual features of the audiogram when referring a child for evaluation. It is also common for

**TABLE 2.2**   Audiologic Checklist

A comprehensive case history is an essential component of any complete audiologic assessment. Listed below are questions that may provide the audiologist with helpful information when making a referral for genetic counseling for a given client. These questions in no way constitute a comprehensive audiological case history. Rather they should be viewed as an addendum to an existing case history form for a pediatric or adult client. Audiologists should keep in mind that most individuals with hereditary deafness will have a negative family history and no other associated findings.

**FAMILY HISTORY**

1. Are there family members with hearing loss? If so, indicate the following for each one:
   • Etiology (or their perception of the cause)
   • Age on onset
   • Degree of loss
   • Progression, if any
2. If more than one family member has hearing loss, is there variable expression in terms of degree and type of loss among family members?
3. Are there any family members with developmental and/or physical disorders?
4. Was there any intermarriage in past generations?
5. Has any family member ever had a genetics work-up?

**MEDICAL HISTORY**

1. Does the client have any of the following conditions?
   _____ Heart defects
   _____ Thyroid problems or enlarged thyroid
   _____ Visual problems (night blindness, tunnel vision, progressive loss of visual acuity, associated balance
          problems)
   _____ Ophthalmologic abnormalities (heterochromia)
   _____ Pigmentary changes of hair, skin (early graying, white patch, vitiligo)
   _____ Musculoskeletal disorders (short stature, arthritis, very tall structure)
   _____ Frequent broken bones
   _____ Orofacial malformations/defects (cleft palate, dysmorphic features)
   _____ Malformations/defects of the ear (congenital atresia, ear pits or tags)
   _____ History of miscarriages or stillbirths
   _____ Kidney disease, frequent urinary tract infections, blood in urine
   _____ Fainting spells, seizures
2. Does any family member have any of the above conditions?

geneticists who work regularly with clients with hearing loss to ask for the audiologist's assistance with the comparison of audiometric features between family members or over time for one individual. When the hearing loss has been progressive, it is often helpful for the audiologist to provide and assist with interpreting serial audiograms that document the progression.

*Physical Examination*

The physical examination is a critical part of the genetic counseling process and should be performed by a board certified clinical (M. D.) geneticist. The clinical geneticist is trained to recognize specific traits and features in order to make a diagnosis of a syndromic or nonsyndromic type of hearing loss. This person will take standard craniofacial measurements and will evaluate structural or functional changes involving other organs or systems. Following the examination, a diagnosis will be made based on this information together with the family and medical history. Occasionally, this physician may recommend additional x-rays, laboratory testing, or evaluations by other specialists. In some situations, the clinical geneticist may decide to perform a chromosome study or other biochemical, metabolic, or genetic studies of the client with hearing loss. The results of these studies may assist with the diagnosis and will be explained to the family.

*Counseling, Follow-Up, and Support Services*

Once the diagnosis has been made, complete information will be provided to the individual or family in a way that is sensitive to their individual emotional and family needs. A variety of issues may be discussed during a counseling session, including exact medical information about the diagnosis and any accompanying conditions if it is syndromic, the mode of inheritance, prognosis, implications for future children or other family members, treatment options, options for prenatal diagnosis, and research efforts that may be underway. The focus of the genetic counseling session is to provide information in an atmosphere that is supportive of the clients' psychosocial needs and cultural differences that may influence decision making. The counseling process may take place during one visit or may require several follow-up visits to assess changing psychosocial concerns or medical aspects. Follow-up visits also allow the geneticists to inform the family about new advances in this rapidly changing field that may di-

rectly benefit them. The genetics team may make referrals to assist individuals and families with educational issues or concerns. Additionally, many families may benefit from a referral to an appropriate professional or organization for additional support and information. There are many local and national support groups and organizations for individuals with hearing loss and their families. There are also numerous groups that have been developed for specific genetic conditions. Many of these organizations provide literature, brochures, newsletters, and opportunities for parents to network with one another. Genetic centers or the Alliance of Genetic Support Groups (See Appendix 7) can assist individuals and parents in locating these organizations.

The audiologist can play an important role in reinforcing the information provided by the genetics evaluation by reviewing the summary letter or report with the family and by ensuring that the client or family takes advantage of the referrals that are made. Additionally, audiologists can refer the family back to the genetics team when necessary. Follow-up may be indicated when future children are planned, if there is a change in a client's audiologic, medical, or family history, or if the family has new or additional questions (which may indicate to the audiologist that the family does not have a clear understanding of the information) and would benefit from a review by the geneticist.

## CASE HISTORIES

Two cases are presented here to illustrate the components of the genetic evaluation, and counseling process for a child with hearing loss and the role of the audiologist in referral, evaluation, and follow-up. These cases represent composites of several case histories.

### Case 1

BL is a 4-year-old female with a moderately severe sensorineural hearing loss who was referred to a genetics center for evaluation and counseling by an audiologist from a local hospital. BL's hearing loss was diagnosed at 3 years of age and the parents are now questioning the cause of hearing loss, chance of progression, and implications for their daughter's medical care. Additionally, the parents may be considering more children depending on the information that they receive in genetic counseling.

### Medical and Audiologic History

BL was born full-term weighing 7 lbs. 8 oz. without any complications during delivery. Pregnancy history was negative. Specifically, her mother could not recall any illnesses, fevers, or complications and denied the use of alcohol, drugs, and medications with the exception of Tylenol for headaches on two occasions. No problems were noted in the neonatal period, and BL went home with her mother from the hospital. Neonatal and infant history were benign. However, mother recounted a time that BL had a fever of 103 degrees resulting from an ear infection. A routine antibiotic was prescribed, and the fever subsided within a few hours. Around this same time, the family became concerned with speech development but formal testing did not occur until 3 years of age. Audiologic evaluation performed on two occasions confirmed a moderately severe sensorineural hearing loss. Binaural hearing aids were prescribed, and the parents noticed a significant change in her sound awareness and speech and language development.

### Family History

BL's family history is shown in Figure 2.9. BL has a 2-year-old brother, who has not yet had formal audiologic testing, although the parents are pleased with his speech development and believe he has normal hearing. The parents have been healthy without evidence of hearing loss. Maternal grandmother developed a high frequency loss at 65 years of age and has been told that this is related to her age. Otherwise the family history is negative for early-onset hearing loss, known genetic conditions, or birth defects. Mother does report, however, that her first cousin is said to have been born with a "dimple on the outside of her ear." The parents denied consanguinity.

### Physical Examination

Prior to the examination, BL's parents were asked several questions about her medical history. No history of visual impairment, syncopal spells (fainting), seizures, birthmarks, cardiac abnormalities, or kidney disease were reported. Examination on BL revealed height and weight to be at the fiftieth percentile. Ocular measurements were within normal limits with no evidence of dystopia canthorum (increased distance between the inner corners of the eyes). Eye color was blue. Eye examination was normal and fundoscopic examination showed no evidence of eye disease. Ears lengths were within normal limits, and the ears were well-formed with no evidence of preauricular pits (dimples, holes) or tags (extra skin). Thyroid was not enlarged. Cardiac, abdominal, genital, and neurologic evaluations were negative. No birthmarks or other pigmentary changes were noted. Muscle strength and coordination were good, and the remainder of the examination was unremarkable.

The parents were briefly examined as well. Examination included measurements of the eyes, ears, and evaluation for the presence of any structural changes of the external ear. Based on the suspected ear pit in mother's first cousin, the geneticist looked for signs of branchio-oto-renal syndrome, characterized by ear pits or tags, hearing loss, branchial (neck) cysts, kidney abnormalities, and other findings in the parents. These findings may be variably expressed in family members. Results of the physical examinations in both parents revealed normal measurements with no traits associated with a syndromic cause of hearing loss.

### Clinical Diagnosis

In the absence of any identifiable traits associated with hearing loss in BL or her parents, it was be-

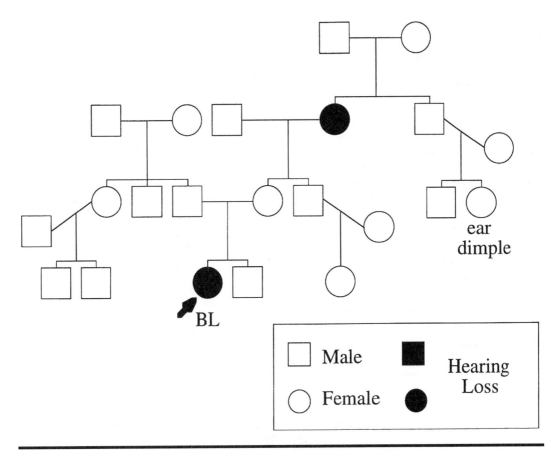

**FIGURE 2.9**   Pedigree of BL (Case 1).

lieved that she has isolated, nonsyndromic sensorineural hearing loss, most likely autosomal recessive.

### Genetic Counseling Issues

A general discussion of all causes of early-onset hearing loss was reviewed with BL's parents. It was explained that at least 50 percent of children who have early-onset hearing loss have a genetic cause. In one-third of these individuals, a specific syndromic cause can be identified, but the majority of individuals with genetic hearing loss have an isolated type, as seen in BL. The most common mode of inheritance for genetic hearing loss is autosomal recessive. Based on BL's negative family history and medical history, this seemed to be the most likely diagnosis for BL. The parents were reassured that the Tylenol use during pregnancy and high fever associated with an ear infection were not the cause of BL's sensorineural hearing loss.

It was explained to BL's parents that in this case, there would be a 25 percent or 1/4 chance for future children to have a similar degree of hearing loss. Prenatal testing for isolated hearing loss is not available through current technology. The parent's feelings about this possible recurrence chance and their reproductive options (including "taking their chances," adoption, donor insemination, or choosing not to have more children) were discussed in detail.

### Recommendations and Follow-Up

Because BL was found to have an "unknown" cause of hearing loss, the geneticist recommended a baseline ophthalmologic exam with follow-up every few years to look for eye diseases that are associated with hearing loss. BL's parents informed the geneticist that an eye examination had been previously performed and the results were normal. These records were requested and reviewed to confirm that BL had a funduscopic examination by an ophthalmologist who was familiar with eye disease associated with hearing loss. Additionally, the parents were informed that any changes in their child's medical history should be reported to the genetics center so that the geneticist could determine if a follow-up examination or other testing (metabolic, cardiac, etc.) was needed. The family was encouraged to maintain contact with the genetics center periodically to learn if any new information was available to them as technologies in the field of genetics improved. Also, opportunities to participate in research projects may be available at a later time.

Other recommendations to the family included follow-up audiologic assessment on BL to monitor the status of the hearing loss and to manage issues related to the hearing loss, such as amplification use. Additionally, BL's brother, as well as any new siblings in the family, would need periodic audiologic monitoring. If hearing loss was documented in other siblings, this would provide strong evidence for a recessive type of hearing loss. In this case, audiologic assessment showed that BL's brother had normal hearing. Lastly, for completeness, audiologic evaluations were recommended for both parents and the maternal grandmother's audiology report was requested. These records were received and reviewed with staff audiologists. The parent's audiograms were considered within normal limits and the maternal grandmother had an audiologic pattern consistent with presbycusis. The family was contacted and the above information was reviewed; a letter was sent to the family summarizing the information discussed in genetic counseling.

## Case 2

RY is a 2-month-old male who was referred by his pediatrician for genetic counseling. At birth, RY was noted to have several unusual facial characteristics including very widely spaced eyes and a flat nasal bridge. Based on these characteristics, ABR testing was done that confirmed the presence of a profound unilateral sensorineural hearing loss. The parents had questions about the cause of the hearing loss and the chance for future children to have a similar hearing loss.

### Medical and Audiologic History

A review of the pregnancy history revealed that the mother was healthy and denied any exposure to drugs, alcohol, prescription medications, or illnesses during pregnancy. RY was born at 40 weeks gestation by a normal vaginal delivery, although the labor was long. After birth, he was found to be in good health and went home from the hospital with his mother. At the first visit to the pediatrician's office at 2 weeks of age, the pediatrician noticed that RY had very widely spaced eyes and a flat nasal bridge. His father had very similar characteristics. The pediatrician discussed a referral to the genetics clinic with the parents, telling them that these features can sometimes be associated with more serious medical conditions. He also recommended a hearing screen for the baby. ABR testing was performed at 1 month of age, and the parents were surprised to learn that RY had a profound unilateral sensorineural hearing loss. This prompted them to follow through with the pediatrician's recommendation to have their baby evaluated by a geneticist.

### Family History

During the initial visit with the geneticist a complete family history was taken. RY has one sister who is 3 years of age and in good health, as are the parents. The father, however, has several distinctive characteristics, including widely spaced eyes, graying of his hair in his teenage years, patches of vitiligo (very light skin pigmentation), and a history of digestive disorders. The father reported that he looked very similar to his own father, and that all of his brothers and sisters, and several aunts, uncles, and cousins had similar features. The family was questioned about the occurrence of heterochromia (different colored eyes), white forelock (a white streak of hair on the front of the head), or hearing loss in other family members. Deafness was reported in only one distant cousin, and no relatives were reported to have white forelock. RY's family history is shown in Figure 2.10.

### Physical Examination

RY, his sister, and both of his parents were examined by the clinical geneticist. Eye measurements on RY and his father confirmed the presence of dystopia canthorum (an increased distance be-

tween the inner corners of the eyes). Both of these individuals also had a flat nasal bridge. The father had extensive vitiligo on his back, arms, and legs, and at age 35 was completely gray-haired. The remainder of the examination was normal. The physical examination of the mother and sister did not reveal the presence of any features associated with syndromic causes of hearing loss.

### Clinical Diagnosis

Based on the physical features present in RY and his father, and the reported family history, a diagnosis of Waardenburg syndrome, type 1, was made. Even though several family members were suspected to have Waardenburg syndrome, this diagnosis had not previously been made in any family members. Only one distant cousin was

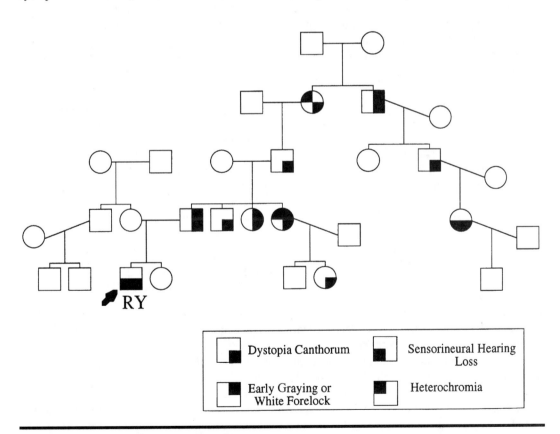

**FIGURE 2.10**  Pedigree of RY (Case 2).

known to have hearing loss. Waardenburg syndrome is an autosomal dominant trait that is characterized by pigmentary changes such as white forelock, heterochromia, and vitiligo as well as a flat nasal bridge, synophrys (eyebrows that grow together across the top of the nose), and sensorineural hearing loss. The hearing loss can be unilateral or bilateral, but occurs in only 20 to 50 percent of individuals with Waardenburg syndrome. The other features associated with Waardenburg syndrome are also variable within families. There are at least two types of Waardenburg syndrome. Dystopia canthorum occurs in type 1 Waardenburg syndrome, but not in type 2, while the occurrence of hearing loss is higher in type 2 Waardenburg syndrome (about 50 percent of individuals) than it is in type 1 Waardenburg syndrome (about 20 percent of individuals). Recent gene mapping studies have identified a gene for type 1 Waardenburg syndrome on chromosome 2 (Baldwin et al., 1992; Tassabehji et al., 1992).

Recent case reports of infants with Waardenburg syndrome who also have spina bifida have suggested that neural tube defects may be part of the spectrum of features of Waardenburg syndrome (Carezani-Gavin, Clarren, and Steege, 1992). This association has not yet been confirmed. A small percentage of individuals with Waardenburg syndrome also have an intestinal blockage called Hirschsprung's megacolon, which usually requires surgical correction at an early age. Many families also report digestive problems such as chronic constipation and heartburn.

### Genetic Counseling Issues

RY's parents were given complete information on the physical characteristics of Waardenburg syndrome and the variability in these features that can occur. A complete explanation of autosomal dominant inheritance was also given. They were told that although their chance for future children to have Waardenburg syndrome was 50/50, there would be only a 20 percent chance for the child to have significant hearing loss, either unilateral or

bilateral. The parents had very few concerns about the other physical features of Waardenburg syndrome, since many of the family members had the same characteristics and had always considered them to be "normal" for their family. However, they did express concern about informing other family members about the chance for hearing loss in future children and the possible association between Waardenburg syndrome and spina bifida. Other family members were referred to geneticists in their own home areas who could provide them with this information face-to-face.

### Recommendations and Audiologic Issues

The parents were also given information about recent research on Waardenburg syndrome and the identification of the gene for Waardenburg syndrome, type 1. Because of their interest in participating in this research, they were referred to one of the geneticists performing this research. The parents also had several questions regarding accommodation for RY's unilateral hearing loss. They were referred back to the audiologist for regular audiologic follow-up and continued management of the hearing loss, including the use of any assistive technology, if appropriate. In addition, as the child approaches school age, the audiologist will be in the position to make referrals and recommendations to handle the issues arising from the educational, developmental, and social implications of the hearing loss.

## APPLICATIONS OF NEW RESEARCH AND TECHNOLOGY TO HEREDITARY HEARING LOSS

Great progress has been made in the last decade in understanding the molecular and biochemical nature of genes that cause hearing loss. Recent genetics technology for the mapping, cloning, sequencing, and characterization of genes and their protein products have been applied to several types of hearing loss. For example, a gene that causes type 1 Waardenburg syndrome has been localized to chromosome 2, and several mutations at this locus have been characterized (Baldwin et al., 1992; Tassabehi et al., 1992). At least four different genetic locations for Usher syndrome have been identified on chromosomes 1, 11, and 14 (Kaplan et al., 1992; Kimberling et al., 1990; Smith et al., 1992). Even more heterogeneity within Usher syndrome is likely to be found in the future. Branchio-oto-renal syndrome has been mapped to chromosome 8 (Smith et al., 1992). Although it is technically much more difficult to localize genes for nonsyndromic hearing loss, recent progress in this area has included the mapping of a gene for autosomal dominant low-frequency hearing loss to chromosome 5 (Leon et al., 1992) and a form of autosomal recessive sensorineural deafness to chromosome 13 (Guilford et al., 1994).

Clinical applications of this technology are potentially wide-ranging. The development of simple methods to identify genes for hearing loss will allow more accurate diagnosis of the cause of hearing loss both postnatally and prenatally, carrier testing for recessive forms of hearing loss, and treatment options for the hearing loss or for the related conditions associated with syndromic types of hearing loss. The recent establishment of the Human Genome Project (HGP), an international effort to identify all of the human genes (United States Department of Health and Human Services, 1991), will certainly speed progress in the identification of genes, diagnosis, treatment, and prevention for different hereditary conditions, including hearing loss. An important adjunct of the HGP is the Ethical, Legal and Social Issues program (ELSI). Considerable funding has been devoted to researching the ethical, legal, and social questions that may arise as technological advances are made through the HGP. Through research projects, training sessions, discussion groups, and workshops, professionals and consumers will seek ideas, develop guidelines, and offer professional and public policy options.

These projects will continue to focus on the areas of public and professional education, genetic service delivery (developing standards for clinical and counseling practice, research, and public health goals) and developing policies that protect individuals and society against unfair access to and use of genetic information (Juengst, 1994). Among the many questions that will be addressed include: (1) Will the Human Genome Project unfairly benefit certain cultures or points of view? (2) Will health and life insurance companies be allowed to use new genetic information to deny coverage to certain individuals or families? (3) Will genetic screening in the workplace lead to employment discrimination? and (4) Will genetic testing continue to be voluntary or who will decide what choices are available? In addition, projects will address how scientists can best educate the general population about complicated new technologies and their applications when few people in the general population have basic knowledge of genetics and the biologic sciences. The ethical implications of genetics technology are of particular concern to many members of the deaf community, most of whom would welcome the birth of a deaf child in their own family and the preservation of deaf culture. As discussed in Chapter 10, this reflects a cultural view of deafness rather than a medical or pathological view that is more familiar to health care professionals. Many of these issues will be discussed in the public forum in the coming years, making it even more important for health care professionals, including audiologists, to learn as much as possible about genetics and the implications for future health care.

## SUMMARY

Genetic factors cause over half of all moderate to profound hearing loss present at birth or in early life. There are over 200 different kinds of genetic hearing loss, many associated with other physical or medical features as part of a syndrome. Hereditary hearing loss can be inherited through nuclear genes in autosomal recessive, autosomal dominant, or x-linked inheritance patterns; mitochondrial genes for several forms of hearing loss have also been identified. Autosomal recessive inheritance, however, accounts for approximately 80 percent of hereditary hearing loss in children. Therefore, most children with genetic hearing loss will have no other family members with hearing loss, making the cause of the loss difficult to identify in many cases.

Genetic counseling is a process that emphasizes accurate diagnosis of hereditary conditions and communication of information to families in a sensitive fashion. Genetic counseling is performed by a team of genetics professionals and involves the collection of family and medical history, a physical examination by a certified clinical geneticist, and follow-up and support services. The issues that arise in genetic counseling differ for every family with hearing loss are often dependent on the degree of hearing loss present in the family, the age at onset, and the family's linguistic and cultural orientation.

Recent developments in genetics technology has led to the identification and characterization of an increasing number of genes for hearing loss. The clinical implications of these developments for the diagnosis and treatment of hereditary hearing loss will be wide-ranging, yet controversial. It is important for audiologists to have a basic understanding of genetic concepts, the contribution of genetic factors to hearing loss, the heterogeneity of hereditary hearing loss, and their role in referring families for genetic counseling.

## REFERENCES

Arnos, K. S., Cunningham, M., Israel, J., and Marazita, M. (1992). Innovative approach to genetic counseling services for the deaf population. *American Journal of Medical Genetics, 44*, 345–351.

Arnos, K. S., Israel, J., and Cunningham, M. (1991). Genetic counseling for the deaf: Medical and cultural considerations. *Annals of the New York Academy of Sciences, 630,* 212– 222.

Ashizawa, T., Anvret, M., Baiget, M., Barcelo, J. M., Brunner, H., Cobo, A. M., and Dallapiccola, B. (1994). Characteristics of intergenerational contractions of the CTG repeat in myotonic dystrophy. *American Journal of Human Genetics, 54,* 414–423.

Baldwin, C. T., Hoth, C. F., Amos, J. A., da-Silva, E. O. and Milunsky, A. (1992). An exonic mutation in the HuP2 paired domain gene causes Waardenburg's syndrome. *Nature, 355,* 637–638.

Ballinger, S. W., Shoffner, J. M., Hedaya, E. V., Trounce, I., Polak, M. A., Koontz, D. A., Wallace, D.C. (1992). Maternally transmitted diabetes, deafness associated with 10.4 kb mitochondrial DNA deletion. *Nature Genetics, 1,* 11–15.

Barker, D. F., Hostikka, S. L., Zhou, J., Chow, L. T., Oliphant, A. R., Gerken, S. C., Gregory, M. C., Skolnick, M. H., Atkin, C. L. and Tryggvason, K. (1990). Identification of muations in the COL4A5 collagen gene in Alport syndrome. *Science, 248,* 1224–1227.

Berger, W., van de Pol, D., Warburg, M., Gal, A., Bleeker-Wagemakers, L., de Silva, H., Meindl, A., Meitinger, T., Cremers, F., and Ropers, H. (1992). Mutations in the candidate gene for Norrie disease. *Human Molecular Genetics, 1,* 461–465.

Bieber, F. R.(1981). Genetic studies of questionnaire data from a residential school for the deaf, unpublished doctoral dissertation, Medical College of Virginia, Richmond, Virginia.

Brunner, H. G., van Bennekom, C. A., Lambermon, E. M., Oei, T. L., Cremers, C. W., Wieringa, B., and Ropers, H. H. (1988). The gene for X-linked progressive mixed deafness with perilymphatic gusher during stapes surgery (DFN3 is linked to PGK). *Human Genetics, 80,* 337–340.

Carezani-Gavin, M., Clarren, S. K., Steege, T. (1992). Letter to the Editor: Waardenburg syndrome associated with meningomyelocele. *American Journal of Medical Genetics, 42,* 135–136.

Dixon, M. J., Read, A. P., Donnai, D., Colley, A., Dixon, J., and Williamson, R. (1991). The gene for Treacher Collins syndrome maps to the long arm of chromosome 5. *American Journal of Human Genetics, 49,* 17–22.

Fraser, G. R., Froggatt, P., and James, T. N. (1964). Congenital deafness associated with electrocardiographic abnormalities, fainting attacks and sudden death. *Quarterly Journal of Medicine, 33,* 361–385.

Gorlin, R. J., Cohen, M. M., and Levin, L. S. (1990). *Syndromes of the Head and Neck,* 3rd ed. (pp. 519–529, 649–652). New York: Oxford University Press.

Guilford, P., Arab, S. B., Blanchard, S., Levilliers, J., Weissenback, J., Belkahia, A., and Petit, C. (1994).

A non-syndromic form of neurosensory, recessive deafness maps to the pericentromeric region of chromosome 13q. *Nature Genetics, 6,* 24–28.

Hall, J. G. (1990). Genomic imprinting: Review, relevance to human diseases. *American Journal of Human Genetics, 46,* 857–873.

Hopwood, J. J., Bunge, S., Morris, C. P., Wilson, P. J., Steglich, C., Beck, M., Schwinger, E., and Gal, A. (1993). Molecular basis of mucopolysaccharidosis type II: Mutations in the iduronate-2-sulphatase gene. *Human Mutation, 2,* 435–442.

Hu, D., Qiu, W., Wu, B., Fang, L., Zhou, F., Gu, Y., Zhang, Q., Yan, J., Ding, Y. & Wong, H. (1991). Genetic aspects of antibiotic induced deafness: mitochondrial inheritance. *Journal of Medical Genetics, 28,* 79–83.

Jones, K. L. (1988). *Smith's Recognizable Patterns of Human Malformation* 4th ed. (pp. 10–13, 364–369, 372–375). Philadelphia: W. B. Saunders Company.

Jordan, I. K. (1991). Ethical issues in the genetic study of deafness. *Annals of the New York Academy of Sciences, 630,* 236–239.

Juengst, E. T. (1994). Human genome research and the public interest: Progress noted from an American science policy experiment. *American Journal of Human Genetics, 54,* 121–128.

Jung, J. H. (1989). *Genetic Syndromes in Communication Disorders.* Boston: College-Hill Press.

Kaplan, J., Gerber, S., Bonneau, D., Rozet, J. M., Delrieu, O., Briard, M. L., Dollfus, H., Ghazi, I., Dufier, J. L., Frezal, J., and Munnich, A. (1992). A gene for Usher syndrome type I (USH1A) maps to chromosome 14q. *Genomics, 14,* 979–987.

Kimberling, W. J., Weston, M. D., Moller, C., Davenport, S. L. H., Shugart, Y. Y., Priluck, I. A., Martini, A., Milani, M., and Smith, R. J. (1990). Localization of Usher syndrome type II to chromosome 1q. *Genomics, 7:* 245–249.

Konigsmark, B. W., and Gorlin, R. J. (1976). *Genetic and Metabolic Deafness.* Philadelphia: W. B. Saunders Company.

Knowlton, R. G., Weaver, E. J., Struyk, A. F., Knobloch, W. H., King, R. A., Norris, K., Shamban, A., Uitto, J., Jimenez, S. A., and Prockop, D. J. (1989). Genetic linkage analysis of hereditary arthro-ophthalmopathy (Stickler syndrome) and the type II procollagen gene. *American Journal of Human Genetics, 45,* 681–688.

Leon, P. E., Raventos, H., Lynch, E., Morrow, J., and King, M. C. (1992). The gene for an inherited form of deafness maps to chromosome 5q31. *Proceedings of the National Academy of Sciences, 89,* 5181–5184.

Marazita, M. L., Ploughman, L. M., Rawlings, B., Remington, E., Arnos, K. S., and Nance, W. E. (1993). Genetic epidemiological studies of early-onset deafness in the U.S. school-age population. *American Journal of Medical Genetics, 46,* 286–491.

McKusick, V. A. (1992). *Mendelian Inheritance in Man,* 10th ed. Baltimore: The Johns Hopkins University Press.

Narod, S. A., Parry, D. M., Parboosingh, J., Lenoir, G. M., Ruttledge, M., Fischer, G., Eldridge, R., Martuza, R. L., Frontali, M., Haines, J. Gusella, J. F., and Rouleau, G. A. (1992). Neurofibromatosis type 2 appears to be a genetically homogeneous disease. *American Journal of Human Genetics, 51,* 486–496.

Padden, C., and Humphries, T. (1988). *Deaf in America—Voices From a Culture.* Cambridge: Harvard University Press.

Prezant, T. R., Agapian, J. V., Bohlman, M. C., Bu, X., Oztas, S., Hu, D., Arnos, K. S., Cortopassi, G. A., Jaber, L., Rotter, J. I., Shohat, M. and Fischel-Ghodsian, N. (1993). Mitochondrial ribosomal RNA mutation associated with antibiotic-induced and nonsyndromic deafness. *Nature Genetics, 4,* 289–294.

Reardon, W. (1992). Genetic deafness. *Journal of Medical Genetics, 29,* 521–526.

Rose, S. P., Conneally, P. M., and Nance, W. E. (1977). Genetic analysis of childhood deafness. In F. H. Bess (Ed.). *Childhood Deafness* (pp. 19–35). New York: Grune and Stratton.

Rotig, A., Cormier, V., Chatelain, P., Francois, R., Saudubray, J., Rustin, P. and Munnich, A. (1993). Deletion of mitochondrial DNA in a case of early onset diabetes mellitus, optic atrophy and deafness (Wolfram syndrome, MIM 222300). *Journal of Clinical Investigation, 91,* 1095–1098.

Ruben, R. J. (1991). The history of the genetics of hearing impairment. *Annals of the New York Academy of Sciences, 630,* 6–15.

Schein, J. D. (1989). *At Home Among Strangers* (pp. 106–134). Washington, DC: Gallaudet University Press.

Scott, H. S., Ashton, L. J., Eyre, H. J., Baker, E., Brooks, D. A., Callen, D. F., Sutherland, G. R., Morris, C. P., and Hopwood, J. J. (1990). Chromosomal localization of the human alpha-L-iduronidase gene (IDUA) to 4p16.3. *American Journal of Human Genetics, 47,* 802–807.

Sill, A. M., Stick, M. J., Prenger, V. L., Phillips, S. L., Boughman, J. A., and Arnos, K. S. (1994). A genetic epidemiologic study of hearing loss in an adult population. *American Journal of Medical Genetics, 54,* 149–153.

Smith, R. J. H., Berlin, C. I., Hejtmancik, J. F., Keats, B. J. B., Kimberling, W. J., Lewis, R. A., Moller, C. G., Pelias, M. Z., and Tranebjaerg, L. (1994). Clinical diagnosis of the Usher syndromes. *American Journal of Medical Genetics, 50,* 32–38.

Smith, R. J. H., Coppage, K. B., Ankerstjerne, J. K. B., Capper, D. T., Kumar, S., Kenyon, J., Tinley, S., Comeau, K., and Kimberling, W. J. (1992). Localization of the gene for branchiootorenal syndrome to chromosome 8q. *Genomics, 14,* 841–844.

Smith, R. J. H., Lee, E. C., Kimberling, W. J., Daiger, S. P., Pelias, M. Z., Keats, B. J. B., Jay, M., Bird, A., Reardon, W., Guest, M., Ayyagari, R., and Hejtmancik, J. F. (1992). Localization of two genes for Usher syndrome type I to chromosome 11. *Genomics, 14,* 995–1002.

Spence, J. E., Perciaccante, R. G., Greig, G. M., Willard, H. F., Ledbetter, D. H., Hejtmancik, J. F., Pollack, M. S., et al. (1988). Uniparental disomy as a mechanism for human genetic disease. *American Journal of Human Genetics, 42,* 217–226.

Sutherland, G. R., and Richards, R. I. (1994). Dynamic mutations. *American Scientist, 82*(2), 157–163.

Sykes, B., Ogilvie, D., Wordsworth, P., Wallis, G., Mathew, C., Beighton, P., Nicholls, A., Pope, F. M., Thompson, E., Tsipouras, P., Schwartz, R., Jensson, O., Arnason, A., Borresen, A. L., Heiberg, A., Frey, D., and Steinmann, B. (1990). Consistent linkage of dominantly inherited osteogenesis imperfecta to the type I collagen loci: COL1A1 adn COL1A2. *American Journal of Human Genetics, 46,* 293–307.

Tassabehji, M., Read, A. P., Newton, V. E., Harris, R., Balling, R., Gruss, P., and Strachan, T. (1992). Waardenburg's syndrome patients have mutations in the human homologue of the Pax-3 paired box gene. *Nature, 355,* 635–636.

Thompson, M. W., McInnes, R. R., and Willard, H. F. (1991). *Thompson and Thompson Genetics in Medicine,* (5th ed.). Philadelphia: W. B. Saunders Company.

United States Department of Health and Human Services, Public Health Services, National Institutes of Health (1991). *The Human Genome Project. New Tools for Tomorrow's Health Research.*

van Wouwe, J. P., Wijnands, M. C., Mourad-Baars, P. E., Geraedts, J., Beverstock, G. C., and van de Kamp, J. (1986). A patient with dup(10p)del(8q) and Pendred syndrome. *American Journal of Medical Genetics, 24,* 211–217.

Wallace, D. C. (1987). Maternal genes: Mitochondrial diseases. *Birth Defects: Original Article Series, March of Dimes Birth Defects Foundation, 23*(3), 137–190.

Wolf, B., Heard, G. S., Jefferson, L. G., Proud, V. K., Nance, W. E. and Weissbecker, K. A. (1985). Clinical findings in four children with biotinidase deficiency detected through a statewide neonatal screening program. *New England Journal of Medicine, 313,* 16–19.

# CHAPTER 3

# CONDUCTIVE HEARING LOSS IN CHILDREN: ETIOLOGY AND PATHOLOGY

*JOHN GREER CLARK AND MICHAEL JAINDL*

## INTRODUCTION

Advances in audiologic assessment and management leads to greater reliance of the otolaryngologist on the judgment and expertise of the audiologist. Similarly, the otolaryngologist's role in the establishment of the etiology of pediatric hearing loss and the efficacious treatment of otic pathology make possible the subsequent management endeavors that the audiologist pursues with the pediatric patient.

This chapter and the one that follows present discussions of many of the pathologies that underlie pediatric hearing loss from combined otologic and audiologic perspectives. It is intended that these two chapters will help the reader form a framework for audiologic evaluation and subsequent management of hearing loss.

## EMBRYOLOGIC DEVELOPMENT OF THE EAR

A review of the embryologic development of the ear not only enhances our understanding of some of the pathological occurrences that may develop, but also increases our appreciation of the miraculous sense we call hearing. For a more in-depth discussion of this topic than is presented here, the reader is referred to Arey (1965), Anson and Davies (1980), Kenna (1990), Zemlin (1988) or to a basic text on developmental anatomy.

### The Sensory Organ

Development of the ear begins during the early life of the human embryo. By the middle of the third week of gestation thickening in the superficial ectoderm along the sides of the open neural tube mark the beginnings of the auditory or otic placodes. This stage is quickly followed by the appearance of distinct auditory pits that close into otocysts, or auditory vesicles (Figure 3.1). Before the embryo is five weeks old the beginnings of the vestibular portion of the labyrinth are recognizable, and the outcroppings of the semicircular canals are visible by the end of the sixth week. The cristae and maculae, sense organs for maintaining equilibrium and detecting direction and extent of movement, differentiate during the seventh week. Early within the eighth week the endolymphatic duct and the three semicircular canals are well-defined.

During this same period, the main endolymphatic sac divides into the utricle and saccule, and the cochlear duct begins to take on its coiled appearance. The coils of the cochlea are completed by the eleventh week. Early in the third month the general adult form of the inner ear is attained although the sensory and supporting cells will not reach full maturation until the fifth month. The newly distinguished otocyst, along with its subdivisions and fibrous support, comprise the membranous labyrinth. Although speculative, the sensorineural system may be sufficiently mature to permit sound sensation by the end of the sixth or beginning of the seventh month of normal gestation (Peck, 1994).

Because the development of the vestibular end organ precedes full maturation of the cochlea, the latter structure is more susceptible to developmental anomalies. In many invertebrates the utri-

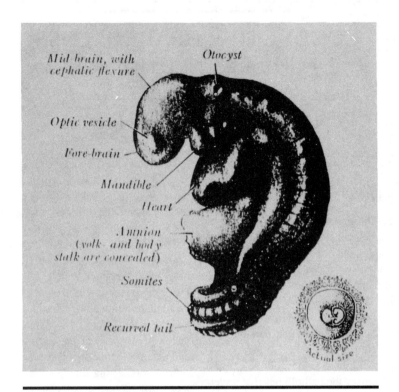

**FIGURE 3.1** Human embryo of 26 days, viewed from the left. (From Arey, L. B. (1965). *Developmental Anatomy*. Philadelphia: W. B. Saunders. Used with permission).

cle and saccule make up the entire "ear," functioning solely for equilibrium. The cochlear duct is historically a secondary outgrowth of this older portion. The mammalian cochlea developed into a coiled structure in contrast to the straight or uncoiled "cochlea" of birds and reptiles. Paleontologic study reveals that the Jurassic vestibular systems over 150 million years ago are virtually indistinguishable from present day reptiles and mammals, bearing witness to an excellent design (McCandless, 1994).

## The Middle and Outer Ears

The conductive portions of the ear evolve simultaneous to the development of the sensory organs of the auditory mechanism. The development of the jaw, neck, and structures of the middle ear are related to the branchial arches, more recently re-

ferred to as the pharyngeal arches. These five arches are ridge-like structures, separated by four ectodermal branchial or pharyngeal grooves, which appear on the two ventrolateral surfaces of the embryo's head during the fourth week (Figure 3.2). The pharyngeal arches correspond to the gill-arches of fish and some amphibians, which subsequently develop into gills through which respiratory water flows.

By the end of the fourth week the endoderm of the pharynx bulges outward to form the pharyngeal pouches at the level of the external branchial grooves. The first pharyngeal arch on each side divides into a maxillary and mandibular process. The fates of the endodermal pouches are varied. In particular, the first pouch retains its lumen and by the eighth week differentiates into the eustachian tube and the tubotympanic recess or tym-

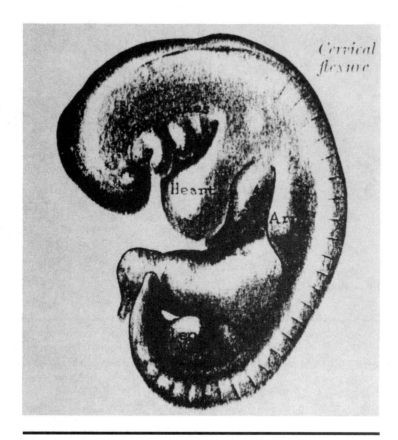

**FIGURE 3.2**    Five-week embryo viewed from the left. Branchial arches
are posterior to the nasal pit and superior to the heart. (From Arey, L. B.
(1965). *Developmental Anatomy*. Philadelphia: W. B. Saunders. Used with
permission.)

panic cavity of the middle ear. At this same time,
the overlying ectodermal groove deepens to become the external auditory meatus. This canal
continues inward to the closing plate, which re-
gains a middle layer of mesoderm and comprises
the tympanic membrane (Figure 3.3). Arising
from a thinning of the mesodermal tissue (middle
layer of cells of an embryo) in the region in which
the deepening external meatus butts against the
wall of the tympanic cavity, the tympanic membrane is covered externally by ectodermal epithelium and internally by endoderm. At birth, the
tympanic membrane is set so obliquely as to almost lie upon the meatal floor (superior edge most

laterally placed), gradually erecting itself as the
canal lengthens during the first three years.

The tympanic cavity is surrounded by loose
connective tissue within which the auditory ossicles develop. In the last fetal months, this spongy
connective tissue degenerates and the tympanic
cavity begins to expand to occupy the resultant
space. The malleus and incus primarily develop
from the condensed mesenchymal tissue (diffuse
network of cells forming the embryonic mesoderm) of the first pharyngeal arch, while the
stapes evolves from that of the second arch. By
the ninth week, the ossicles are miniature models
of their adult counterparts, beginning ossification

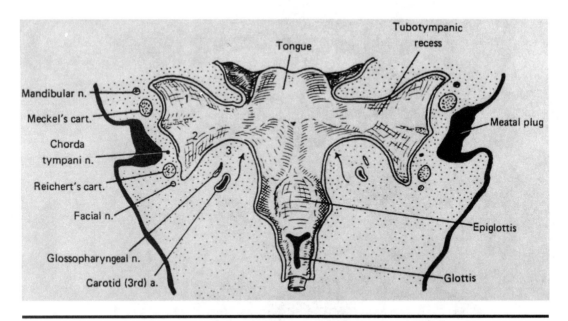

**FIGURE 3.3** Floor of the pharynx of an embryo showing the formation of the tubotympanic recess. The recess arises as a lateral expansion of the pharyngeal lumen at the level of the first three internal pharyngeal grooves and pouches. The external auditory meatus is shown as a solid "meatal plug" of ectoderm growing deeply into the mesoderm from the upper end of the first external pharyngeal groove to make contact with the tubotympanic recess, the "drum" being formed at the area of contact. (From Anson, B. J. and Davies, J. (1980). Embryology of the ear. In M. M. Paparella and D. A. Shumrick (eds.), *Otolaryngology* (vol. 1, 4th ed.) Philadelphia: W. B. Saunders and Company. Used with permission).

between the twelfth and eighteenth week. These bones soon lose connection with their respective arches, and articulations develop where they touch each other. The malleus attaches to the tympanic membrane; the stapes fits into the oval window of the perilymphatic space, and the incus articulates with the malleus and stapes. Corresponding to the developmental origins of the ossicles, the tensor tympani muscle derives from the first pharyngeal arch, and the stapedial muscle from the second arch. The auricle develops around the first pharyngeal groove with tissue arising from both the first and second pharyngeal arches. During the sixth week, six hillocks (tissue thickenings) appear on these parts, which evolve into the adult-shaped auricle by the eighth week (Figure 3.4 [B–E]).

At birth, the newborn child hears imperfectly, as the external auditory canal is not completely free of detritis (remaining tissue), and the middle ear cavity is largely filled with a gelatinous tissue. A progressive resorption of this material leaves the infant with normally acute hearing in the first weeks after birth.

### Developmental Anomalies

Congenital hearing loss may result from imperfect neural connections, imperfect development of the membranous labyrinth, ossicles, or tympanic membrane, or an atresia of the tympanic cavity and/or the external meatus. The temporal proximity of arrested or aberrant development to conception is directly related to the extent and severity of the resultant hearing disorder. However, a complete agenesis of the inner, middle, or outer ear is very rare. As these structures arise from different embryonal tissues, a disorder in one does not necessarily herald the presence of a disorder in an-

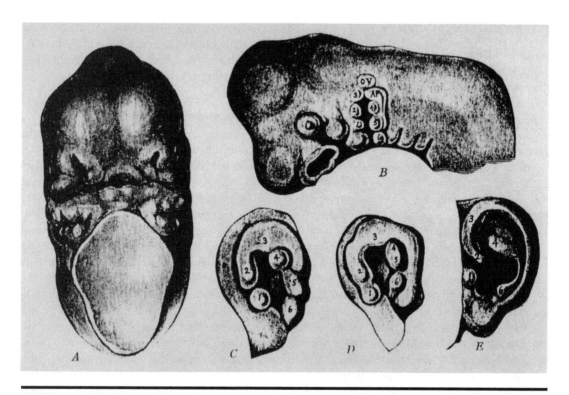

**FIGURE 3.4** Development of the human auricle. *A,* Front view of the head, at 12.5 mm (× 13). Below the face are the ear hillocks grouped about the first branchial grooves. *B-E,* Side views of the auricle at 11 mm, 13.5 mm, 15 mm, and in adult. *AF,* Auricular fold; *OV,* otic vesicle; 1–6, elevations on the mandibular and hyoid arches that respectively become 1, tragus; 2, 3, helix; 4, 5, antihelix; 6, antitragus. (From Arey, L. B. (1965). *Developmental Anatomy.* Philadelphia: W. B. Saunders. Used with permission).

other. Their general proximity, however, does lend to this possibility. In addition, outer and middle ear disorders will coexist more frequently with each other than with inner ear disorders given their similar origins from the first and second pharyngeal arches (Peck, 1994).

Hearing loss from damage to the organ of Corti secondary to maternal rubella (German measles) in the second month of pregnancy was a frequent occurrence in the 1960s. Today, sensorineural hearing loss is more common secondary to high-risk birth and developmental factors.

The auricles may fail to develop appreciably, resulting in the fetal-type auricles occasionally seen in adults. This inhibited development may result in some immeasurable decrease in the pinna's ability to contribute to sound localization and the pinna's natural resonance of sound that adds to the reception of higher frequencies. Complete absence of the auricles may result in significant decreases in these abilities that may not be clearly reflected when measuring hearing with earphones. Pits, or fistulae, sometimes occur in areas of the ear in early stages of development, especially in front of the base of the helix. However, a complete fistula connecting into the middle ear cavity is extremely rare.

An appreciation of the developmental anatomy of the embryonic ear leaves us in awe of the complexity of this organ. This, coupled with an understanding of the physiologic mechanisms of hearing, can greatly enhance our understanding and evaluation of the conductive hearing mechanism and its pathologies.

## OTOLOGIC INSPECTION

When evaluating conductive hearing loss the audiologist's assessment provides documentation of the extent of hearing loss presented by a disorder and of the improved hearing status that may be experienced following any prescribed medical or surgical intervention. In addition, audiologic assessment provides baseline data around which decisions will be made regarding audiologic management if hearing impairment persists following treatment or continues for a protracted time during treatment.

Prior to the audiologic evaluation the audiologist should begin with a close inspection of the patient's ears and the physical relation of the ears to the head. The audiologist should note any abnormalities observed including ear formation, position of the ears, visible asymmetries between the two ears, ear canal stenosis or aural atresia, ear canal blockage, and intactness of the tympanic membrane. Statements of the appearance of these structures is appropriate within subsequent reports. However, diagnostic statements of presumed pathologies that are observed should be left to the physician.

### Auricle

The visible portion of the ear, the auricle or pinna, consists of a single convoluted cartilage covered by a thin layer of loose connective tissue and skin. Knowledge of the normal configuration of the external ears is beneficial to the examination of the auricle (Figure 3.4E). During this examination, the position of the auricle should be observed. Normally, the top of the helix is at the same level as the eyebrow. The lobule, which is devoid of cartilage support, is superior to the angle of the mandible, and the external auditory meatus should be in line with the nasal ala. By age 5 years, the external ear is almost adult size, measuring 3.5 to 4.5 cm from the tragus to the superior helical rim and 3 to 4 cm from the tragus to the posterior helical rim (Kenna, 1990).

During fetal development, the ear begins in a position caudal (inferior) to the mandible and mi-

grates superiorly. Low-set ears are common in congenital disorders in which arrest in the cephalad migration of the auricles occurs (migration upward from the neck and toward the head).

### External Auditory Canal

The external auditory canal extends from the meatal opening to the annulus (outer ring) of the tympanic membrane. The lateral and movable part of the canal is cartilaginous and is usually less than 50 percent of the total length. The meatus (passage) is slightly concave anteriorly and the canal tracks posteriorly and superiorly. The bony external canal angles slightly anteriorly with the temporomandibular joint (TMJ) protruding into the anterior canal wall in varying degrees. Sometimes the protrusion of the TMJ will obscure visibility of the tympanic membrane. The size and shape of the external canal also varies according to individual differences and age. In some infants, particularly those with craniofacial anomalies, the external canal may be extremely small (Figure 3.5), requiring binocular microscopic examination (Figures 3.6).

Collapse of the external auditory canal may occur when the pinna is compressed against the side of the head, as may be experienced when standard supra-aural earphones are placed on the ears. Such collapse is different from a prolapsed ear canal that may result from trauma or inflammatory disorders. As many as 4 percent of a typical audiology caseload may have collapsing ear canals (Jerger and Jerger, 1981). One may expect this more often in a pediatric population as the outer portion of the ear canal is less rigid before age 7 years. The narrow ear canals seen in children with Down syndrome also leads to a greater chance of canal collapse during hearing testing. Jerger and Jerger note that the effect on air-conduction hearing thresholds is typically 10 to 15 dB but may range as high as 50 dB depending on the amount of occlusion produced by the collapsing canal.

Inspection for meatal collapse should be done routinely before proceeding with a hearing evalu-

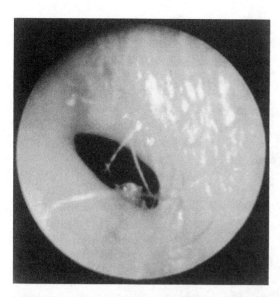

**FIGURE 3.5** External auditory canal stenosis may be congenital or acquired. This congenitally stenotic canal was 1 mm × 2 mm in size and associated with ossicular fixation. Canal stenoses may follow recurrent external otitis or trauma. (From Chole, R. A. (1982). *Color Atlas of Ear Disease.* New York: Appleton-Century Crofts. Used with permission.)

ation or any time the presence of an air-bone gap does not agree with the case history or subsequent test findings. Pressing the pinna against the side of the patient's head while inspecting the external canal lumen will reveal a collapsing ear canal. A verification that the canals have not collapsed during testing can easily be attained by repeating a portion of the threshold assessment in the sound field for comparison to the earphone results. Similarly, Reiter and Silman (1993) recommend a routine screen for meatal collapse by comparing air-conduction thresholds at 4000 Hz obtained with the jaw/mouth closed and the jaw/mouth open. If the threshold with the jaw/mouth open is better by 15 dB or more, collapse is present. The use of either insert ear phones or circumaural earphone cushions can help avoid the problem of collapsing canals, although the latter may create calibration difficulties. If such transducers are not available, air-conduction thresholds should be measured with the jaw and mouth open in the presence of collapsed canals.

### Tympanic Membrane

Examination of the ear drum, or tympanic membrane, is best performed with a hand-held otoscope or examining binocular microscope with the patient in a sitting or supine position. Visibility of the tympanic membrane is made easier when the canal is straightened by pulling the pinna posteriorly and superiorly while holding counter traction on the preauricular skin. The tympanic membrane of infants may be more easily seen by pulling the pinna downward because their ear canals have a more downward angle. The speculum of the otoscope is then inserted first in a slightly anterior direction to clear the tragus, then rotated slightly posteriorly as the speculum is advanced into the canal. It is important to use the *largest* speculum that will pass into the meatus to allow visibility of as much of the tympanic membrane as possible in the viewing area.

For purposes of standardizing nomenclature, the tympanic membrane is oriented like a clock with 12 o'clock being cephalad (toward the head, or top) and 3 o'clock being posterior on the left ear. Examination of the tympanic membrane begins with identification of the landmarks (Figure 3.7). The annulus is present inferiorly from the 10 o'clock to the 2 o'clock positions and identifies the perimeter of the pars tensa. The annulus is absent superiorly where the tympanic membrane drapes from the lateral process of the malleus. This area, the pars flaccida, should be carefully inspected because of its high propensity for disease, such as retraction pockets and cholesteatoma.

The pars tensa is attached to the manubrium of the malleus forming the umbo at the tip of the malleus, a common landmark. The slightly conical shape of the tympanic membrane comes to its apex at the umbo. The frequently noted light reflex can be seen as a triangle of reflected light extending from the umbo to the annulus in an anteroinferior direction due to the anteromedial angulation of the tympanic membrane. The blood supply to

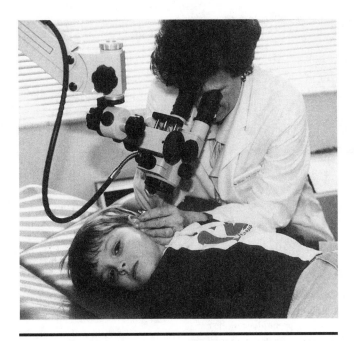

**FIGURE 3.6**    Binocular microscopic inspection of the ear canal and the tympanic membrane (Courtesy of HearCare, Inc.)

the tympanic membrane can sometimes be seen coursing along the manubrium and radiating outwards at the umbo, meeting the blood vessels at the annulus. These are especially pronounced during inflammation owing to the intense erythema seen on examination.

Often a healthy tympanic membrane is very transparent and middle ear structures can be easily seen. In the posterior superior quadrant the long process of the incus and the stapedial tendon may appear as a white elbow (Figure 3.8). Occasionally the dark shadow of the oval window is apparent just inferior to the stapedial tendon. The pale promontory (basal turn of the cochlea) and round window niche may also be seen posteriorly. Note that the incus and stapes are vulnerable in the posterior superior quadrant of the pars tensa. A penetrating injury to this region could result in violation of the inner ear. In addition to possible perforations, several disease processes can be identified early by careful inspection of the posterior superior quadrant.

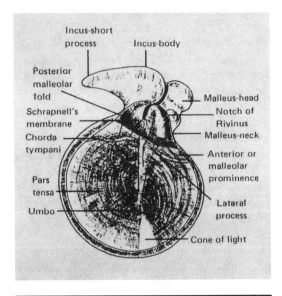

**FIGURE 3.7**    Schematic of tympanic membrane and associated structures. (From Zemlin, W. R. (1982). *Speech and Hearing Science* (3rd ed.). Englewood Cliffs, NJ: Prentice Hall. Used with permission.)

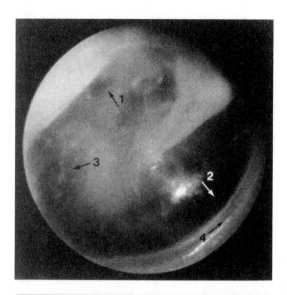

**FIGURE 3.8**   The translucency of this normal right tympanic membrane allows visibility of the underlying incus (1), eustachian tube orifice (2), and the round window niche (3). The anterior part of the tympanic sulcus (4), is often hidden from view during routine otoscopy. (From Chole, R. A. (1982). *Color Atlas of Ear Disease*. New York: Appleton-Century Crofts. Used with permission.)

## EXTERNAL EAR DISORDERS

### Congenital Malformation

Table 3.1 presents a list of congenital disorders of the external ear. Of these, only the first two, congenital aural atresia and microtia, present a potential for significant hearing loss and challenges with amplification. The congenital aural atresia complex can consist of any degree of microtia accompanied by external canal atresia, an atretic middle ear, varying degrees of ossicular involvement, and anomalies of the cochlea and vestibular labyrinth. Although the auricle, external canal, ossicles and labyrinth all are almost completely developed in the first three months, as discussed earlier, their embryologic origin and development are mostly independent.

Although the formation of the ear structures appears to occur independently, it is estimated that

**TABLE 3.1**   Congenital Disorders of the External Ear

| | |
|---|---|
| Microtia | Periauricular attachments |
| Atresia of the external auditory canal | Pre- and postauricular and prehelical sinuses |
| Appendages | Fusion of auricle with scalp |
| Fistula | |
| Cryptotia | Large auricle |
| Macrotia | Absence of auricle |
| Anotia | Displacement of ear onto the neck |
| Synotia | |
| Melotia | Displacement of ear onto cheek |
| Low set ears | |
| Lobular anomalies | Lack of aural migration |
| Antihelical anomalies | Absence, split, thickened, or nodular |
| Tragal anomalies | |
| Underdeveloped auricle | Absence or poor development |
| Underdeveloped canal | |

30 percent of congenital aural atresia is associated with inner ear malformation and most cases of total canal atresia are associated with some degree of microtia (Altman, 1950; Naunton and Valvassor, 1968). This suggests a high propensity for conductive and sensorineural hearing loss. In fact, hearing loss may range from maximally conductive at 50 to 60 dB to complete anacusis. It is important to note that radiological evaluation of the labyrinth may not be predictive of the functional status of the cochlea. In cases of congenital aural atresia, a complete hearing evaluation must be performed very early and amplification provided as indicated.

### Acquired External Ear Disorders

Mechanical obstruction of the external canal is the most common cause of immediately reversible hearing loss and cerumen is the most common cause of mechanical obstruction. The most common cause of cerumen impaction in the pediatric population results from parent's inappropriate use of cotton swabs. Not only are cotton swabs ineffective in cleaning the ear canal, their use can create problems ranging from minor canal lacerations to more serious complications including tympanic membrane perforation and sensorineural hearing loss secondary to ossicular displacement through the oval window of the inner ear. Audiologists should be direct with parents in advocating proper ear hygiene.

Complete obstruction of the canal may mimic otitis media producing a conductive hearing loss, flat tympanogram, and a sensation of pressure or pain. Any foreign body large enough to obstruct the canal can produce similar findings. Young children frequently place small objects in their ear canals including small toys or beads, pieces of food, or portions of crayons. Probably the most common foreign body found in children's ears is an extruded ventilation, or pressure equalization, tube (PE tube). If not removed an extruded tube will often collect cerumen and debris until the canal is blocked.

The 1990s have brought many changes to the profession of audiology, in professional academic preparation and continuing education requirements, as well as in the scope of practice. Arising from these changes, the audiologist's role in cerumen management has been frequently examined (ASHA, 1992; Roeser, Adams, Roland, and Wilson, 1992). While the removal of cerumen from a patient's ear canal is often expeditious to the audiologist's testing and management, these procedures must be approached with extreme caution when working with the pediatric population. Very young children are prone to be frightened during cerumen removal leading to unexpected and undesired movements that may seriously impede and complicate the procedure. Before attempting cerumen removal with children, audiologists should feel highly comfortable with the degree of training and experience they have received in this area. The rapport and comfort level reached between the child and the audiologist should be similarly high. Otherwise, to avoid possible injury to the ear canal, the tympanic membrane, or the middle ear ossicles, cerumen removal for children should be deferred to the otolaryngologist.

If a physician is not on site, the audiologist may question how much cerumen precludes the continuation of assessment. If any portion of the tympanic membrane remains visible, the audiologist may proceed with testing. If the audiologist is uncertain if a complete blockage is present, the presence of normal tympanometry will rule out a blocked ear canal. In most cases, the ear canal must be completely occluded before an appreciable change in hearing sensitivity will be noted on the hearing test.

Inflammatory disorders of the external canal most commonly include otitis externa (swimmer's ear), otomycosis (fungal infection), eczema, herpes zoster oticus, and herpes simplex oticus. These disorders are easily observed on otoscopic inspection and often produce swelling and erythema sometimes accompanied by intense pain, discharge and blisters localized to the external canal and/or the conchal bowl (Figure 3.9). Conductive

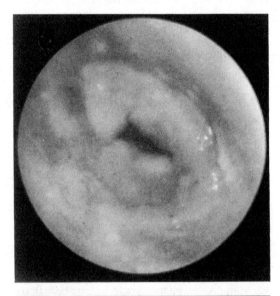

**FIGURE 3.9** In this case of acute bacterial external otitis, purulent debris totally occludes the external canal. (From Chole, R. A. (1982). *Color Atlas of Ear Disease.* New York: Appleton-Century Crofts. Used with permission.)

hearing loss is common from blockage of the external canal and from any resultant tympanic membrane and middle ear involvement.

Benign tumors of the external ear are common and may be a cause of conductive hearing loss or may obstruct proper fitting of assistive devices. Keloids are growths that occur in areas of penetrating trauma or surgery, most commonly in dark skin populations. Although rare in the conchal bowl or external canal, it is not uncommon for a keloid to develop in a postauricular incision after surgery, making a behind-the-ear hearing instrument difficult to fit. External canal cysts of the sebaceous and cerumenous glands may occur in the cartilaginous portion of the canal. These, too, can become quite large, totally obstructing the canal, and require surgical resection.

Osteomas and exostoses are benign bony neoplasms of the bony external canal. Osteomas are sessile (broad-based) and usually occur as a single growth on the floor of the ear canal at the bony-cartilaginous junction. Exostoses may occur in multiples and can be sessile or become quite long like an appendage, impinging on the tympanic membrane producing pain and even hearing loss. Exostoses are common but rarely occur before 10 years of age (Figure 3.10). In contrast, osteomas are rare and can occur at any age. Both can become large enough to obstruct the canal and produce a conductive hearing loss.

Soft tissue neoplasms (Table 3.2) including adenomas, hemangiomas, papillomas, and fibromas are uncommon but can present with a conductive hearing loss. Polyps seen in the external canal may arise from an infectious or inflammatory site on the canal wall or tympanic membrane and often represent significant middle ear disease.

Malignant tumors of the external ear are rare in children. However, a variety of sarcomas (soft tissue tumors) and skin cancers have been reported in the pediatric population. These children generally present with an enlarging mass, chronic bloody drainage, and/or pain, and occasionally facial paralysis. Symptoms may at first mimic infection and produce conductive hearing loss from

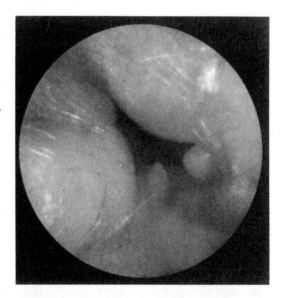

**FIGURE 3.10** This external canal is almost occluded by multiple sessile exostoses of the bony canal. Exostoses of this type are often seen in cold water swimmers. Some patients with multiple exostoses experience recurrent external otitis, necessitating surgical removal of the lesions. (From Chole, R. A. (1982). *Color Atlas of Ear Disease.* New York: Appleton-Century Crofts. Used with permission.)

**TABLE 3.2**  Neoplasms of the External Ear

| BENIGN | MALIGNANT |
| --- | --- |
| Papilloma | Squamous cell carcinoma |
| Ceruminoma | Rhabdomyosarcoma |
| Pilomatrixoma | Basal cell carcinoma |
| Lymphangioma | |
| Hemangioma | |
| Fibroma | |
| Dermatofibroma | |
| Neurofibroma | |
| Adenoma | |

canal obstruction. Treatment is often radical surgery, and hearing restoration without amplification can be a difficult challenge.

## MIDDLE EAR DISORDERS

### Congenital Malformations of the Middle Ear

Congenital middle ear anomalies associated with craniofacial syndromes are not uncommon and may be accompanied by hearing loss. Table 3.3 presents a list of the more common craniofacial anomalies and their associated middle ear defects. Nonsyndromic ossicular anomalies may occur alone or with congenital aural atresia as previously discussed. Reported isolated ossicular anomalies have included absence of, or fusion of, part or all of each of the ossicles with a resultant nonprogressive mild to moderately severe conductive hearing loss. *Otosclerosis* is a familial disorder that is inherited as an autosomal-dominant trait with a 40 to 50 percent penetrance. The clinical onset is usually postpuberty, suggesting a hormonal influence. Although it is more common in young adults otosclerosis is occasionally seen in children under 17 years of age.

Congenital cholesteatoma is a rare lesion thought to be produced by entrapment of epidermal tissue in the middle ear during fetal development. These cystic growths are insidious in nature and often are not discovered until there is ossicular involvement. They typically appear as a white spherical mass in the middle ear usually seen in the anterior superior quadrant (Figure 3.11). A conductive hearing loss can occur when the enlarging mass becomes compressed between the manubrium of the malleus and the promontory of the middle ear. The degree of hearing loss, however, is not predictive of the extent of the cholesteatoma. For example, a large cholesteatoma filling the middle ear space, compressed between the incudostapedial joint and the tympanic membrane, will transmit sound waves very well and may produce little to no conductive hearing loss.

### Acquired Disorders of the Middle Ear

Infectious processes of the middle ear are well described in the literature; however, the classification and terminology of various infectious and inflammatory conditions are sometimes confusing because of a lack of universal consensus. The classification scheme employed in this section is consistent with that described by Bluestone (1984) and is in common usage today.

Acute otitis media, also referred to as acute suppurative otitis media or purulent otitis media, is a rapid-onset bacterial infection characterized by three stages: inflammation, followed by suppuration, and finally resolution or complication. During the inflammatory stage, the blood vessels are dilated and the tympanic membrane appears injected and is often painful (Figure 3.12). The tympanic membrane may be transparent, the middle ear space clear of fluid, and hearing normal, although negative pressure may be noted on tympanometry.

Suppuration is the exudative process that results in a purulent (pus-filled) fluid filling the middle ear space. The tympanic membrane begins to bulge under pressure producing increased pain and a 30- to 40-dB hearing loss with a flat tympanogram. Resolution occurs by destruction of the bacteria and mucosal resorption of the exudate or drainage of the middle ear either through the eustachian tube, or rupture of the tympanic membrane. Occasionally after resolution of the infection a clear effusion will be present in the middle ear space for varying periods of time. If the infection escapes the protective boundaries of the middle ear other than through a perforation in the tympanic membrane, complications such as meningitis and brain abscess can occur.

Otitis media with effusion is an inflammatory condition of the middle ear with fluid present behind an intact tympanic membrane (Figure 3.13). Commonly encountered terminology for this condition are secretory otitis, serous otitis media, nonsuppurative otitis media, mucoid ear, glue ear, and others. Examination of the tympanic membrane reveals a number of possible visual presentations including a retraction of the tympanic membrane with a dish-shaped appearance, a bulging or fullness of the tympanic membrane, a thickened opacified tympanic membrane with complete loss

**TABLE 3.3**   Middle Ear Anomalies of Congenital Origin

| CHROMOSOMAL DEFECTS | |
|---|---|
| *Syndrome* | *Middle Ear Defect* |
| Turner's syndrome (gonadal aplasia) | Middle ear hypoplasia, stapes malformation |
| Goldenhar's syndrome | Malformed or absent ossicles<br>Oval window hypoplasia |
| Patau's syndrome (trisomy 17–15) | Small tympanic membrane, thickened manubrium, distorted IS joint |
| Down syndrome (trisomy 21) | Deformed stapes |
| Trisomy 22 | Nonpneumatized middle ear, absence of stapes and oval window, bony closure of round window niche |

| FAMILIAL (INHERITED) DISORDERS | | |
|---|---|---|
| *Syndrome* | *Pattern of inheritance* | *Middle Ear Defect* |
| Achondroplasia | Autosomal dominant | Fusion of ossicles, undeveloped ossicular mass |
| Apert's syndrome | Autosomal dominant | Fixation of footplate |
| Atresia auris congenital | Autosomal dominant | Absence or fusion of ossicles<br>Abnormal IS and/or MI joint |
| Kippel-Feil syndrome | Autosomal recessive | Stapes footplate fistula |
| Pierre Robin syndrome | Autosomal dominant | Thick stapes and footplate<br>Absence of middle ear |
| Cleidocranial dysostosis | Autosomal dominant | Small ossicles, absence of manubrium and long process of incus, stapes fixation |
| Mobius syndrome | Autosomal | Undeveloped ossicular mass |
| Crouzons | Autosomal dominant | Absence of T. M., malleus fixation/deformation, stapes fixation, narrow middle ear, narrow round window niche |
| Duane's syndrome | Autosomal/X-linked | Ossicular fusion, disarticulation |
| Hurler's disease | Autosomal recessive | Absence of IM joint, deformed stapes, fibrous invasion of middle and inner ear |
| Letterer Siwe | Autosomal recessive | Bony destruction of canal and middle ear structures |
| Treacher-Collins syndrome | Autosomal dominant | Ossicles deformed, absence of stapes/tensor tympani muscle |

| CONGENITAL SYNDROMES WITH ASSOCIATED MIDDLE EAR DEFECTS | | |
|---|---|---|
| *Syndrome* | *Pattern of Inheritance* | *Middle Ear Defect* |
| Fanconi's syndrome | Autosomal recessive | Stapes fixation |
| Mohr syndrome | Autosomal recessive | Absence of IS joint |
| Osteitis deformans (Padgett's) | Autosomal dominant | Abnormal stapes ossification |
| Osteopetrosis | Autosomal | Abnormal ossicles, small middle ear space |
| Otopalatal digital syndrome | Autosomal recessive | Immature ossicles, fixed stapes, absence of oval window |

*(continued)*

**TABLE 3.3   continued**

### CONGENITAL SYNDROMES WITH ASSOCIATED MIDDLE EAR DEFECTS

| | | |
|---|---|---|
| DiGeorge syndrome | Unknown | Absence of ossicles and oval window |
| Osteogenesis imperfecta | Autosomal dominant | Abnormal stapes |
| Sickle cell anemia | Autosomal dominant | Resorption of incus and head of stapes |

### DISEASES ASSOCIATED WITH PRENATAL INFECTIONS

| | |
|---|---|
| Rubella syndrome | Malleus fixation, abnormal stapes, stapes footplate fixation, persistant fetal mesenchymal tissue |
| Congenital syphillis | Thickening of malleus, IM joint fusion, osteitis of incus and stapes. |

of landmarks, a transparent tympanic membrane with fluid visible (usually amber, blue, clear, or white in appearance), bubbles, or an air fluid level in the middle ear. On occasion, even an absolutely normal appearing tympanic membrane will demonstrate a flat tympanogram and conductive hearing loss, and myringotomy will reveal the presence of a serous fluid.

Otitis media with effusion is clinically distinguished from acute otitis media by the usual lack of fever and significant otalgia (ear pain). A conductive hearing loss may be present to varying degrees up to approximately 40 dB. The tympanogram is usually flat, but may be of nearly any shape including normal tympanometric results depending on middle ear volume, the quantity of fluid present, and the characteristics of the fluid (Gates, Avery, Cooper, Hearne and Holt, 1986; Orchik, Dunn, and McNutt, 1978). Chronic otitis media is a commonly used term with variable meanings but usually implies a chronic tympanic membrane perforation with otorrhea. This can occur with chronic infections of the middle ear and mastoid and is commonly seen with cholesteatoma.

Atelectasis, a condition due to a persistent negative pressure on the tympanic membrane, may occur in conjunction with or independent of inflammatory and infectious processes of the middle ear. Severe atelectasis (collapse) from long-standing eustachian tube dysfunction may lead to hearing loss, chronic otitis media, cholesteatoma,

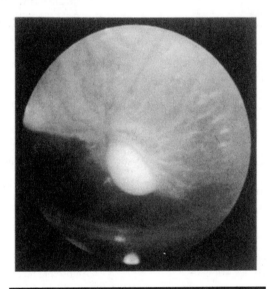

**FIGURE 3.11**   A congenital cholesteatoma appears as a small keratin pearl in the center of this four-year-old's right tympanic membrane. There was no history of trauma or otitis media. These congenital keratin inclusion cysts may be the result of epithelial rests in the tympanic membrane. (From Chole, R. A. (1982). *Color Atlas of Ear Disease.* New York: Appleton-Century Crofts. Used with permission.)

and ossicular discontinuity. Findings on otoscopic examination vary with the degree of severity. Early or mild cases may appear as a medial displacement of the tympanic membrane. Severe atalectasis can result in massive stretching and thinning of the

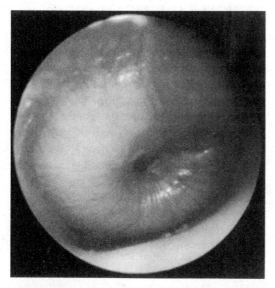

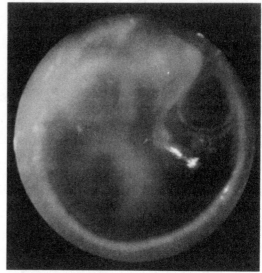

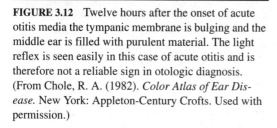

**FIGURE 3.12**  Twelve hours after the onset of acute otitis media the tympanic membrane is bulging and the middle ear is filled with purulent material. The light reflex is seen easily in this case of acute otitis and is therefore not a reliable sign in otologic diagnosis. (From Chole, R. A. (1982). *Color Atlas of Ear Disease.* New York: Appleton-Century Crofts. Used with permission.)

**FIGURE 3.13**  Serous otitis media (otitis media with effusion) is often seen as a sequelae of acute otitis media. In this case of a chronic effusion in a 9-year-old child, an amber-colored fluid is visible behind a normal tympanic membrane. Gas bubbles are seen just anterior to the malleus. The light reflection is normal as it is in most cases of otitis media with effusion. (From Chole, R. A. (1982). *Color Atlas of Ear Disease.* New York: Appleton-Century Crofts. Used with permission.)

tympanic membrane with adhesion of the majority of the tympanic membrane to the ossicles and walls of the middle ear (Figure 3.14). Blind retraction pockets occur when the tympanic membrane retracts into unexposed areas of the middle ear such as the epitympanum, hypotympanum, protympanum, tympanic sinus, and facial recess.

The tympanogram is almost always abnormal but may be of nearly any configuration, including normal. The audiogram may demonstrate a conductive hearing loss, but the severity may not be predictive of the severity of disease. For example, a severe anterior retraction pocket with cholesteatoma may be present with a normal posterior tympanic membrane and functioning ossicles. In this scenario the hearing may be minimally affected. Similarly, a retracted tympanic membrane that is adhered to the incus, stapedius tendon, and head

of the stapes (functional stapediomyringopexy) may elicit only a 10- to 15-dB conductive loss. In contrast, a retracted tympanic membrane may present a 30-dB conductive hearing loss if it is adhered to the promontory, thus tethering the manubrium and stiffening the ossicular chain. Adhesive otitis with a completely retracted tympanic membrane adhered to all middle ear structures is generally accompanied by a severe conductive loss.

There is a high incidence of middle ear disease among children with cleft palate most likely related to eustachian tube dysfunction secondary to developmental anomalies of the tensor palatini and levator palatini muscles (Schuknecht, 1993). Bluestone (1971) reports that approximately 50 percent of children with cleft palate exhibit conductive hearing loss. Children with a cleft lip who

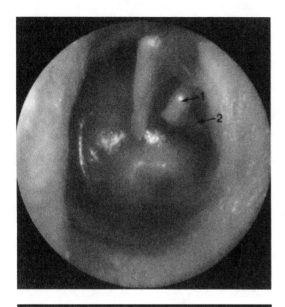

**FIGURE 3.14**    Chronic serous otitis and recurrent acute otitis media have resulted in atalectasis of the middle ear. The thin tympanic membrane is adherent to a partially eroded incus (1) (spontaneous myringoincudopexy) and the stapedial tendon is visible behind it (2). (From Chole, R. A. (1982). *Color Atlas of Ear Disease.* New York: Appleton-Century Crofts. Used with permission.)

do not exhibit an overt cleft palate may subsequently be found to have a submucous cleft of the palate. The recurrent otologic and hearing problems associated with both overt and submucous cleft palate make it imperative that these children be monitored through immittance measures with otologic follow-up as indicated. Similarly, children with Down syndrome have a higher incidence of recurrent otitis media, middle ear anomalies, and congenital ossicular malformations than the general pediatric population. As with children with other pathologies of the conductive mechanism, when hearing impairment persists following otologic intervention, aggressive audiologic follow-up is imperative to keep hearing at its optimum levels for these children. This may include assistive listening devices, or sound field amplification within the classroom.

## MEDICAL COMPLICATIONS OF OTITIS MEDIA

Prior to antibiotics, the natural course of acute otitis media usually followed one of two paths. Usually resolution occurred facilitated by the body's immune system and drainage of the middle ear through the eustachian tube or a spontaneous tympanic membrane rupture. In the absence of spontaneous resolution, complications could occur such as mastoiditis, meningitis, and brain abscess, sometimes necessitating radical surgical treatment and occasionally resulting in death. Today, with the frequent use of antibiotics, the more common complications associated with otitis media are more insidious in nature (Table 3.4).

### Extracranial Complications of Otitis Media

Conductive hearing loss occurs transiently with the middle ear effusion that accompanies otitis media. The degree of hearing loss is directly proportional to the amount of fluid present and inde-

**TABLE 3.4**    Complications of Otitis Media

| EXTRACRANIAL COMPLICATIONS | INTRACRANIAL COMPLICATIONS |
| --- | --- |
| Conductive hearing loss | Meningitis |
| Sensorineural hearing loss | Extradural abscess |
| Tympanic membrane perforation | Subdural abscess |
| Chronic otitis media | Brain abscess |
| Retraction pocket/ cholesteatoma | Lateral sinus thrombosis |
| Ossicular discontinuity | Otic hydrocephalus |
| Adhesive mastoiditis | |
| Granulomatous otitis media | |
| Tympanosclerosis | |
| Coalescent mastoiditis | |
| Serous/suppurative labyrinthitis | |
| Sclerosing labyrinthitis | |

pendent of its viscosity. Average hearing loss ranges from 15 dB to 45 dB. Resolution of the effusion should reverse the conductive hearing loss.

Sensorineural hearing loss may occur with acute otitis media or otitis media with effusion. The etiology probably results from inflammation and thickening (decreasing the compliance) of the round window membrane and is usually mild and transient. Inflammatory toxins may also diffuse through the round and oval window membranes producing a serous labyrinthitis. This phenomenon is often accompanied by vestibular symptoms ranging from mild unsteadiness to severe vertigo. Invasion of bacteria through the round and oval windows may lead to labyrinthitis. Other pathways may also exist for neuronal and organ of Corti damage without bacterial labyrinthitis or meningitis.

Tympanic membrane perforation secondary to acute otitis media can be part of the natural course of the disease (Figure 3.15). Rupture usually occurs in the pars tensa, releasing purulent material under pressure and relieving much of the associated pain. These perforations usually heal spontaneously within several days or weeks. Persistence of the perforation is more likely to occur with larger perforations and with chronic otorrhea. Some infectious agents such as group A beta hemolytic strep (the streptococci type pathogenic to humans) and *Mycobacterium* (a genus of acid-fast organisms that include the causative organisms of tuberculosis and leprosy) have been known to aggressively attack the tympanic membrane producing large or multiple defects. Perforations present for greater than 2 to 3 months are considered chronic and often require surgical correction.

The size and location of the perforation will influence the severity of the associated conductive hearing loss. Conductive hearing loss may be undetectable for small perforations and progress to approximately 35 dB for complete absence of the tympanic membrane. The timing of surgical correction varies depending on size of the perforation, age of the patient, infectious history, and other health and social factors. The intervening

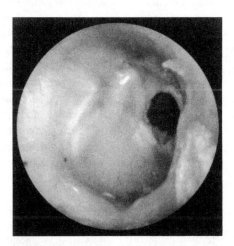 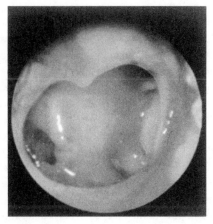

**FIGURE 3.15** The photo on the left is an asymptomatic simple perforation of the right tympanic membrane anterior to the long process of the malleus. This tympanic membrane is thickened due to repeated infections many years previous; hearing was normal. The photo on the right displays a large central infected perforation. Purulent material is seen in the middle ear of this patient with chronic otitis and otorrhea. (From Chole, R. A. (1982). *Color Atlas of Ear Disease.* New York: Appleton-Century Crofts. Used with permission.)

conductive hearing loss may necessitate educational or audiologic intervention.

Cholesteatoma forms from keratinizing (hardening) squamous (scale-like) epithelium present in the middle ear space or other air-containing spaces of the temporal bone. Congenital cholesteatomas are thought to occur from rests (a remnant of embryonic tissue that persists in the adult) of epithelium trapped in the air space of the temporal bone during embryonic development, however, their existence is a topic of debate and are considered by some to occur as a complication of otitis media. If discovered early, they often appear as a white mass behind a transparent intact tympanic membrane. (See Figure 3.11.) Hearing loss occurs if left untreated or undiscovered until the cholesteatoma enlarges enough to produce mechanical obstruction of the ossicles or tympanic membrane.

Acquired cholesteatomas probably occur by several mechanisms. Traumatic or iatrogenic (treatment-induced) displacement of epithelium into the middle ear space is commonly accepted as an etiology for middle ear cholesteatomas. Foreign body penetration, surgical manipulation and implosion of the tympanic membrane from barotrauma, can contaminate the middle ear space with keratinizing squamous epithelium from the external canal or lateral surface of the tympanic membrane. The keratinizing epithelium is the seed that eventually produces the cholesteatoma or "keratoma" by continuous growth and desquamation.

Epithelial migration is probably another mechanism for cholesteatoma formation (Brandow, 1977). This theory suggests that keratinizing squamous epithelium from the external surface of the tympanic membrane or external canal migrates by division and growth through an existing perforation in the tympanic membrane to gain access to the middle ear space. The annulus is probably a protective barrier to migrating epithelium. However, disruption of the annulus may occur from ear surgery, penetrating injuries, or slag injuries (known to occur in welders from small balls of molten metal entering the external ear and rolling onto the annulus and tympanic membrane).

Chronic infection and inflammation are a theorized mechanism for formation of cholesteatoma but is difficult to prove because of the high incidence of tympanic membrane perforation that occurs with otitis media (Tumarkin, 1938). In this controversial theory, severe metaplasia (conversion of one kind of tissue into a form that is not normal for that tissue) of pluripotential cells (embryonic cells with the potential to develop in one of several ways) results in transformation of nonkeratinizing mucosal cells into keratinizing squamous epithelium.

Acquired cholesteatoma in children most commonly occur coincidental to retraction pockets in the posterior superior quadrant and occasionally in the pars flaccida (Bluestone and Klein, 1990). The suggested mechanism begins with eustachian tube dysfunction resulting in wide fluctuations in middle ear pressure. The tympanic membrane becomes stretched, resulting in a retraction pocket that can adhere to the ossicles and other middle ear structures. The exact mechanism for transformation from retraction pocket to cholesteatoma is not understood, but may result from infection and entrapment of debris in the retraction pocket or from perforation within the retraction pocket with epithelial hyperplasia (excessive proliferation of normal cells) and migration. Extensive cholesteatoma migration and growth is more common in children than adults. The reason for this is the more extensive pneumatization of the temporal bone in children. Adults with chronic ear disease typically have poorly developed mastoid air cells.

Hearing loss is common with cholesteatoma but is often not noticed or not present until late in the disease process. Cholesteatoma involving the ossicles may produce erosion, fixation, or disarticulation resulting in mild to severe conductive loss. An infected cholesteatoma may produce a serous labyrinthitis resulting in vertigo or unsteadiness and mixed hearing loss. Destruction and invasion of the labyrinth is uncommon except in very advanced disease and could result in ana-cusis, vertigo, and intracranial complications.

Adhesive otitis media is an inflammatory condition that yields a proliferation of fibrous tis-sue within the middle ear and mastoid producing a thickening of the tympanic membrane with fixa-tion of the ossicles, ossicular discontinuity, and possibly cholesteatoma formation. The etiology of this condition is probably due to recurrent otitis media with eustachian tube dysfunction and atelectasis. The tympanogram is typically flat and a maximum conductive hearing loss up to 55 dB may be present.

Tympanosclerosis appears as a chalky white patch on the tympanic membrane resulting from a pathologic condition involving the abnormal dep-osition of calcium and phosphate crystals in the submucosal layers of the tympanic membrane and middle ear (Figure 3.16). It is a common occur-rence in children with a history of frequent otitis media. Tympanosclerosis probably occurs more

readily at sites of tympanic membrane perforation or tympanotomy. When isolated to the tympanic membrane, it usually produces no additional prob-lems and warrants no treatment. Tympanosclero-sis less commonly involves the ossicular chain where it can produce fixation with significant conductive hearing loss.

Ossicular discontinuity most commonly oc-curs due to erosion of the long process of the in-cus resulting in incudostapedial disarticulation. Complete resorption of one or more of the ossi-cles can also occur with cholesteatoma, retraction pockets, and adhesive otitis media. Ossicular dis-continuity in the presence of an intact tympanic membrane produces a maximum conductive hear-ing loss of 50 to 60 dB due to the poor impedance matching interface between the tympanic mem-brane and the round and oval windows. However, hearing loss may be mild or nonexistent if conti-nuity is maintained with the stapes or footplate such as when a cholesteatoma is pressed between

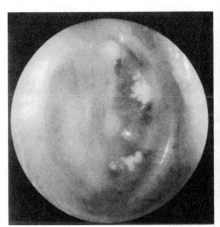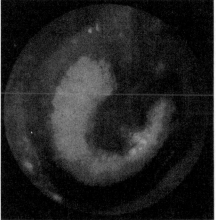

**FIGURE 3.16**  A common sequel of acute otitis media, tympanosclerosis is recognized by chalky white deposits in the tympanic membrane. The photo on the left reveals two small patches of tympanosclerosis in the anterior quadrants of this right tympanic membrane. Con-trastingly, there is scarring and collagen formation in the posterior quadrants. The photo on the right reveals a more extensive tympanosclerosis. This patient was observed for 15 years with no change in the plaques or the hearing levels. (From Chole, R. A. (1982). *Color Atlas of Ear Disease.* New York: Appleton-Century Crofts. Used with permission.)

the stapes and the tympanic membrane or a retracted tympanic membrane adheres to the stapes superstructure (stapediomyringopexy) therefore bypassing the malleus and incus.

Mastoiditis, by definition, is inflammation of the mucosal lined air-containing spaces of the mastoid portion of the temporal bone. Because the mastoid air cells usually communicate with the middle ear space through the antrum, infection in the middle ear space may produce an inflammatory response in the mastoid air cells. Resolution usually occurs with successful treatment of the otitis media. However, an unresolved infection may invade the mastoid bone producing an osteitis referred to as coalescing mastoiditis that may present as a painful, protruding ear with postauricular erythema and tenderness. Conductive hearing loss would be expected, with possible vertigo and sensorineural hearing loss from a concomitant labyrinthitis. In addition, coalescing mastoiditis may lead to intracranial complications.

Labyrinthitis, an inflammatory or toxic insult to the cochlea, the contents of the vestibule and/or the semicircular canals and ampulla, is commonly classified into four types: serous labyrinthitis, acute bacterial labyrinthitis, chronic labyrinthitis, and sclerotic labyrinthitis. Serous labyrinthitis is by far the most common form. Also known as acute toxic labyrinthitis, it is not an uncommon occurrence with acute or chronic otitis media and may occur with meningitis. Toxins probably enter the labyrinth through the oval or round window producing alterations in the perilymph. According to Schuknecht (1993), mild serous labyrinthitis produces the same principal pathologic findings as endolymphatic hydrops; vertigo with sensorineural hearing loss. In the mild form, complete recovery is expected. In the more severe form precipitates are present in the endolymph and cytotoxic changes to the membranous labyrinth may produce permanent sensorineural hearing loss (Schuknecht, 1993).

Acute bacterial labyrinthitis is caused by bacterial invasion of the inner ear from surrounding regions of the temporal bone or meningeal extension. When associated with middle ear infection,

bacteria most likely enter through the oval and round window membranes or through fistula in the bony labyrinth. Symptoms are indistinguishable from severe serous labyrinthitis but recovery is much less likely to occur. Due to the common use of antibiotics, bacterial labyrinthitis of middle ear origin is unusual. More common is bacterial labyrinthitis secondary to meningitis. The route of bacterial invasion is probably through the internal auditory canal following the eighth cranial nerve or through the cochlear aqueduct. Destruction of the membranous labyrinth produces irreversible profound sensorineural hearing loss and loss of vestibular function.

## Intracranial Complications of Otitis Media

Meningitis is the most common intracranial complication of ear disease in children. A study by Gower and McQuirt (1983) of eighty-four children with intracranial complications of otitic origin revealed a 77 percent rate of meningitis. Meningitis and ear infections may be related by three mechanisms: direct extension of infection from the middle ear through the dura into the subdural or subarachnoid space; inflammation of the meninges from a suppurative focus adjacent to the dura; or hematogenous spread (through blood circulation) of bacteria from an upper respiratory source with a concomitant otitis media produced by contiguous spread of bacteria from the same source. Since the widespread use of antibiotics, direct spread of infection to the meninges is unusual. Hematogenous spread is probably the most common.

Extradural abscess, subdural empyema, dural sinus thrombosis, brain abscess, and otitic hydrocephalus are rare but serious complications of middle ear disease. Extradural abscess is the most common because of its association with cholesteatoma. Erosion of the adjacent bone by cholesteatoma can produce a collection of granulation tissue or pus between the dura and the cranium. Symptoms are usually severe earache, headache, and low-grade fever. Intracranial signs are uncommon. Sometimes asymptomatic extradural abscesses are found at the time of surgery for cholesteatoma.

Subdural empyema, dural sinus thrombosis, and brain abscess may occur by direct invasion of bacteria or less commonly through retrograde thrombophlebitis (bacterial invasion and propagation through penetrating venous pathways). Otitic hydrocephalus is a vary rare condition of increased intracranial pressure associated with otitis media. The originating mechanism is unknown but it has been associated in some cases with lateral sinus thrombosis (blood clot). Although visual disturbances may occur due to optic atrophy, we know of no reports of associated hearing loss.

## DEVELOPMENTAL COMPLICATIONS OF OTITIS MEDIA

### Developmental Theories

Controversy still continues regarding the effects of middle ear effusion in children. For more than 30 years the consequences of middle ear disease have been investigated, often through studies with significant research flaws. However, there clearly appear to be developmental consequences to otitis media beyond its medical or audiologic sequelae. It has been hypothesized that children's minds are not "blank slates" as the empiricist theory would hold, but rather that children possess a biologic endowment that permits them to select organized aspects of information from the diversity of sensory input in their environment. This hypothesis further holds that critical periods exist for the development of specific functions, including speech and language proficiency (Lennenberg, 1967) and auditory comprehension (Northern and Downs, 1991). According to this theory of critical periods, an organism can best use stimuli for further growth and development during a specific time period and if stimuli are not received optimally during this critical period, permanent adverse effects will result. The precepts of the critical period theory may be particularly alarming since otitis media with effusion is one of the most common diseases in young children and coincides with the age span most critical to input for cognitive development.

Feldman and Gelman (1986) present a theory that disagrees with the precept of irreversible changes when input is disrupted during the critical period for auditory language development. They take the critical period theory one step further. Their rational-constructionist theory holds that infants and young children are not passive, but have an active role in their own cognitive development. As such, infants are motivated to seek out relevant inputs that will stimulate developing structures.

If we accept the rational-constructionist theory, which follows much of Piaget's (1953) findings of infant and children's cognitive development, then we must begin to question some of the critical period theory, so much of which is based on animal sensory deprivation studies. In contrast to the critical period theory, the rational-constructionist theory predicts that some high-level abilities will develop normally even when auditory input is limited, as in recurrent conductive hearing loss. Feldman and Gelman suggest that the resilience of cognitive or language functions in the presence of repeated bouts of hearing loss will depend, in part, on whether the given function relies on auditory input alone for its development. These authors posit that children take an active role in the creation of their own environments and may gravitate toward areas of improved signal-to-noise ratio, or, may prefer favorable styles of communication such as face-to-face interaction, frequent repetitions, and simplified linguistic style.

### Implications of Fluctuating Hearing Loss

A large number of studies have looked at the effects of middle ear effusion on child development (for review see Clark, 1980b; Kavanagh, 1986; Menyuk, 1992). In spite of the myriad weaknesses in methodological and experimental design present in most of these studies, the repetition of the consequential findings is nevertheless noteworthy. Studies have found that otitis-prone children lag behind their peers with negative otologic histories in articulatory and phonological development, in the ability to receive and express thoughts through spoken language, in the use of grammar and syntax, in the acquisition of vocabulary, in the development of auditory memory and auditory perception skills, and in social maturation.

Eisen (1962) was possibly the first to report on the adverse effects of middle ear disease on child maturation. It took over thirty years to unequivocally verify this report. Brown (1994) reported diagnostic speech audiometric findings on a pair of 4-year-old twin girls, only one of whom had experienced recurrent episodes of chronic otitis media. As the two subjects were identical twins, the research flaws of past investigations were eliminated as relating to subject differences in age, race, socioeconomic background, intelligence, experiential differences in language exposure and child-rearing practices, and other immeasurable contributing environmental factors. In Brown's investigation the twin with a positive history of otitis media showed a striking drop in word recognition in the presence of a background speech competition. No significant differences between these two children were found for speech recognition measures in quiet. This finding highlights the observation that clinically routine speech recognition measures employing acoustically redundant speech materials within ideal listening conditions are insufficient in taxing auditory processing skills for the purpose of identifying some performance deficiencies.

It would appear almost certain that protracted or frequent bouts of middle ear effusion can have deleterious effects on a child within a number of developmental areas. The child with fluctuating hearing loss during the first several years of life receives distortions in speech input that can weaken reception of the subtle acoustic differences that lead to the perception of phonetic contrasts. While contextual cues and the shear redundancy of the acoustic speech signal may salvage speech comprehension, children with fluctuating conductive hearing loss may progress more slowly in the formation of phonemic categories. The "interpretation" that these children bring to multiple acoustic parameters may also differ from that of their peers

with more stable hearing levels (Strange, 1986). Indeed, as Strange points out, children with recurrent fluctuations in hearing are left with an unreliable speech signal, and a difficult and error-prone decoding task that may often prove too difficult for them. In her opinion, the resultant inattention to auditory input may expand to more favorable listening situations, thus leading to the patterns of auditory inattention characteristic of some learning disabled children.

Clearly there is a need for early identification and effective management of recurrent middle ear effusions in children because of the potential for severe and adverse effects of this condition. Intervention would appear necessary regardless of whether these effects are permanent or whether there is in fact a high degree of developmental resiliency as suggested in the rational-constructionist theory. Although Needleman (1977) concluded that children's phonological abilities do indeed catch-up developmentally as age increases, more recent studies yield conflicting findings in this area (Grievenk, Peters, Van Bon, and Schilder, 1993; Roberts, Burchinal, Davis, Collier, and Henderson, 1991; Silva, Chalmers, and Stewart, 1986). A good deal of controlled and longitudinal research may be needed to prove the permanent disruption to higher level functioning implied by a rigid adherence to the precepts of the critical period theory. However, regardless of the permanency of these effects, we should consider otitis-prone children at risk for the development of learning problems. The fact that some children with positive histories of otitis develop no speech, language, or educational delays suggests that additional factors to fluctuating hearing loss may also be involved in the learning process (Davis, 1986) but in no way reduces the need for intervention.

## MEDICAL/SURGICAL MANAGEMENT OF OTITIS MEDIA

The controversial subject of medical versus surgical therapy has been the target of many studies and has been hotly debated in the pediatric and otolaryngology literature. The most widely accepted treatments for recurrent acute otitis media, otitis media with effusion, and eustachian tube dysfunction include episodic antibiotic therapy, prophylactic antibiotic therapy, myringotomy and drainage, myringotomy with ventilation tube placement, adenoidectomy, tonsillectomy, and any combination of the above. Other less widely used treatments include, but are not limited to, autoinflation and the Politzer method of inflating the middle ear space, saline lavage (irrigation) of the nasopharynx, decongestants, expectorants, steroids, and allergy evaluation and treatment. The last two may have a significant role in the treatment of otitis media with effusion.

The purpose of treating otitis media is to shorten the course of the infectious process and to minimize the risk of complications. The goal in treating children with recurrent or persistent otitis media is to minimize the time in which a pathologic process is present in the middle ear space.

Otitis media starting in early infancy usually decreases in frequency with age due to maturation of the nasopharynx, eustachian tubes, and middle ear space. A small subset of children will continue to have middle ear disease into early childhood and beyond. This subset gets progressively smaller as the child progresses through puberty into adulthood.

Although there are pros and cons of the use of chronic antibiotic therapy versus ventilation tube placement (Tables 3.5 and 3.6), ventilation tubes have been demonstrated to be very effective in eliminating middle ear fluid and decreasing the number of infectious episodes (Lildholt, 1979; Shah, 1971). These devices are typically shaped like a grommet, rivet, or sewing bobbin and are inserted through a myringotomy incision in the tympanic membrane much like a rivet through sheet metal (Figure 3.17). The hole in the tube provides pressure equalization of the middle ear space thus bypassing the presumably dysfunctioning eustachian tube.

Ventilation tubes are generally placed as a temporizing procedure in children in anticipation that after extrusion of the tubes, the eustachian

**TABLE 3.5** Chronic Antibiotic Treatment of Otitis Media

| PROS | CONS |
|---|---|
| May shorten the course of acute otitis media | May result in resistant bacteria |
| May prevent recurrent acute otitis media | May precipitate allergic reactions |
| May prevent complications of acute otitis media | Side effects of medication including diarrhea, yeast infections, etc |
| May prevent progression of OME to acute otitis media | Pseudomembranous colitis |
| | Expensive, up to $200 for a 2-week course |
| | May not eliminate effusions |
| | May require refrigeration |
| | Some have only 2-week shelf life |
| | Compliance may be a problem |
| | Does not eliminate eustachian tube dysfunction and pressure changes |
| | Does not eliminate the pain associated with acute otitis media |
| | Risk of spontaneous perforation of the tympanic membrane |

**TABLE 3.6**  Treatment of Otitis Media with Ventilation Tube Placement

| PROS | CONS |
|---|---|
| Eliminates pressure and pain | General anesthesia |
| May decrease incidence of acute otitis media | Risk of permanent perforation |
| Eliminates OME | Risk of cholesteatoma |
| Decreases risk of complications | Risk of chronic otorrhea |
| Decreases need for antibiotics | Risk of tympanosclerosis |
| Establishes normal hearing | |

tube and nasopharynx will have matured and will be functioning normally. While some practitioners are more conservative about recommending surgical treatment for otitis media, Bluestone and Klein (1990) recommend placement of ventilation tubes in several specific instances: recurrent bouts of acute otitis media occuring at a rate of three or more in a 6-month period, or four or more in a year; or failure of antibiotic prophylaxis; persistent otitis media with effusion remaining unre-sponsive to antibiotic therapy for 3 months or more; or pain, significant and symptomatic hearing loss, vertigo, or tinnitus produced by eustachian tube dysfunction. Tonsillectomy and/or adenoidectomy may be further helpful for a subset of children who require multiple sets of ventilation tubes.

An interdisciplinary panel of the U.S. Public Health Service's Agency for Health Care Policy and Research (AHCPR) has released a clinical practice guideline for treatment of otitis media with effusion (Stool et al., 1994). It should be noted that application of these guidelines (Table 3.7) are specifically intended only for children 1 to 3 years of age with no neurologic or craniofacial anomalies or sensory deficits that would place the child at greater risk for developmental delay. In addition, the guidelines are not applicable for other forms of otitis media. It is not within the audiologist's province to dictate, or even suggest, a management approach for resolution of otitis media. However, when more aggressive treatment appears indicated based on Bluestone and Klein's recommendations, or the AHCPR guidelines, it may be in the child's best interest to encourage parents to ask their pediatrician for referral for an otolaryngologic consult.

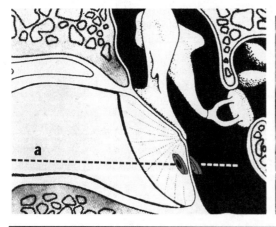 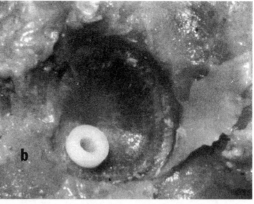

**FIGURE 3.17**  Middle ear ventilation (pressure equalization) tube. (*A*) Illustration of tube in position in the tympanic membrane. (*B*) Surgical photograph of the same. (Courtesy of XOMED®, Jacksonville, Florida.)

TABLE 3.7   Clinical Practice Guidelines for Otitis Media with Effusion in Young Children

**CLINICAL DIAGNOSIS**

1. It is strongly recommended that the diagnostic evaluation include pneumatic otoscopy.
2. Tympanometry is recommended as a test for conformation of OME.
3. For children with less than 3 months of effusion hearing evaluation is a clinical option. Hearing evaluation is recommended for effusions that have been present for a total of three months[*] or longer.

**TREATMENT PROTOCOL**

1. Environmental factors (i.e., passive smoking, group child-care, feeding method [reclined bottling]) should be controlled as part of the treatment process.
2. Anytime hearing is 15 dB HL or better in at least one ear, or before effusion is present for a total of 3 months,[*] observation or use of antibiotics remains a clinical option.
3. When effusion has been present for 3 months[*] *and* hearing is 20 dB HL or worse in the better ear, bilateral myringotomy with tubes is a clinical option.
4. When effusion has been present 4 to 6 months[*] *and* hearing is 20 dB HL or worse in the better ear, bilateral myringotomy with tubes is recommended.
5. The use of steroids, decongestants, and antihistamines is not recommended for treatment of OME. Decongestants and antihistamines have been found to be ineffective treatment agents in the absence of any underlying allergic airway disease.
6. Given a present lack of evidence of benefits that significantly outweigh surgical risk, tonsillectomies and adenoidectomies are not recommended as a treatment for OME in young children, although they may be performed for coexisting tonsil or adenoid pathology.

[*]Cumulative days, not consecutive days.

From Stool et al. (July 1994). *Managing Otitis Media with Effusion in Young Children. Quick Reference Guide for Clinicians.* AHCPR Publication No. 94–0623. Rockville, MD: Agency for Health Care Policy and Research, Public Health Service, U.S. Department of Health and Human Services, with restrictions to age and comorbid conditions as specified.

## AUDIOLOGIC/EDUCATIONAL MANAGEMENT OF OTITIS MEDIA

The educational implications of a mild, fluctuating, conductive hearing loss may be quite significant in a system heavily dependent upon language as a primary teaching tool. A perceptual constancy within the human sensory system is necessary to keep sensations in the perspective necessary for maintaining a sense of reality among auditory and visual stimuli. It may be that the organism's need for perceptual consistency underlies Katz's (1979) view that the child with fluctuating conductive hearing loss is at a comparative disadvantage to the child with a stable sensorineural hearing loss of similar degree.

We have often questioned the wisdom of the continued use of the term "mild" hearing loss. The impact of such a loss is far from benign for children and is even more than the term implies when used for adults. Better terms may be "educationally significant" or "developmentally significant" for children and "socially significant" for adults. Persistence in our indiscriminate use of the term mild may actually undermine the very intervention efforts we are trying to promote.

Davis (1986) presents one of the only indepth discussions of the remediation of hearing, speech, and language deficits that may arise from otitis media. She reminds us that this condition seriously compromises a child's ability to learn through the auditory channel. First, given the relationship between the intensity of a sound and the perception of loudness, a reduction of 10 dB in sound intensity creates perception of sound as only half as intense as it would be otherwise. One can quickly calculate that a 30-dB conductive hearing loss causes sounds to be perceived as only one-eighth of their original intensity. Second, auditory processing deficiencies commonly reported among children with early recurrent otitis media require enhanced signal-to-noise ratios for adequate understanding. As discussed in Chapter 14, many of life's communication exchanges, including classroom instruction, present less than ideal signal-to-noise ratios.

Since hearing loss is the critical factor in predicting the effects of otitis with effusion, Davis correctly notes that hearing impairment must become the focal point of any remediation for children with middle ear disease. Certainly not all children who suffer recurrent bouts of otitis media with effusion will experience adverse developmental consequences. However, when present, the negative effects of otitis media far outlast the active stages of ear disease and continue well beyond the temporary hearing loss. We do not believe personal hearing aids provide the needed signal-to-noise ratio to be of benefit to children with developmental otitis sequelae. However, mild gain FM systems or classroom amplification (see Chapter 14) can be of benefit to these children even after hearing has returned to normal levels.

Gravel and Wallace (1992) contend that chronic otitis media with effusion results in a lack of development of higher order auditory listening skills necessary to success in the classroom. Given this frequently reported consequence of early and recurrent otitis, Clark (1980b) suggests it may prove advisable to use previously published suggestions for the classroom management of children with central auditory dysfunction (Clark, 1980a).

## SUMMARY

Congenital conductive hearing loss must be identified as early as possible so that appropriate intervention may be employed to offset the effects of decreased hearing sensitivity. Acquired conductive hearing pathologies are a common occurrence in young children. These too must be resolved early and as fully as possible as their presence will not only decrease hearing sensitivity of children with otherwise normal hearing, but will also decrease the utility of residual hearing for those children with sensorineural hearing loss.

Given present-day antibiotics, many serious sequela to acquired conductive pathologies can now be avoided. However, given the potential long-term implications of fluctuating hearing loss with otitis media, audiologists must strive to achieve effective identification of conductive hearing loss and early referral to their otolaryngology colleagues and to provide suggestions for developmental/educational intervention for persistent conductive hearing loss when indicated.

## REFERENCES

Altman, F. (1950). Normal development of the ear and its mechanics. *Archives of Otolaryngology, 52,* 725.

American Speech-Language-Hearing Association. (ASHA). (1992). External auditory canal examination and cerumen management. *ASHA, 35*(5), 65–66.

Anson, B. J. and Davies, J. (1980). Embryology of the ear. In M. M. Paparella and D. A. Shumrick (eds.) *Otolaryngology* (vol. 1, 4th ed.) Philadelphia: W. B. Saunders Company.

Arey, L B. (1965). *Developmental Anatomy.* Philadelphia: W. B. Saunders Company.

Bluestone, C. D. (1971). Eustachian tube obstruction in the infant with cleft palate. *Annals of Otology, Rhinology, and Laryngology, 80* (Suppl. 2), 1–30.

Bluestone, C. D. (1984). State of the art: Definitions and classifications. In D. S. Lim, C. D. Bluestone, Klein, J. O., and Nelson, J. D. (eds.). *Recent Advances in Otitis Media with Effusion.* Toronto: B. C. Decker.

Bluestone, C. D. and Klein, J. O. (1990). Intratemporal complications and sequelae of otitis media. In C. D. Bluestone and S. E. Stool (eds.), *Pediatric Otolaryngology.* Philadelphia: W. B. Saunders Company.

Bluestone, C. D. and Klein, J. O. (1990). Otitis media, atelectasis, and eustachial tube dysfunction. In C. D.

Bluestone and S. E. Stool (eds.), *Pediatric Otolaryngology.* Philadelphia: W. B. Saunders Company.

Brandow, E. C., Jr. (1977). Implant cholesteatoma in the mastoid. In B. F. McCabe, Sade, J., and M. Abramson (eds.), *Cholesteatoma: First International Conference.* New York: Aesculapius.

Brown, D. P. (1994). Speech recognition in recurrent otitis media: Results in a set of identical twins. *Journal of the American Academy of Audiology, 5,* 1–6.

Chole, R. A. (1982). *Color Atlas of Ear Disease.* New York: Appleton-Century-Crofts.

Clark, J. G. (1980a). Central auditory dysfunction in school children: A compilation of management suggestions. *Speech, Language, and Hearing Services in Schools, 11*(4), 208–213.

Clark, J. G. (1980b). The effects of middle ear disease on early child development: A literature review. *Seminars in Speech, Language and Hearing, 1*(2), 149–157.

Davis, J. (1986). Remediation of hearing, speech, and language deficits resulting from otitis media. In J. F. Kavanagh (ed.), *Otitis Media and Child Development* (pp. 182–191). Parkton, MD: York Press.

Eisen, N. H. (1962). Some effects of early sensory deprivation on later behavior: The quondam hard-of-hearing child. *Journal of Abnormal and Social Psychology, 65,* 338–342.

Feldman, H. and Gelman, R. (1986). Otitis media and cognitive development: Theoretical perspectives. In J. F. Kavanagh (ed.), *Otitis Media and Child Development* (pp. 27–41). Parkton, MD: York Press.

Gates, G. A., Avery, C., Cooper, J. C., Hearne, E. M., and Holt, G. R., (1986). Predictive value of tympanometry in middle ear effusion. *Annals of Otology, Rhinology and Laryngology, 95,* 46–50.

Gower, D. and McQuirt, W. F. (1983). Intracranial complications of acute and chronic ear disease: A problem still with us. *Laryngoscope, 93,* 1028

Gravel, J. S. and Wallace, I. F. (1992). Listening and language at 4 years of age: Effects of early otitis media. *Journal of Speech and Hearing Research, 35,* 588–595.

Grievink, E. H., Peters, S. A., Van Bon, W. H. J., and Schilder, A. G. M. (1993). The effects of early bilateral otitis media with effusion on language ability: A prospective cohort study. *Journal of Speech and Hearing Research, 36,* 1004–1012.

Jerger, S. and Jerger, J. (1981). *Auditory Disorders: A Manual for Clinical Evaluation.* Boston: Little, Brown and Company.

Katz, J. (1979). Auditory perception and learning. Presented at the Sixth Annual Conference on Communicative Disorders, Louisiana Tech.

Kavanagh, J. F. (1986). *Otitis Media and Child Development.* Parkton, MD: York Press.

Kenna, M. (1990). Embryology and developmental anatomy of the ear. In C. D. Bluestone and S. E. Stool (eds.), *Pediatric Otolaryngology.* Philadelphia: W. B. Saunders Company.

Lennenberg, E. H. (1967). *Biological Foundations of Language.* New York: John Wiley and Sons.

Lildholt, T. (1979). Unilateral grommet insertion and adnoidectomy in bilateral secretory otitis media: Preliminary report of the results of 91 children. *Clinical Otolaryngology, 4,* 87–93.

Martin, F. N. (1994) *Introduction to Audiology* (5th ed.). Englewood Cliffs, NJ: Prentice-Hall.

McCandless, G. A. (1994). Hearing in Jurassic Park: A dinosaur's ear. *Audiology Today, 6*(2), 10–12.

Menyuk, P. (1992). Relationship of otitis media to speech and language development. In J. Katz, N. A. Stecker, and D. Henderson (eds.), *Central Auditory Processing: A Transdisciplinary View* (pp. 187–197). St. Louis: Mosby Year Book.

Naunton, R. F. and Valvassor, G. E. (1968). Inner ear anomalies: Their association with atresia. *Laryngoscope, 78,* 1042.

Needleman, H. (1977). Effects of hearing loss from early recurrent otitis media on speech and language development. In B. F. Jaffe (ed.), *Hearing Loss in Children* (pp. 640–649). Baltimore: University Park Press.

Northern, J. L. and Downs, M. P. (1991). *Hearing in Children.* Baltimore: Williams and Wilkins.

Orchik, D. J., Dunn, J. W., and McNutt, L. (1978). Tympanometry as a predictor of middle ear effusion. *Archives of Otolaryngology, 104,* 4–6.

Peck, J. E. (1994). Development of hearing. Part II. Embryology. *Journal of the American Academy of Audiology, 5,* 359–365.

Piaget, J. (1953). *The Origins of Intelligence in the Child.* London: Routledge & Kegan Paul.

Reiter, L. A., and Silman, S. (1993). Detecting and remediating external meatal collapse during audiology assessment. *Journal of the American Academy of Audiology, 4,* 264–268.

Roberts, J. E., Burchinal, M. R., Davis, B. P., Collier, A. M., and Henderson, F. W. (1991). Otitis media in early childhood and later language. *Journal of Speech and Hearing Research, 34,* 1158–1168.

Roeser, R., Adams, R., Roland, P., and Wilson, P. (1992). A safe and effective technique for cerumen management. *Audiology Today, 4*(3), 26–30.

Schuknecht, H. F. (1993). *Pathology of the Ear,* (2nd ed.) Malvern, Pennsylvania: Lea & Febiger.

Shah, N. (1971). Use of grommets in "glue" ears. *Journal of Laryngology and Otology, 85,* 283–287.

Silva, P. A., Chalmers, D., and Stewart, J. (1986). Some audiological, psychological, educational and behavioral characteristics of children with bilateral otitis media with effusion: A longitudinal study. *Journal of Learning Disabilities, 19,* 165–169.

Stool, S. E., Berg, A. O., Berman, S., Carney, C. J., Cooley, J. R., Culpepper, L., Eavey, R. D., Feagans, L. V., Finitzo, T., Friedman, E., et al. (July, 1994) *Managing Otitis Media with Effusion in Young Children. Quick Reference Guide for Clinicians.* AHCPR Publication No. 94–0623. Rockville, MD: Agency for Health Care Policy and Research, Public Health Service, U. S. Department of Health and Human Services.

Strange, W. (1986). Speech input and the development of speech perception. In J. F. Kavanagh (ed.), *Otitis Media and Child Development* (pp. 12–26). Parkton, MD: York Press.

Tumarkin, A. (1938). A contribution to the study of middle ear supparation with special reference to the pathology and treatment of cholesteatoma. *Journal of Laryngology and Otology, 53,* 685.

Zemlin, W. R. (1988). *Speech and Hearing Science* (3rd ed.). Englewood Cliffs, NJ: Prentice-Hall.

# CHAPTER 4

# SENSORINEURAL HEARING LOSS IN CHILDREN: ETIOLOGY AND PATHOLOGY

*PATRICIA A. CHASE, JAMES W. HALL III, AND JAY A. WERKHAVEN*

## INTRODUCTION

Sensorineural hearing loss in children is generally categorized as being congenital or acquired and further classified according to etiology, either genetic or nongenetic. A classification system that Paparella, Fox, and Schachern (1989) have found clinically useful will be followed in this discussion (Table 4.1). Congenital and delayed sensorineural hearing loss of genetic etiology, in which hearing loss occurs alone or as part of a syndrome, has been addressed in Chapter 2 of this text and will not be covered here. This chapter addresses the medical assessment of sensorineural hearing loss in children and will provide present and future audiologists with essential information on pediatric sensorineural hearing loss. Extensive references have been provided to guide readers seeking more thorough coverage of specific etiologies.

## ETIOLOGIES OF CONGENITAL HEARING LOSS

### Ototoxic Drugs

About 200 drugs have been labeled ototoxic due to their ability to cause toxic reactions to inner ear structures (Govaerts, Claes, Van De Heyning, Jorens, Marquet, and De Broe 1990). Aminoglycoside antibiotics and the cancer chemotherapeutic agents cisplatin and carboplatin may cause permanent ototoxic effects while the ototoxic effects of loop diuretics, salicylates, and quinine are generally temporary (Brummett, 1980).

Acknowledgments: The authors wish to express appreciation to the following graduate audiology students for their assistance with some of the research for this chapter: B. Cihocki, J. Kang, T. Kelly, and M. Middleton.

Aminoglycosides are the most vestibulotoxic of the ototoxic drugs (Cass, 1991) and include streptomycin, gentamicin, tobramycin, and netilmicin (Govaerts et al. 1990). Kanamycin, amikacin, neomycin, and dihydrostreptomycin are cochleotoxic (ASHA, 1994). Gentamicin can cause both vestibular and cochlear damage and appears to equal kanamycin in terms of cochleotoxicity with tobramycin and netilmicin less ototoxic than kanamycin or gentamicin (ASHA, 1994). The ototoxic effects of aminoglycosides may be latent, resulting in initial or progressive hearing loss after treatment has ended (Meyerhoff, Malle, Yellin, and Roland, 1989) because aminoglycosides take a longer time to clear from inner ear fluids than from blood serum (Rederspil, 1981).

Reports of clinical studies of aminoglycoside ototoxicity in neonates have been variable. Matz (1993) notes that aminoglycoside cochleotoxicity is more common in adults than in neonates and children, possibly due to the difficulty of obtain-

**TABLE 4.1** Nongenetic Etiologies Associated with Sensorineural Hearing Loss in Children

| CONGENITAL LOSS | ACQUIRED LOSS |
|---|---|
| Ototoxic poisoning | Bacterial infection |
| Teratogenic drugs | Spirochetal infection |
| Viral infection | Viral infection |
| Protozoan infection | Ototoxic poisoning |
| Metabolic disorders | Neoplastic disorders |
| Erythroblastosis fetalis | Traumatic injury |
| Radiation (first trimester) | Metabolic disorders |
| Prematurity | Sudden deafness |
| Anoxia, birth trauma | |

Source: Paparella, Fox, and Schachern, 1989.

ing reliable audiometric data in young patients. McCracken (1986) reviewed aminoglycoside ototoxicity studies involving 1300 newborns and concluded that aminoglycoside antibiotics had been used safely and efficaciously with neonates and infants for twenty years. Henley and Rybak (1993) report that preterm infants appear to be hypersensitive to the ototoxic effects of aminoglycosides.

Cisplatin, used in the treatment of cancers in children, is highly ototoxic producing irreversible hearing loss initially observed in the high frequencies (Fausti, Henry, Schaffer, Olson, Frey, and Bagby, 1993). Carboplatin, a less toxic drug than its parent cisplatin, is used for treating a variety of pediatric tumors (Wake, Takeno, Ibrahim, Harrison, and Mount, 1993).

Loop diuretics inhibit the ascending Henle loop in the kidney and alter cochlear function (Elidan, Lin, and Honrubia, 1986) though their effects on the vestibular system are controversial (Elidan et al., 1986). Temporary hearing losses are produced by furosemide, bumetanide, and ethacrynic acid (Matz, 1976); however, synergistic cochleotoxicity is produced when loop diuretics and aminoglycosides are administered at the same time (Hoffman, Whitworth, Jones, and Rybak, 1987). Ototoxic potentiation may occur when loop diuretics are administered with many other drugs including cisplatin (Brummett, Fox, Russell, and Davis, 1981) and carboplatin (Brummett, Guitjens, Vestergaard, and Johnson, 1993). Furosemide is widely used in neonatal intensive care units for the treatment of bronchopulmonary dysplasia, which is common among very-low-birthweight premature infants treated for respiratory distress syndrome (Wells, 1990). Blood level monitoring to avoid the accumulation of furosemide to ototoxic levels may be necessary in newborns receiving repeated doses (Henley and Rybak, 1993).

Acetylsalicylic acid (aspirin) and sodium salicylate are commonly used ototoxic salicylates that are available without prescription (Miller, 1985). Salicylate-induced hearing loss usually manifests as high-pitched tinnitus accompanied by hearing loss and occasional vestibular dysfunction (Cass, 1991). Most salicylate-induced losses are reversible, bilateral, and symmetrical (Miller, 1985) with partial hearing improvement 24 to 48 hours after taking the drug and normal hearing within 7 to 10 days (ASHA, 1994). Noise can potentiate the cochleotoxic effects of salicylates (McFadden and Plattsmier, 1983), aminoglycosides (Brown, Brummett, Meikle, and Vernon, 1978), and cisplatin (Sharma and Edwards, 1983).

## Teratogenic Drugs

Teratogenic drugs (tending to produce anomalies of formation) cross the placenta and cause direct damage to the developing fetal ear, and in some instances, such as thalidomide-induced embryopathy, produce a wide variety of other abnormalities in the infant (Chan, 1994; Lenz and Knapp, 1962; Paparella et al., 1989). Thalidomide was used in Europe in the late 1950s and early 1960s, but it was never released in the United States. Infants of mothers who used thalidomide while pregnant have varying degrees of hearing loss, usually moderate to severe, and vestibular deficits have been reported (Chan, 1994). Hypoplasia (incomplete development) of the cochlea and congenital hearing loss have been reported in infants whose mothers received chloroquine or quinine during pregnancy (Hart and Naunton, 1964).

Isoretinoin (Accutane), a vitamin A derivative used in the treatment of severe cystic acne, can have major teratogenic effects on the offspring of women taking it during pregnancy (Westerman, Gilbert, and Schondel, 1994). Isoretinoin is especially damaging during the first trimester, resulting in a variety of malformations primarily of the central nervous system and head and neck region (Jahn and Ganti, 1987). Otologic management, if the infant survives the perinatal period, includes documentation of external malformations and assessment of cochlear function followed by intense auditory habilitation (Jahn and Ganti, 1987). Westerman and colleagues (1994) recommend the evaluation of vestibular function as well.

## Viral Infections

The acronym TORCHES has long been used as a reminder of a number of prenatal infections that can result in a group of clinically indistinguishable illnesses in the neonate. TORCHES refers to toxoplasmosis, rubella, cytomegalovirus (CMV), herpes simplex, and syphilis. Because many other agents can cause similar illnesses, and diagnostic workups should not be limited to the original four agents (not including syphilis), Freij and Sever (1994) recommend that use of the mnemonic be limited or completely abandoned.

### *Maternal Rubella*

Maternal rubella (German measles) during the first trimester of pregnancy can result in congenital cataracts or glaucoma, congenital heart disease, central nervous system problems, mental retardation, microcephaly and/or sensorineural hearing loss (Chan, 1994; Paparella et al., 1989). More than 12,000 infants were born with congenital rubella and hearing loss after the last United States epidemic in 1964 (Trybus, Karchmer, and Kerstetter, 1980). Maternal rubella infection causes hearing loss in 60 to 80 percent of cases with the characteristic loss being severe to profound, symmetric or asymmetric, with a flat configuration, and possibly progressive (Meyerhoff, Cass, Schwaber, Sculerati, and Slattery, 1994).

Sheraton (1964) studied 227 children exposed to rubella during the first trimester of pregnancy and found that about 20 percent developed hearing loss by age 8 to 11 years though their hearing was initially thought to be normal. Barr and Wedenberg (1965) followed 23 children with hearing loss caused by maternal rubella infection and observed progression of the losses during the observation periods, which lasted from 5 to 11 years. More recently, Newton and Rowson (1988) reported hearing deterioration prior to the age of 7 years in three children whose hearing losses were associated with maternal rubella infection. Cochleosaccular dysplasia is the distinguishing otopathologic feature (Chan, 1994; Pappas, 1985). Hayes and Pashley (1991) report that the rubella

vaccination program has essentially eliminated congenital rubella as a significant etiology of pediatric sensorineural hearing loss.

### *Cytomegalovirus*

Cytomegalovirus is the most common congenital infection in newborns (Alford, Stagno, Pass, and Britt, 1990) with about 40,000 infected infants born each year in the United States (Hall, Prentice, Byrn, Smiley, and Davidson, 1995; Meyerhoff et al., 1994). Serious health problems result when CMV is transmitted to the fetus during the prenatal or perinatal period with the greatest risk for symptomatic congenital CMV disease occurring when the fetus is infected during the first half of pregnancy (Chan, 1994). More than 90 percent of infants infected with CMV are asymptomatic as neonates while the other 10 percent of congenital CMV cases present as multiorgan systemic infections with a 20 to 30 percent mortality rate (Chan, 1994). Manifestations of congenital CMV include microcephaly, chorioretinitis, mental retardation, neuromuscular disorders, hepatosplenomegaly, hyperbilirubinemia, petechiae, thrombocytopenia, cerebral calcifications, and hearing impairment (Paparella et al., 1989; Stagno, 1990).

Thirty to 60 percent of those children symptomatic at birth will have congenital or late-onset hearing loss that may continue to deteriorate (Meyerhoff et al., 1994). The frequency of hearing loss in asymptomatic children ranges from 6 to 24 percent with losses often unilateral and varying from mild to profound. These losses may continue to progress through middle childhood (Williamson, Demmler, Percy, and Catlin, 1992). Schildroth (1994) compares the effects of the CMV-induced hearing loss, often accompanied by mental retardation and cerebral palsy, to those of the 1964–1965 rubella epidemic and encourages the development of a vaccine and subsequent CMV immunization program.

Children with congenital CMV infection need periodic audiologic monitoring regardless of their initial hearing status, since hearing loss may be of delayed onset and is likely to deteriorate during early childhood (Hall et al., 1995). The pathophysiology of CMV hearing loss is uncertain, and it has been hypothesized that the audiological changes documented in congenitally infected infants may be linked to the periods of dormancy and reactivation characteristic of CMV infections (Meyerhoff et al., 1994).

The hearing loss associated with CMV may be progressive and severe. In general, children with symptomatic CMV present a significant clinical challenge to the audiologist for at least six reasons: (1) CMV-related hearing loss may be unilateral or highly asymmetric. For early detection to be effective, hearing assessment must be ear specific. (2) Because of the delayed onset and progressive nature of the sensorineural hearing loss, conscientious monitoring of auditory status is required, even for infants passing the initial screening. (3) The audiologist must strive to implement prompt management, such as amplification, while keeping in mind that hearing status is subject to change. (4) The marked neurologic deficits that characterize some patients with symptomatic CMV can compromise valid behavioral audiometry. (5) There is little published information on the audiometric configurations of hearing loss associated with CMV. (6) In view of the central nervous system pathology that is often a feature of CMV, central auditory dysfunction and processing disorder would not be unlikely in some patients.

*Herpes Simplex Virus*
Herpes simplex virus (HSV) infects a significant number of newborns with 50 to 85 percent of infected neonates dying. Surviving infants are left with severe, generalized complications (Stagno, Pass, and Alford, 1981). Neonatal HSV, usually caused by HSV-2, is often acquired during delivery from infected maternal genital secretions (Whitley and Alford, 1981). Clinical outcomes appear similar for newborns infected with either HSV-1 or HSV-2 (Nahmias and Visintine, 1976).

Limited information is available on the effects of HSV on the auditory system; however,

Dahle and McCollister (1988) suggest that HSV and CMV, both members of the herpes virus family and structurally similar (Wilson, 1986), may have nearly the same effects. These investigators studied twenty children diagnosed with symptomatic neonatal HSV and found eighteen of the children to have normal hearing while two had sensorineural hearing impairments. One of these children had a moderate to severe bilateral loss while the other loss, also of moderate to severe degree, was unilateral. Both children with hearing impairments were infected in utero while the other eighteen with normal hearing were thought to be infected during delivery. Dahle and McCollister (1988) note the similarity to congenital CMV in which a high prevalence of hearing impairment is also reported as compared to children infected with CMV during delivery or postnatally. Both HSV and CMV appear more likely to cause hearing loss when infection is prenatal rather than perinatal or postnatal.

*Human Immunodeficiency Virus*
Epidemiologic changes in the adult population have resulted in rapid spread of the human immunodeficiency virus (HIV) into the pediatric population (Chanock and McIntosh, 1989). Approximately 6000 newborns are exposed to HIV every year (MaWhinney, Pagano, and Thomas, 1993) with 85 percent of infants infected by perinatal transmission from mother to child (Scott, 1992). Ample evidence exists to support intrauterine acquisition of HIV as well as transmission of the virus during the birth process (Chanock and McIntosh, 1989). HIV-infected children may be referred to the otolaryngologist with a variety of complaints, many of which are associated with bacterial infections and parotid gland enlargement (Chanock and McIntosh, 1989). Several studies (Chow, Stern, Kaul, Pincus, and Gromisch, 1990; Principi, Marchisio, Tornaghi, Onorato, Massironi, and Picco 1991; Williams, 1987) have reported a greater incidence of middle ear disease in HIV-infected children than in noninfected children.

The most common serious opportunistic infection among children that is HIV-associated is *Pneumocystis carinii* pneumonia (PCP) (Chow et al., 1990). PCP, usually diagnosed between 3 and 6 months of age (Centers for Disease Control, 1991), rapidly progresses from acute respiratory illness to respiratory failure in infants (Chow et al., 1990). Because these children are immunocompromised, secondary opportunistic infections such as HSV, varicella-zoster (chicken pox) virus, and measles constitute major health threats and may result in life-threatening conditions (Chanock and McIntosh, 1989; Rarey, 1990). Although middle ear and mastoid infections are well recognized in HIV-infected persons, sensorineural hearing loss, though obvious, is poorly understood (Kohan, Rothstein, and Cohen, 1988). Pappas, Sekhar, Lim, and Hillman (1994) report cochlear pathology based on ultrastructural findings in adult temporal bone investigations.

## Toxoplasmosis

Toxoplasmosis, caused by a protozoan parasite *Toxoplasmosa gondii,* is an acquired, asymptomatic infection in humans generally traceable to improper handling of cat litter pans or ingestion of contaminated raw or undercooked meat (Stein and Boyer, 1994). Congenitally acquired toxoplasmosis is transmitted in utero resulting in permanent damage to the eyes and central nervous system as well as other organ systems. Approximately 3000 to 3300 affected infants are born yearly in the United States with most asymptomatic at birth (McCleod, Wisner, and Boyer, 1992; Remington and Desmonds, 1990). Ophthalmic signs of the infection often develop in the first few months of life with definitive diagnosis accomplished through specific *Toxoplasma* serologic tests (Stein and Boyer, 1994). Several studies have reported sensorineural hearing loss, unilateral or bilateral, in approximately 15 to 20 percent of congenitally infected children who received little or no treatment (e.g., Stein and Boyer, 1994). McGee, Walters, Stein, Kraus, Johnson, Boyer, Mats, Roizen, Beckman, and Meier (1992) report less frequent hearing loss and less severe manifestations of toxoplasmosis in infants receiving early and prolonged treatment with a combination of pyrimethamine and sulfonamide.

## Erythroblastosis Fetalis

Erythroblastosis fetalis is a hemolytic disease caused by Rh incompatibility between a mother and fetus that presents clinically as jaundice (Paparella et al., 1989). Bilirubin is toxic to cochlear nuclei and other central auditory pathways (Robbins, Aotran, and Kumar, 1984). Hyperbilirubinemia causing sensorineural hearing loss may be the result of several etiologies including erythroblastosis fetalis and other forms of hemolytic disease or hemorrhage (Chan, 1994). Kernicterus can cause mild-to-severe high-frequency sensorineural hearing loss though mild hyperbilirubinemia less frequently produces hearing loss (Barr and Wedenberg, 1965).

## Prematurity-Anoxia-Birth Trauma

Sensorineural hearing loss occurs in approximately 9 percent of infants born weighing less than 1500 grams (Paparella et al., 1989). Anoxia, hypothermia, traumatic delivery, need for resuscitation, and ambient noise (Barr and Wedenberg, 1965; Paparella et al., 1989) may be factors in this loss that generally affects the high frequencies resulting in a steeply sloped audiogram (Davey, 1962).

Severe perinatal asphyxia results in sensorineural hearing loss, which is generally bilaterally symmetrical and most severe in the high frequencies (Paparella et al., 1989). Damage to the organ of Corti may be the result of intracerebral hemorrhage due to cranial injury at birth (Paparella et al., 1989). Schumacher, Spak, and Kileny (1990) report a high incidence of decreased hearing sensitivity after extracorporeal membrane oxygenation (ECMO) treatment of severe respiratory failure in term newborns.

Infants with persistent pulmonary hypertension (PPHN) or persistent fetal circulation have a history of severe hypoxemia (patent ductus arteriosus) following birth asphyxia (Northern and Downs, 1991). An increased incidence of sensorineural hearing loss ranging from mild to severe, unilateral or bilateral, and sometimes progressive has been documented in these infants (e.g., Walton and Hendricks-Munoz, 1991). Walton and Hendricks-Munoz (1991) found sensorineural hearing loss in nineteen of fifty-one infants (37 percent) diagnosed with PPHN. Of these nineteen infants, sixteen had bilateral hearing losses, three had unilateral impairments, and in five progressive sensorineural hearing losses were identified. Audiometric profiles were typically downward sloping, and degree of hearing loss varied considerably. Walton and Hendricks-Munoz (1991) correlated duration of hyperventilation with hearing outcome and reported an incidence of hearing loss twenty-five times greater for infants with PPHN than for at-risk infants in the same neonatal intensive care unit. Marron, Crisafi, Driscoll, Wung, Driscoll, Fay, and James (1992) treated thirty-four infants diagnosed with PPHN without paralysis or hyperventilation. Twenty-seven of these received audiological testing between 10 months of age and 6 years of age, and none demonstrated sensorineural hearing loss. These findings suggest that conservative management of PPHN may decrease the incidence of sensorineural hearing loss and optimize neurologic outcome (Marron et al., 1992).

The most common respiratory problem encountered by newborns, both premature and full term, is respiratory distress syndrome (RDS) or hyaline membrane disease (Konkle and Knightly, 1993). Severe-to-profound delayed-onset sensorineural hearing loss has been reported in several cases of infants diagnosed with RDS (Konkle and Knightly, 1993).

## Other Causes

CHARGE (C-coloboma, H-congenital heart disease, A-atresia choanae, R-retarded growth and development, G-genital anomalies in males, E-ear anomalies and deafness) association refers to a collection of congenital malformations of unknown etiology occurring in nonrandom association with choanal atresia (Brown and Israel, 1991). Association rather than syndrome is used because the physical anomalies may not all occur together; however, the mnemonic CHARGE reminds clinicians that a logical management approach must consider each systemic anomaly (Hall, 1992). External ear malformations are wide-ranging with small ears being the most commonly described abnormality (Oley, Baraitser, and Grant, 1988). Kaplan (1989) reports that the highly unusual appearance of the external ears and the facial nerve palsy suggest a facial "gestalt" in CHARGE. Estimates of hearing impairment range from 20 to 85 percent with the majority of the hearing losses being sensorineural, although malformations of the middle ear and associated conductive hearing impairments have been identified (Dobrowski, Grundfast, and Rosenbaum 1985; Goldson, Smith, and Stewart, 1986; Kaplan, 1985; Oley et al., 1988; Pagon, Graham, and Zonana, 1981). A high-frequency sloping sensorineural hearing loss is characteristic of CHARGE though the loss may range from mild to profound (Meyerhoff et al., 1994). Progression of the hearing loss is common although it may be slow or intermittent (Thelin, Mitchell, Hefner, and Davenport, 1986). Brown and Israel (1991) report audiologic findings from a set of fraternal twins that demonstrate the variability and asymmetry of hearing losses associated with CHARGE. In a review of 150 patients from the literature as well as 13 from their own center, Byerly and Pauli (1993) document the frequency of cranial nerve dysfunction in CHARGE association and suggest multiple cranial nerve abnormalities as a primary cause for the facial paralysis, feeding difficulties, and sensorineural hearing loss characteristic of this disorder.

Congenital hearing loss can result from maternal exposure to other substances or conditions that may be toxic to fetal development including drugs, alcohol, and severe maternal diabetes (Bergstrom, 1987; Gerkin, 1984; Gerkin and

Church, 1987). Fetal alcohol syndrome (FAS) describes a pattern of congenital malformations that are occasionally observed in children of women who abused alcohol while pregnant (Smith, 1982). Church and Gerkin (1988) report audiologic findings on fourteen children with FAS noting that thirteen of the fourteen had histories of hearing disorders in childhood. Thirteen were otitis prone, and four had bilateral sensorineural hearing loss suggesting hearing disorders as characteristic of FAS. Berman, Beare, Church, and Abel (1992) report additive effects of acoustic trauma on rats prenatally exposed to alcohol resulting in greater sensorineural hearing loss than either condition alone. Converging evidence from both human and animal studies suggests that infants and children prenatally exposed to alcohol are at increased risk for otitis as well as sensorineural hearing loss (Church and Gerkin, 1988). In animal studies of prenatal cocaine exposure, Church and Overbeck (1991) reported auditory brain-stem response findings consistent with sensorineural hearing loss.

## ETIOLOGIES OF ACQUIRED HEARING LOSS

### Bacterial Infections

#### Labyrinthitis

Bacterial meningitis is an acute infectious disease of the central nervous system, whose most common complication is sensorineural hearing loss, which affects 30 to 40 percent of surviving infants and children (Dodge, Davis, Feigin, Holmes, Kaplan, Jubelirer, Stechenberg, and Hirsh, 1984; Lindberg, Rosenhall, Nylen, and Ringner, 1977; Ozdamar, Kraus, and Stein, 1983; Sell, Merrill, Doyne, and Zimsky, 1972). When bacteria invade the cochlea, acute suppurative labyrinthitis occurs resulting in hearing loss (Stein and Boyer, 1994). *Streptococcus pneumoniae, Neisseria meningitidis,* and *Hemophilus influenzae* type b (Hib) are the most common organisms associated with meningitis, with hearing loss occurring in 30 per-

cent of pneumococcal, 10 percent of meningococcal, and 4 to 18 percent of cases with Hib meningitis (Dodge et al., 1984; Lindberg et al., 1977; Ozdamar et al., 1983; Sell et al., 1972). During the prenatal period, *Escherichia coli* and Group B streptococci infections predominate (Stein and Boyer, 1994); however, meningococcal labyrinthitis caused by Hib accounts for about 18,000 cases of meningitis each year in the United States (Eskola, Peltola, Takala, Kayhty, Hakulinen, Karanko, Kela, Rekola, Ronnberg, Samuelson, Gordon, and Makela, 1987). Attack rates are highest for young infants less than 1 year of age (Schlech, Ward, Band, Hightower, Fraser, and Broome, 1985). *Hemophilus influenzae* is the most common cause of bacterial meningitis in children older than 1 month; however, sensorineural hearing loss more commonly follows pneumococcal meningitis than Hib meningitis (Meyerhoff et al., 1994).

The hearing loss can occur some time after the infection has been treated and can progress several years after treatment for meningitis (Epstein and Reilly, 1989). Postmeningitic children with an existing hearing loss often demonstrate additional hearing deterioration during adolescence that may be secondary to cochlear ossification (Epstein and Reilly, 1989). Meningitic hearing losses are predominately bilateral sensorineural losses of severe to profound degree (Guiscafre, Benitez-Diaz, Martinez, and Munoz, 1984). With the introduction of Hib vaccine, the incidence of meningitis caused by this pathogen has decreased (Murphy, White, and Pastor, 1993) and may be eliminated as an important cause of childhood hearing loss (Stein and Boyer 1994).

Unilateral sensorineural hearing loss following meningitis may occur (Ruben, 1983). Rosenhall and Kankkunen (1980) reported mild to moderate hearing loss following meningitis and noted complete or partial hearing recovery in some patients. Fluctuating hearing loss associated with meningitis has also been reported (Rosenhall and Kankkunen, 1981). Brookhouser and Auslander (1989) reported three cases of long-term hearing improvement in children up to 25 months post meningitis. McCormick and colleagues (McCormick, Gibbin, Lutman, and O'Donoghue, 1993) recommend a 6-month delay after meningitis before cochlear implantation for those rare cases in which hearing demonstrates spontaneous recovery. Recently reported reductions in the incidence of moderate to profound sensorineural hearing loss in patients with bacterial meningitis who were treated with dexamethasone (Odio, Faingezicht, and Paris, 1991) may have a very positive effect on the reduction of hearing loss caused by meningitis.

## Syphilis

Syphilis, caused by infection with the spirochete, *Treponema pallidum,* has several stages and affects many body systems. Congenital syphilis results from being born to an infected mother, while acquired syphilis is the result of sexual intercourse with an infected partner (Amenta, Dayal, Flaherty, and Weil, 1992). Congenital syphilis has two stages: early, with symptoms manifesting during the first 2 years of age, and late, with symptoms presenting after 2 years of age (Amenta et al., 1992). Early-stage congenital syphilis results when the fetus is infected transplacentally with 38 to 64 percent of cases asymptomatic (Zenker and Rolfs, 1989) while the others have devastating multisystem disease (Amenta et al., 1992).

Estimates of hearing loss in congenital syphilis range from 3 to 38 percent (Dalsgaard-Neilson, 1938; Fiumara and Lessell, 1970; Karmody and Schuknecht, 1966). Karmody and Schuknecht (1966) report that 37 percent of patients develop hearing loss between 1 and 10 years of age with the remaining 63 percent of patients reporting onset after age 25 years. A flat sensorineural hearing loss is usually characteristic of childhood onset with the loss being sudden, bilateral, symmetric, and profound with no associated vestibular symptoms (Amenta et al., 1992). Other manifestations of congenital syphilis include interstitial

keratitis (Morrison, 1975) and Hutchinson's notched incisors (Hutchinson, 1863). The fluorescent treponemal antibody absorption test (FTA-ABS) is the diagnostic test of choice for congenital syphilis (Zoller, Wilson, Nadol, and Girard, 1978).

## Viral Diseases

Hearing loss in childhood can be the result of viral infections such as mumps, measles, chicken pox, infectious mononucleosis, and HSV. These hearing losses can be partial and gradually progress over time (Meyerhoff et al., 1994). The mumps virus is generally believed to be the most common cause of unilateral acquired sensorineural hearing loss in children (Meyerhoff et al., 1994) even though vaccine is available. The sensorineural hearing loss caused by mumps ranges from a mild high-frequency impairment to a profound one (Chan, 1994). Hearing deficits from measles are generally bilaterally symmetric and of moderate to profound degree (Chan, 1994).

## Neoplastic Disorders

Neoplastic processes such as leukemia, histiocytosis X, and neuroblastoma can invade the temporal bone resulting in increased otologic complications including sensorineural hearing loss (Chan, 1994). Acoustic tumors and pontine glioma may account for unilateral sensorineural hearing loss as well as tinnitus and dizziness (Paparella et al., 1989).

## Traumatic Injury
### Fractures of the Temporal Bone
Temporal bone fractures can be longitudinal, transverse, or combined; however, transverse fractures through inner ear structures more commonly result in sensorineural hearing loss that may be unilateral or bilateral (Paparella et al., 1989). Petrous bone fractures are fairly common in children and are usually diagnosed after collisions and falls (Glarner, Meuli, Hof, Gallati, Nadal, Fisch, and Stauffer, 1994). Transverse fractures generally result from trauma to the fron-

tal or occipital area (Paparella et al., 1989), and the diagnostic method of choice is the computed tomography (CT) scan (Shaffer and Haughton, 1980). Meningitis may be an additional complication that can result in sensorineural hearing deficit (Ward, 1969). Hearing loss from perilymphatic fistula associated with head trauma can be sudden, fluctuating, and progressive (Meyerhoff et al., 1994). In a review of 127 cases of petrous bone fractures, Glarner and colleagues (1994) reported hearing disorder in 69 percent of children receiving audiometrics. Interdisciplinary management is essential to minimize morbidity, and therapeutic measures may include vaccination against *Streptococcus pneumoniae* and subtotal petrosectomy to lower the incidence of post-traumatic meningitis (Glarner et al., 1994). Labyrinthine concussion without temporal bone fracture may result in sudden sensorineural hearing impairment (Pappas, 1985) with audiometric configurations that are notched, sloping, flat, or parabolic (Wofford, 1981).

## Acoustic Trauma

Acoustic trauma resulting in sensorineural hearing loss can be the result of prolonged exposure to noise or sudden injury from excessive noise (Chan, 1994). Premature infants often spend long periods of time in neonatal intensive care nurseries in which noise levels sometimes exceed 80 dB SPL (Pappas, 1985). Stereo headphones and rock concerts contribute to the excessive noise exposure of children and adolescents (Epstein and Reilly, 1989). Brookhouser, Worthington, and Kelly (1992) investigated 114 cases of probable noise-induced hearing loss and found the classical audiometric notch in 70 percent while the other 25 percent had sloping losses. Ninety percent of these 114 cases were males, and hearing loss was identified in three-fourths of the cases by age 16 years. Hearing deterioration was progressive in 70 percent of the 47 cases who received follow-up. Audiometric patterns from this investigation suggest that continued noise exposure may result in a high-frequency loss with gradual disappearance

of the characteristic notch. Appropriate counseling on the hazards of exposure to intense sound levels should always be coupled with hearing monitoring.

## Metabolic Disorders

### Meniere Disease

The pediatric age group comprises approximately 3 percent of all patients with Meniere disease (Paparella et al., 1989). Symptoms in children are identical to those in adults including vertigo, tinnitus, and hearing loss (Chan, 1994). Treatment has included traditional medical therapy and shunt procedures (Chan, 1994). Inner-ear fluid imbalance can be caused by Meniere disease, perilymphatic fistula, and perilymphatic hypertension resulting in fluctuating or progressive sensorineural hearing loss (Meyerhoff et al., 1994).

### Autoimmune Disease

Though most autoimmune diseases associated with sensorineural hearing loss affect adults only, Chan (1994) reported sensorineural hearing loss in children with juvenile rheumatoid arthritis and other collagen diseases. Clinical symptoms in addition to bilateral, progressive sensorineural hearing loss with or without dizziness, include ear pressure and tinnitus, reduced vestibular function, unsteadiness and ataxia in darkness, and temporary facial palsy (Hughes, Moscicki, Barna, and San Martin, 1994). Hughes and colleagues (1994) prefer the term immune inner ear disease and report the disease to be more common in middle-aged females though it can occur in males, and onset can be in childhood. Presently, the two most clinically useful tests for diagnosing immune inner ear disease are the lymphocyte transformation test and the Western blot immunoassay; however, these antigen-specific studies are relatively unavailable (Hughes et al., 1994). In cases where antigen-specific tests cannot be obtained, steroid trials may be initiated with the patient with beneficial treatment response supporting the presumptive clinical diagnosis (Hughes et al., 1994).

## Sudden Deafness

Sudden-onset deafness is relatively rare in the pediatric age group and may sometimes represent the end event in a progressive or fluctuating sensorineural hearing loss (Chan, 1994). Etiology cannot be determined in most patients; however, the three most often cited causes are viral infection, vascular compromise, and labyrinthine membrane breaks (Emmett, 1994). Cole and Jahrsdoerfer (1988) report increasing support for the viral autoimmune etiologies in sudden hearing loss. The hearing loss in sudden-onset deafness is usually unilateral with varying audiometric pattern, may be of cochlear and/or eighth cranial nerve origin, and may sometimes be accompanied by tenderness, tinnitus, and mild vertigo (Silman and Silverman, 1991). Epstein and Reilly (1989) report that early medical intervention, which increases circulation and oxygenation to the inner ear, may restore all or part of the deteriorated hearing. Although numerous conventional medical therapies have been attempted (Grandis, Hirsch, and Wagener, 1993), up to 65 percent of patients recover functional hearing without treatment (Mattox and Simmons, 1977). In a case report of two 19-year-old sisters, identical twins, who listened to loud music at a rock concert and simultaneously experienced idiopathic sudden hearing loss, Emmett (1994) suggested a genetic predisposition for rupture of the intracochlear membranes.

Perilymphatic fistula, leakage of inner ear fluid through the oval or round window into the middle ear space, is a known cause of sudden hearing loss syndrome (Chan, 1994). Perilymphatic fistulas can occur spontaneously in children with existing congenital sensorineural hearing loss and in children with normal hearing due to increased exertion or sudden changes in barometric pressure (Epstein and Reilly, 1989). Signs and symptoms of perilymphatic fistula vary considerably (McCabe, 1989), and surgical exploration is the only reliable diagnostic method (Harvey and Millen, 1994). Harvey and Millen (1994)

surgically explored four children who presented with abrupt decreases in hearing that progressed from mixed to purely sensorineural loss and found these children to have absent round window reflexes rather than perilymphatic fistula. These investigators theorize that the findings indicate altered inner ear fluid dynamics. In an update on 115 patients diagnosed and treated for perilymphatic fistula over an 11-year period, McCabe (1989) reports that closure of the fistula improves vestibular symptoms in 94 percent of patients and stabilizes or improves hearing in 49 percent of patients.

## Monitoring of Dynamic Sensorineural Hearing Loss in Children

Dynamic sensorineural hearing loss, hearing loss that progressively worsens without treatment or improves with treatment, poses special considerations for the audiologic management of infants and young children (Hall, Bratt, Schwaber, and Baer, 1993). Indicators associated with delayed-onset sensorineural hearing loss in infants and young children include family history of hereditary hearing loss in childhood, in utero infections, neurofibromatosis type II, and neurodegenerative disorders (JCIH, 1994). Infants with these indicators should have their hearing assessed at least every 6 months until they are 3 years old with continued hearing evaluation as needed thereafter (JCIH, 1994).

Because young children may be at increased risk for ototoxicity relative to adults (Schell, McHaney, Green, Kun, Hayes, Horowitz, and Meyer, 1989), children receiving treatment with potentially ototoxic drugs require long-term audiologic follow-up to determine whether hearing loss is stable or progressive (ASHA, 1994). After baseline audiologic evaluation, follow-up testing should occur immediately (depending on drug schedules), at 3 months, 6 months, and 1 year after treatment has ended (ASHA, 1994). Ototoxicity monitoring in infants and young children requires that the audiologist and physician work cooperatively to determine an individual protocol appropriate for a sick child (Campbell and Durrant, 1993).

Matkin (1988) emphasizes the importance of systematic monitoring of all children with sensorineural hearing loss. Audiologic reevaluations should be scheduled every 3 months until age 3 years with retesting at 6-month intervals between age 3 and 6. Yearly audiologic reevaluations are appropriate for children who are in school. This ongoing, rigorous monitoring enables the audiologist to identify progressive hearing loss and conductive hearing loss, to assist parents in adjusting to their child's hearing impairment and to optimize the performance of amplification systems used by the child (Matkin, 1988).

## MEDICAL DIAGNOSIS AND TREATMENT

The process of identifying sensorineural hearing loss in an individual child may be initiated by several different sources including parents, pediatricians, primary care physicians, audiologists, neonatologists, and otolaryngologists. Epstein and Reilly (1989) emphasize the need for pediatricians who suspect hearing loss to seek answers through careful history taking and thorough general physical and otoscopic examinations. Pediatricians are encouraged to follow up vigorously to confirm normal hearing, thereby alleviating parental concern about the child's responses to sounds. This follow-up can be accomplished utilizing other specialized health care professionals including pediatric audiologists and pediatric otolaryngologists.

Although there is no specific medical test battery for diagnosing sensorineural hearing loss in children, otolaryngologists generally focus on history, physical examination, audiologic assessment, imaging studies, and additional laboratory testing (Ruth and Lambert, 1991). With the exception of audiologic assessment, which has already been discussed, each of these areas will be addressed in detail.

## History

In recognizing the importance of thorough history taking as an essential component of the medical evaluation process, Chan (1994) recommends the 1990 position statement of the Joint Committee on Infant Hearing (1991) as a model for otolaryngologists. Pertinent factors for identifying neonates and infants at risk for sensorineural hearing impairment are included in the 1990 Joint Committee document. As previously discussed in this chapter, the 1994 Joint Committee on Infant Hearing Position Statement (JCIH, 1994) contains indicators (high-risk factors) associated with sensorineural hearing loss in children that can be used during history taking.

Paparella and colleagues (1989) emphasize obtaining a thorough gestational history with particular emphasis on prenatal infections, drug administrations, and systemic illnesses of the mother. Perinatal history should explore complications at delivery, anoxia at birth, head injuries, meningitis, and central nervous system infections. Family history should include questions about the child's immediate family as well as hearing loss in other relatives (Ruth and Lambert, 1991).

## Physical Examination

A careful physical examination of the head and neck is essential with particular emphasis on the child's eyes, ears, craniofacial growth and development, and cranial nerves (Ruth and Lambert, 1991). Though most children born with congenital sensorineural hearing loss have no associated defects, there are more than seventy known syndromes associated with sensorineural hearing loss in children (Epstein and Reilly, 1989). Because physical findings may occur alone or as part of a syndrome, otolaryngologists must familiarize themselves with key physical findings often associated with sensorineural hearing loss as well as the features characteristically identified with certain syndromes. Selected physical findings pertinent to the assessment of sensorineural hearing loss in children are summarized in Table 4.2.

**TABLE 4.2**   Selected Physical Findings Associated with Sensorineural Hearing Loss in Children

| FINDINGS | DISORDER |
| --- | --- |
| *Ears* | |
| Preauricular pits | — |
| Auricular appendages | — |
| Auricular malformations | — |
| Position/shape combined with maxilla/mandible development | Crouzon's disease Treacher-Collins syndrome |
| *Eyes* | |
| Retinitis pigmentosa | Usher's syndrome |
| Dystopia canthorum | Waardenburg syndrome |
| Heterochromia iridis | Waardenburg syndrome |
| Coloboma | CHARGE association |
| Cataracts | Congenital rubella |
| Keratitis | Cogan's syndrome |
| Corneal opacities | Syphilis |
| Sclera—blue color | Osteogenesis imperfecta |
| *Neck* | |
| Goiter | Pendred syndrome |
| Branchial fistulas | Branchio-oto-renal syndrome |
| *Musculoskeletal* | |
| Fusion of cervical vertebrae | Klippel-Feil syndrome |
| Dwarfism | Achondroplasia |
| *Integumentary* | |
| White forelock | Waardenburg syndrome |
| Hypopigmentation | Albinism |
| Ectodermal dysplasia | Ichthyosis |
| *Neurologic* | |
| Ataxia | — |
| Mental retardation | — |

The ear is thoroughly inspected using a pneumatic otoscope or operating microscope to identify congenital abnormality, infection, trauma, or active disease. Additional information on the hearing loss may be obtained using tuning fork tests. An examination of the hard and soft palate and the eustachian tube orifices completes the ear examination.

## Imaging Studies

The examination of choice for evaluating congenital malformations of the ear and temporal bone is thin-section high-resolution computed tomography (CT) with "bone algorithm" (Fisher and Curtin, 1994). This algorithm provides excellent border definitions between bone, air, fluid, and soft tissues. Magnetic resonance imaging (MRI) is the method of choice for evaluating acoustic neuromas (Fisher and Curtin, 1994). Magnetic resonance imaging can identify perilymph and endolymph in the inner ear; however, the cortical bone and air spaces comprising most middle and inner ear anatomy are indistinguishable (Fisher and Curtin, 1994). Computed tomography studies of patients with sensorineural hearing loss are often normal. Jackler, Luxford, and House (1987) found inner ear malformations in only 20 percent of patients with congenital sensorineural hearing loss.

Computed tomography studies are useful in the evaluation of sensorineural hearing loss in children though Fisher and Curtin (1994) report that infants and young children sometimes require sedation for these radiographic studies. Contrast agents are indicated when there is suspicion of a tumor or vascular abnormality (Eelkema and Curtin, 1989). Information available from CT studies may be invaluable for management of sensorineural hearing loss in children and may assist in counseling parents as well (Chan, 1994).

## Additional Laboratory Testing

Because there is no standard laboratory panel for sensorineural hearing loss and yields from mass screenings are excessively low, the clinician's index of suspicion, based on history and physical findings, determines the need for additional laboratory studies (Chan, 1994). Blood and laboratory studies (Table 4.3) can be used to diagnose a small percentage of cochlear disorders (Chan, 1994) and

TABLE 4.3    Cochlear Disorders That Can Be Investigated with Blood and Laboratory Studies

| DISORDER | BLOOD AND LAB STUDIES |
|---|---|
| Acute ototoxicity | Serum drug levels |
| Congenital rubella | Isolate live virus from body fluids |
| | Cord serum rubella-specific IgM titer |
| | Serial measures of infant serum IgG levels |
| | Fetal IgM via cordocentesis |
| | DNA probe from chorionic villus biopsy |
| Alport's syndrome | Renal function studies |
| Autoimmune disease | Sedimentation rate |
| | Antinuclear antibody |
| | Quantitative immunoglobulins |
| | Lab panel nonspecific though helpful when positive |
| | Distinct signs and symptoms, so not usually a diagnostic problem |
| Metabolic diseases | Lipids |
| | Glucose |
| | Thyroid function tests |
| Syphilis | FTA-ABS test (during neonatal period may get falsely negative results in adequately treated mother) |
| Viral diseases | Herpes |
| | Rubella |
| | Toxoplasmosis |
| Congenital cytomegalovirus | Cytomegalic viral titers |
| | Positive viral culture (first week of life) |
| | Serial measures of IgG |

thus prove helpful in determining the etiology of sensorineural hearing loss in children.

## Medical Evaluation Strategy

Health care cost containment and the medical-legal implications of missed or delayed diagnosis of sensorineural hearing loss in children are critical issues for the pediatric otolaryngologist. Chan (1994) proposes the following reasonable strategy for evaluating sensorineural hearing loss that takes these factors into consideration. After sensorineural hearing loss has been established by audiological testing, a detailed history should be obtained. Though high-risk criteria will generally be identified by the neonatologist prior to otolaryngology referral, appropriate evaluations

should be initiated if unidentified high-risk criteria are suspected. Though most syndromes have been identified prior to the otolaryngology referral, a comprehensive physical examination and consultation with a geneticist may identify syndromal hearing loss in some questionable cases.

After history taking, physical examination, and obtaining indicated diagnostic test results, some children will be left with sensorineural hearing loss of "undetermined etiology." Limited laboratory panels including a thyroid function test, urinalysis, and blood work to rule out syphilis (FTA-ABS) are frequently obtained. In cases of progressive, asymmetric, or fluctuating hearing loss, a temporal bone CT scan is indicated. Rapidly progressive hearing loss necessitates auto-immune sensorineural hearing loss evaluation including sedimentation rate, rheumatoid factor, antinuclear antibody titer, and inner ear autoanti-body assays when available. Patients with vestibular complaints should receive vestibular testing protocols (Chan, 1994) as discussed in Chapter 7.

## SUMMARY

This chapter has reviewed congenital and acquired etiologies of nongenetic sensorineural hearing loss in children. Audiologic assessment strategies have been overviewed, and medical evaluation of pediatric sensorineural hearing loss has been detailed. Extensive references have been provided for those students who desire additional information, and case reports have been included to demonstrate the practical application of current technology in the diagnosis and management of sensorineural hearing loss in children.

## REFERENCES

Alford, C. A., Stagno, S., Pass, R. F., and Britt, W. J. (1990). Congenital and perinatal cytomegalovirus infections. *Reviews of Infectious Diseases, 12,* S745.

Amenta, C. A. III, Dayal, V. S., Flaherty, J., and Weil, R. J. (1992). Luetic endolymphatic hydrops: Diagnosis and treatment. *American Journal of Otology, 13(6),* 516–524.

American-Speech-Language-Hearing Association. (1991). Guidelines for the audiologic assessment of children from birth through 36 months of age. *Asha, 33* (Suppl. 5), 37–43.

American Speech-Language-Hearing Association. (1994). Guidelines for the audiologic management of individuals receiving cochleotoxic drug therapy. *Asha, 36* (March, Suppl. 12): 11–19.

Barr, B. and Wedenberg, E. (1965). Perceptive hearing loss in children with respect to genesis and the use of hearing aid. *Acta Otolaryngology and Rhinology, 59,* 462–474.

Bergstrom, L. (1987). Medical diagnosis of prelinguistic hearing loss. In K. Gerkin and A. Amochaev (eds.), *Hearing in Infants: Proceedings from the National Symposium. Seminars in Hearing* 8:83–88.

Berman, R. F., Beare, D. J., Church, M. W., and Abel, E. L. (1992). Audiogenic seizure susceptibility and auditory brainstem responses in rats prenatally exposed to alcohol. *Alcoholism 10(3),* 400–408.

Brookhouser, P. E. and Auslander, M. C. (1989). Aided auditory thresholds in children with postmeningitic deafness. *Laryngoscope, 99,* 800–808.

Brookhouser, P. E., Worthington, D. W., and Kelly, W. J. (1992). Noise-induced hearing loss in children. *Laryngoscope, 102,* 645–655.

Brown, D. P., and Israel, S. M. (1991). Audiologic findings in a set of fraternal twins with CHARGE association. *Journal of the American Academy of Audiology, 2(3),* 103–108.

Brown, J. J., Brummett, R. E., Meikle, M. B., and Vernon, J. (1978). Combined effects of noise and neomycin: Cochlear changes in the guinea pig. *Acta Oto-Laryngologica, 86,* 394–400.

Brummett, R. E. (1980). Drug-induced ototoxicity. *Drugs, 19,* 412–428.

Brummett, R. E., Fox, K. E., Russell, N. J., and Davis, R. R. (1981). Interaction between aminoglycoside antibiotics and loop-inhibiting diuretics in the guinea pig. In S. A. Lerner, G. J. Matz, and J. E. Hawkins Jr. (eds.), *Aminoglycoside Ototoxicity.* Boston: Little, Brown and Company.

Brummett, R. E., Guitjens, S., Vestergaard, A., and Johnson, T. (1993). The ototoxicity of carboplatin as influenced by furosemide. In D. J. Lim (ed.), *Association for Research in Otolaryngology, Abstracts of the Sixteenth Midwinter Meeting,* St. Petersburg Beach, FL.

Byerly, K. A., and Pauli, R. M. (1993). Cranial nerve abnormalities in CHARGE association. *American Journal of Medical Genetics, 45(6),* 751–757.

Campbell, K. C. M. and Durrant, J. (1993). Audiologic monitoring for ototoxicity. *Otolaryngologic Clinics of North America, 26(5),* 903–914.

Cass, S. P. (1991). Role of medications in otological vertigo and balance disorders. *Seminars in Hearing, 12,* 257–269.

Centers for Disease Control. (1991). Guidelines for prophylaxis against *Pneumocystis carinii* pneumonia for children infected with human immunodeficiency syndrome. *Journal of the American Medical Association, 265,* 1637–1644.

Chan, K. H. (1994). Sensorineural hearing loss in children. *Otolaryngologic Clinics of North America, 27(3),* 473–486.

Chanock, S. J. and McIntosh, K. (1989). Pediatric infection with the human immunodeficiency virus: Issues for the otorhinolaryngologist. *Otolaryngologic Clinics of North America, 22(3),* 637–660.

Chow, J. H., Stern, J. C., Kaul, A., Pincus, R. L., and Gromisch, D. S. (1990). Head and neck manifestations of the acquired immunodeficiency syndrome in children. *Ear, Nose, and Throat Journal, 69,* 416–419, 422–423.

Church, M. W. and Gerkin, M. A. (1988). Hearing disorders in children with fetal alcohol syndrome: Findings from case reports. *Pediatrics, 82(2),* 147–154.

Church, M. W. and Overbeck, G. W. (1991). Sensorineural hearing loss as evidenced by the auditory brainstem response following cocaine exposure in the Long Evans rat. *Teratology, 43(6),* 561–570.

Cole, R. R. and Jahrsdoerfer, R. A. (1988). Sudden hearing loss: An update. *American Journal of Otology, 9(3),* 211–215.

Dahle, A. J. and McCollister, F. P. (1988). Audiological findings in children with neonatal herpes. *Ear and Hearing, 9(5),* 256–258.

Dalsgaard-Neilson, E. (1938). Correlations between syphilitic interstitial keratitis and deafness. *Acta Ophthalmologica, 16,* 635–647.

Davey, P. R. (1962). Hearing loss in children of low birthweight. *Journal of Laryngology and Otolaryngology, 76,* 274–277.

Dobrowski, J. M., Grundfast, K. M., and Rosenbaum, K. N. (1985). Otorhinolaryngologic manifestations of CHARGE association. *Otolaryngology—Head and Neck Surgery, 93,* 798.

Dodge, P. R., Davis, H., Feigin, R. D., Holmes, S. J., Kaplan, S. L., Jubelirer, D. P., Stechenberg, B. W., and Hirsh, S. K. (1984). Prospective evaluation of hearing impairment as a sequela of acute bacterial meningitis. *New England Journal of Medicine, 311*(14), 869–874.

Dunst, C., Trivette, C., and Deal, C. (1988). Help giver and family functioning. In *Enabling and Empowering Families.* Cambridge, MA: Bookline Books.

Education of the Handicapped Act Amendments of 1986, Public Law 99–457, 34 CFR Part 303, Part H. *Federal Register,* 54(119), 119, 26306–26348, June 22, 1989.

Eelkema, E. A. and Curtin, H. K. (1989). Congenital anomalies of the temporal bone. *Seminars in Ultrasound, CT, and MR* 10, 195.

Elidan, J., Lin, J., and Honrubia, V. (1986). The effect of loop diuretics on the vestibular system. *Archives of Otolaryngology—Head and Neck Surgery, 112,* 836–839.

Emmett, J. R. (1994). Simultaneous idiopathic sudden hearing loss in identical twins. *American Journal of Otology, 15(2),* 247–249.

Epstein, S. and Reilly, J. S. (1989). Sensorineural hearing loss. *Pediatric Clinics of North America, 36(6),* 1501–1519.

Eskola, J., Peltola, H., Takala, A., Kayhty, H., Hakulinen, M., Karanko, V., Kela, E., Rekola, P., Ronnberg, P., Samuelson, J., Gordon, L., and Makela, P. (1987). Efficacy of *Haemophilus influenzae* type b polysaccharide-diptheria toxoid conjugate vaccine in infancy. *New England Journal of Medicine, 317,* 717–722.

Fausti, S. A., Henry, J. A., Schaffer, H. I., Olson, D. J., Frey, R. H., and Bagby, G. C. (1993). High-frequency monitoring for early detection of cisplatin ototoxicity. *Archives of Otolaryngology—Head and Neck Surgery, 119,* 661–668.

Fisher, N. A. and Curtin, H. D. (1994). Radiology of congenital hearing loss. *Otolaryngologic Clinics of North America, 27(3),* 511–531.

Fiumara, N. J. and Lessell, S. (1970). Manifestations of late congenital syphilis. *Archives of Otolaryngology, 91,* 474–478.

Friedrich, B. W. (1985). The state of the art in audiologic evaluation and management. In E. Cherow, N. Matkin, and R. J. Trybus (eds.), *Hearing-impaired Children and Youth with Developmental Disabilities: An Interdisciplinary Foundation for Service.* Washington, DC: Gallaudet University Press.

Freij, B. J. and Sever, J. L. (1994). Chronic infections. In G. B. Avery, M. A. Fletcher, and M. G. McDonald (eds.), *Neonatology: Pathophysiology and Management of the Newborn* (4th ed.), Philadelphia: J. B. Lippincott Company.

Gerkin, K. P. (1984). The high risk register for deafness. *Asha, 26,* 17–23.

Gerkin, K. and Church, M. (1987). Fetal alcohol syndrome and hearing loss. In K. Gerkin and A. Amochaev (eds.), *Hearing in Infants: Proceedings from the National Symposium. Seminars in Hearing, 8,* 89–92.

Glarner, H., Meuli, M., Hof, E., Gallati, V., Nadal, D., Fisch, U., and Stauffer, U. G. 1994. Management of petrous bone fractures in children: Analysis of 127 cases. *Journal of Trauma, 36(2),* 198–201.

Goldson, E., Smith, A. C., and Stewart, J. M. (1986). The CHARGE association. *American Journal of Diseases in Childhood, 140,* 918.

Govaerts, P. J., Claes, J., Van De Heyning, P. H., Jorens, P. G., Marquet, J., and De Broe, M. E. (1990). Aminoglycoside-induced ototoxicity. *Toxicology Letters, 52,* 227–251.

Grandis, J. R., Hirsch, B. E., and Wagener, M. M. (1993). Treatment of idiopathic sudden sensorineural hearing loss. *American Journal of Otology, 14(2),* 183–185.

Guiscafre, H., Benitez-Diaz, L., Martinez, M. C. and Munoz, O. (1984). Reversible hearing loss after meningitis: Prospective assessment using auditory evoked responses. *Annals of Otology, Rhinology, and Laryngology, 93*(3, Part 1, 229–232.

Hall, J. W. III. (1992). *Handbook of Auditory Evoked Responses.* Needham Heights, MA: Allyn and Bacon.

Hall, J. W. III, Bratt, G. W., Schwaber, M. K., and Baer, J. E. (1993). Dynamic sensorineural hearing loss: Implications for audiologists: Case reports. *Journal of American Academy of Audiology,* 4, 399–411.

Hall, J. W. III, Prentice, C. H., Byrn, A. M., Smiley, G., and Davidson, L. H. (1995). Auditory findings in congenital cytomegalovirus (CMV): A case report. *Journal of the American Academy of Audiology* (in press).

Hart, C. W. and Naunton, R. F. (1964). Ototoxicity of chloroquine phosphate. *Archives of Otolaryngology,* 80, 407–412.

Harvey, S. A. and Millen, S. J. (1994). Absent round window reflex: Possible relation to step wise hearing loss. *American Journal of Otology, 15(2),* 237–242.

Hayes, D. and Pashley, N. R. T. (1991). Assessment of infants for hearing impairment. In J. T. Jacobson and J. L. Northern (eds.), *Diagnostic Audiology.* Austin: PRO-ED.

Henley, C. M. and Rybak, L. P. (1993). Developmental ototoxicity. *Otolaryngologic Clinics of North America, 26(5),* 857–871.

Hoffman, D. W., Whitworth, C. A., Jones, K. L., and Rybak, L. P. (1987). Nutritional status, glutathione levels, and ototoxicity of loop diuretics and aminoglycoside antibiotics. *Hearing Research, 31,* 217–222.

Hughes, G. B., Moscicki, R., Barna, B. P., and San Martin, J. E. (1994). Laboratory diagnosis of immune inner ear disease. *American Journal of Otology, 15(2),* 198–202.

Hutchinson, J. A. 1863. *A Clinical Memoir on Certain Diseases of the Eye and Ear Consequent on Inherited Syphilis.* London: Churchill.

Jackler, R. K., Luxford, W. M., and House, W. F. (1987). Congenital malformation of the inner ear: A classification based on embryogenesis. *Laryngoscope, 97* (3, Part 2), 2.

Jacobson, J. T. and Hall, J. W. III. (1994). Newborn and infant auditory brainstem response applications. In J. T. Jacobson (ed.), *Principles and Applications in Auditory Evoked Potentials.* Needham Heights, MA: Allyn and Bacon.

Jahn, A. F. and Ganti, K. (1987). Major auricular malformations due to Accutane (isoretinoin). *Laryngoscope, 97* (7 Part 1), 832–835.

Jerger, J. F. and Hayes, D. (1976). The cross-check principle in pediatric audiometry. *Archives of Otolaryngology, 102,* 614–620.

Joint Committee on Infant Hearing. (1991). 1990 Position Statement. *Audiology Today, 3(4),* 14–17.

Joint Committee on Infant Hearing. (1994). 1994 Position Statement. *Audiology Today, 6(6),* 6–9.

Kaplan, L. C. (1985). Choanal atresia and its associated anomalies—further support for the CHARGE association. *International Journal of Pediatric Otorhinology, 8,* 237.

Kaplan, L. C. (1989). The CHARGE association: Choanal atresia and multiple congenital anomalies. *Otolaryngologic Clinics of North America, 22(3),* 661–672.

Karmody, D. S. and Schuknecht, H. F. (1966). Deafness in congenital syphilis. *Archives of Otolaryngology, 83,* 18–27.

Kohan, D., Rothstein, S. G., and Cohen, N. L. (1988). Otologic disease in patients with AIDS. *Annals of Otology, Rhinology, and Laryngology, 97,* 636–640.

Konkle, D. F. and Knightly, C. A. (1993). Delayed-onset hearing loss in respiratory distress syndrome: Case reports. *Journal of American Academy of Audiology, 4,* 351–354.

Lenz, W. and Knapp, K. (1962). Die Thalidomed Embryopathie. *Dtsch Med Ulschr Schweiz Med Wochenschr, 87,* 1232–1242.

Lindberg, J., Rosenhall, U., Nylen, O., and Ringner, A. (1977). Long-term outcome of *Haemophilus influenzae* meningitis related to antibiotic treatment. *Pediatrics, 60,* 1–6.

Marron, M. J., Crisafi, M. A., Driscoll, J. M. Jr., Wung, J. T., Driscoll, Y. T., Fay, T. H., and James, L. S.

(1992). Hearing neurodevelopmental outcome in survivors of persistent pulmonary hypertension of the newborn. *Pediatrics, 90(3),* 392–396.

Matkin, N. D. (1988). Re-evaluating our approach to evaluation: Demographics are changing—are we? In F. H. Bess (ed.), *Hearing Impairment in Children.* Parkton, MD: York Press.

Mattox, D. E. and Simmons, F. B. (1977). Natural history of sudden sensorineural hearing loss. *Annals of Otology, Rhinology, and Laryngology, 86,* 463–480.

Matz, G. J. (1976). The ototoxic effects of ethacrynic acid in man and animals. *Laryngoscope, 86,* 1065–1086.

Matz, G. J. (1993). Aminoglycoside cochlear ototoxicity. *Otolaryngologic Clinics of North America, 26(5),* 705–712.

MaWhinney, S., Pagano, M., and Thomas, P. (1993). Age at AIDS diagnosis for children with perinatally acquired HIV. *Journal of Acquired Immune Deficiency Syndromes, 6,* 1139–1144.

McCabe, B. F. (1989). Perilymph fistula: The Iowa experience to date. *American Journal of Otology* 10, 262.

McCleod, R., Wisner, J., and Boyer, K. (1992). Toxoplasmosis. In S. Krugman, S. Katz, A. Gershon, and C. Wilfert (eds.), *Infectious Diseases of Children.* St. Louis: Mosby.

McCormick, B., Gibbin, L. P., Lutman, M. E., and O'Donoghue, G. M. (1993). Late partial recovery from meningitic deafness after cochlear implantation: A case study. *American Journal of Otology, 14(6),* 610–612.

McCracken, G. H. (1986). Aminoglycoside toxicity in infants and children. *American Journal of Medicine, 80* (Suppl. 68), 172–178.

McFadden, D. and Plattsmier, H. S. (1983). Aspirin can potentiate the temporary hearing loss induced by intense sounds. *Hearing Research, 9,* 295.

McGee, T., Walters, C., Stein, L., Kraus, N., Johnson, D., Boyer, K., Mats, M., Roizen, N., Beckman, J., and Meier, P. (1992). Absence of sensorineural hearing loss in treated infants and children with congenital toxoplasmosis. *Otolaryngology—Head and Neck Surgery, 108(1),* 75–80.

Meyerhoff, W. L., Cass, S., Schwaber, M. K., Sculerati, N., and Slattery, W. H. III. (1994.) Progressive sensorineural hearing loss in children. *Otolaryngology—Head and Neck Surgery, 110(6),* 560–570.

Meyerhoff, W. L., Malle, G. E., Yellin, W., and Roland, P. (1989). Audiologic threshold monitoring of patients receiving ototoxic drugs. *Annals of Otology, Rhinology, and Laryngology, 98,* 950–954.

Miller, J. J. (1985). *Handbook of Ototoxicity.* Boca Raton: CRC Press.

Morrison, A. W. (1975). *Management of Sensorineural Deafness.* Boston: Butterworths.

Murphy, T., White, K., and Pastor, P. (1993). Declining incidence of *Haemophilus influenzae* type b disease since introduction of vaccination. *Journal of American Medical Association, 269,* 246–248.

Nahmias, J. J. and Visintine, A. M. (1976). Herpes simplex. In J. S. Remington and J. O. Klein (eds.), *Infectious Diseases of the Fetus and Newborn Infant.* Philadelphia: WB Saunders Company.

Newton, V. E. and Rouson, V. J. (1988). Progressive sensorineural hearing loss in childhood. *British Journal of Audiology, 22(4),* 287–295.

Northern, J. L. and Downs, M. P. (1991). *Hearing in Children* (4th ed.), Baltimore: Williams & Wilkins.

Odio, C., Faingezicht, I., and Paris, M. (1991). The beneficial effects of early Dexamethasone administration in infants and children with bacterial meningitis. *New England Journal of Medicine, 324,* 1525–1531.

Oley, C. A., Baraitser, M., and Grant, D. B. (1988). A reappraisal of the CHARGE association. *Journal of Medical Genetics, 25,* 147.

Ozdamar, O., Kraus, N., and Stein, L. (1983). Auditory brainstem responses in infants recovering from bacterial meningitis. *Archives of Otolaryngology, 322,* 141–147.

Pagon, R. A., Graham, J. M., and Zonana, V. (1981). Coloboma, congenital heart disease, and choanal atresia with multiple anomalies: CHARGE association. *Journal of Pediatrics, 99,* 223.

Paparella, M. M., Fox, R. Y., and Schachern, P. A. (1989). Diagnosis and treatment of sensorineural hearing loss in children. *Otolaryngologic Clinics of North America, 22(1),* 51–74.

Pappas, D. G. (1985). *Diagnosis and Treatment of Hearing Impairment in Children: A Clinical Manual.* San Diego: College-Hill Press.

Pappas, D. G. Jr., Sekhar, H. K. C., Lim, J., and Hillman, D. E. (1994). Ultrastructural findings in the cochlea of AIDS cases. *American Journal of Otology, 15(4),* 456–465.

Principi, N., Marchisio, P., Tornaghi, R., Onorato, J., Massironi, E., and Picco, P. (1991). Acute otitis media in human immunodeficiency virus-infected children. *Pediatrics, 88,* 566–571.

Rarey, K. E. (1990). Otologic pathophysiology in patients with human immunodeficiency virus. *American Journal of Otolaryngology, 11,* 366–369.

Rederspil, P. (1981). Pharmacokinetics of aminoglycoside antibiotics in the perilymph. In S. A. Lerner, G. J. Matz and J. E. Hawkins (eds.), *Aminoglycoside Ototoxicity.* Boston: Little, Brown and Company.

Remington, J. and Desmonds, G. (1990). Toxoplasmosis. In J. Remington and J. Klein (eds.), *Infectious Diseases of the Fetus and Newborn, Third Edition.* Philadelphia: WB Saunders Co.

Robbins, S. L., Aotran, R. S., and Kumar, V. (1984). *Pathologic Bases of Disease.* Philadelphia: W. B. Saunders Company.

Rosenhall, U. and Kankkunen, A. (1980). Hearing alterations following meningitis: hearing improvement. *Ear and Hearing, 1,* 185–190.

Rosenhall, U. and Kankkunen, A. (1981). Hearing alterations following meningitis, II—variable hearing. *Ear and Hearing, 2,* 170–176.

Ruben, R. J. (1983). Diseases of the inner ear and sensorineural deafness. In C. D. Bluestone and S. E. Stool (eds.), *Pediatric Otolaryngology.* Philadelphia: W. B. Saunders Company.

Ruth, R. A. and Lambert, P. R. (1991). Evaluation and diagnosis of cochlear disorders. In J. T. Jacobson and J. L. Northern (eds.), *Diagnostic Audiology.* Austin: PRO-ED.

Schell, M. J., McHaney, V. A., Green, A. A., Kun, L. E., Hayes, A. F., Horowitz, M., and Meyer, W. H. (1989). Hearing loss in children and young adults receiving cisplatin with or without prior cranial irradiation. *Journal of Clinical Oncology, 7,* 754–760.

Schildroth, A. N. (1994). Congenital cytomegalovirus and deafness. *American Journal of Audiology, 3(2),* 27–38.

Schlech, W., Ward, J., Band, J., Hightower, A., Fraser, D., and Broome, C. (1985). Bacterial meningitis in the United States, 1978 through 1981. *Journal of the American Medical Association, 253,* 1749–1754.

Schumacher, R. E., Spak, C., and Kileny, P. R. (1990). Asymmetric brain stem auditory evoked responses in infants treated with extracorporeal membrane oxygenation. *Ear and Hearing, 11(5),* 359–362.

Scott, G. B. (1992). Pediatric HIV-1 infection: A clinical overview. *Pediatric Dermatology 9,* 323–325.

Sell, S., Merrill, R., Doyne, E., and Zimsky, E. (1972). Long-term sequelae of *Haemophilus influenzae* meningitis. *Pediatrics, 49,* 206–211.

Shaffer, K. A. and Haughton, V. M. (1980). Thin section computed tomography of the temporal bone. *Laryngoscope, 90,* 1099–1105.

Sharma, R. P. and Edwards, I. R. (1983). Cis-platinum: Subcellular distribution and binding to cytosolic ligands. *Biochemical Pharmacology, 32,* 2665–2669.

Sheraton, M. D. (1964). Final report of a prospective study of children whose mothers had rubella in early pregnancy. *British Medical Journal, 2,* 536–539.

Silman, S. and Silverman, C. A. (1991). *Auditory Diagnosis: Principles and Applications.* San Diego: Academic Press.

Smith, D. W. (1982). *Recognizable Patterns of Human Malformation* (3rd ed.), Philadelphia: W. B. Saunders Company.

Stagno, S. (1990). Cytomegalovirus. In J. S. Remington and J. O. Klein (eds.), *Infectious Diseases of the Fetus and Newborn Infant* (3rd ed.), Philadelphia: W. B. Saunders.

Stagno, S., Pass, R., and Alford, C. (1981). Perinatal infections and maldevelopment. *Birth Defects, 17,* 31–50.

Stein, L. K. and Boyer, K. M. (1994). Progress in the prevention of hearing loss in infants. *Ear and Hearing, 15(2),* 116–125.

Thelin, J. W., Mitchell, J. A., Heffner, M. A., and Davenport S. L. H. (1986). CHARGE syndrome. *International Journal of Pediatric Otolaryngology, 12,* 145–163.

Trybus, R., Karchmer, M. A., and Kerstetter, P. P. (1980). The demographics of deafness resulting from maternal rubella. *American Annals of the Deaf, 125,* 977–984.

Wake, M., Takeno, S., Ibrahim, D., Harrison, R. V., and Mount, R. J. (1993). Carboplatin ototoxicity: An animal model. In D. J. Lim (ed.), *Association for Research in Otolaryngology, Abstracts of the Sixteenth Midwinter Meeting,* St. Petersburg Beach, FL.

Walton, J. P. and Hendricks-Munoz, K. (1991). Profile and stability of sensorineural hearing loss in persistent pulmonary hypertension of the newborn. *Jour-*

nal of Speech and Hearing Research, 34, 1362–1370.

Ward, D. H. (1969). The histopathology of auditory and vestibular disorders in head trauma. *Annals of Otology, Rhinology, and Laryngology, 78,* 227–238.

Wells, T. G. (1990). The pharmacology and therapeutics of diuretics in the pediatric patient. *Pediatric Clinics of North America, 37,* 463–504.

Westerman, S. T., Gilbert, L. M., and Schondel, L. (1994). Vestibular dysfunction in a child with embryonic exposure to Accutane. *American Journal of Otology, 15(3),* 400–403.

Whitley, R. J. and Alford, C. A. (1981). Preventive and therapeutic approaches to the newborn infant with perinatal viral and toxoplasma infections. *Clinical Perinatology* 8, 591–603.

Williams, M. A. (1987). Head and neck findings in pediatric acquired immune deficiency syndrome. *Laryngoscope, 97,* 713–716.

Williamson, W. D., Demmler, G. J., Percy, A. K., and Catlin, F. I. (1992). Cytomegalovirus: Progressive hearing loss in infants with asymptomatic congenital cytomegalovirus infection. *Pediatrics, 90(6),* 862–866.

Wilson, W. (1986). The relationship of the herpes virus family to sudden hearing loss: A prospective clinical study and literature review. *Laryngoscope, 96,* 870–877.

Wofford, M. (1981). Audiological evaluation and management of hearing disorders. In F. N. Martin (ed.), *Medical Audiology: Disorders of Hearing.* Englewood Cliffs, NJ: Prentice-Hall.

Zenker, P. N. and Rolfs, R. T. (1989). Treatment of syphilis. *Rev Infect Dis, 12*(Suppl. 6), S590–S609.

Zoller, M., Wilson, W. R., Nadol, J. B., Jr., and Girard, K. F. (1978). Detection of syphilitic hearing loss. *Archives of Otolaryngology, 104(2),* 63–65.

# PART TWO

# IDENTIFICATION AND EVALUATION

# CHAPTER 5

# PEDIATRIC HEARING SCREENING

*ROBERT J. NOZZA*

## INTRODUCTION

For the child with hearing loss, who must acquire language and who must perform in the auditory–verbal environment of school, early identification and intervention are critical. It is clear that early identification and intervention will minimize disability and will increase the likelihood that a child with a hearing impairment will achieve academically regardless of the academic path chosen. The early identification, diagnosis, and habilitation of sensory disabilities is a national priority. Federal legislation and other federal documents related to people with disabilities attest to the growing national interest in providing every opportunity to people with disabilities to develop into productive members of society. For example, recent legislation has seen the enactment of Public Law 99-457 Amendment to the Education for All Handicapped Children Act and Pulic Law 101-476 Individuals with Disabilities Education Act, or IDEA, both reauthorizations and amendments to Public Law 94-142, Education of Handicapped Children Act. Also, The Americans with Disabilities Act and Healthy People 2000: National Health Promotion and Disease Objectives became rallying points for those with disabilities as well as for those involved in identification, assessment, and management of those with disabilities.

Estimates of the incidence of significant bilateral hearing impairment vary depending on a variety of factors. Obtaining an accurate estimate of incidence and prevalence is difficult because of differences among investigations in how hearing impairment is defined, in the population that is sampled, in the test methods that are used, and in the way data are analyzed (Davidson, Hyde, and Alberti, 1989). For example, one study might consider mild and unilateral hearing loss in the hearing-impaired group, while another might count only those with bilateral hearing losses of more than a mild degree. Otitis media with effusion is a major cause of mild conductive hearing loss in children, but may or may not be counted because it is usually transient in nature. Davidson and colleagues (1989) and Mauk and Behrens (1993), in reviewing epidemiological studies of hearing impairment, show that typical prevalence figures in childhood are between 1/1000 and 2.5/1000, depending on age and definition of impairment. Clearly, there are sufficient numbers of children with auditory dysfunction that can affect the normal process of language acquisition and educational achievement to warrant early identification and remediation.

One concern regarding hearing loss in children is that, in many cases, identification occurs only after symptoms appear and long-term consequences of the hearing loss have already occurred. Symptoms are more apparent with profound hearing impairment, and identification may come from observations of parents or relatives. However, profound hearing loss accounts for only about 10 percent of hearing impairments. Most children with hearing impairment have some hearing and, as a result, often show some response to sound, albeit inconsistent, which serves to delay identification. The infant born with a hearing loss and not screened at birth will often go undiagnosed for many months or years. Infants and children with late-onset hearing impairment may be even more difficult to identify. The solution to such a situation is to have audiologic screening for children of all ages, from birth through school age, so that children with hearing impairment can be identified as early as possible.

Audiologists working in medical centers, speech and hearing centers, schools and other settings may at one time or another be asked to organize and/or direct a hearing screening program. To have a successful screening program, the audiologist must work together with administrators, other professionals, and those who will be targeted for the screening. To be effective, the audiologist must be knowledgeable about the principles of screening, about selection and measurement of screening tests, about the effects of the choice of the test criterion, and about the effects of population characteristics on test performance. The objective of this chapter is to provide information on the basic concepts and principles of screening as they pertain to early identification of audiologic disorders at all stages of childhood.

## HEARING SCREENING GUIDELINES

There are many guidelines, reports, and articles available to audiologists charged with the development or direction of a screening program. The American Academy of Audiology (AAA) and the American Speech-Language-Hearing Association (ASHA), two of several professional organizations for audiologists, have provided information on audiologic screening in the form of position statements, guidelines, and reports. Both associations are strongly committed to the prevention and early identification of audiologic disorders in people of all ages. For example, the ASHA Position Statement on Prevention of Communication Disorders (1988) states that "...audiologists should...play a significant role in the development and application of prevention strategies." Prevention, according to the position statement, includes not only "the elimination or inhibition of the onset and development of a communication disorder" (primary prevention), but also "the early detection and treatment of communication disorders" (secondary prevention). In that regard, the position statement goes on to state that audiologists and speech-language pathologists should "demonstrate the ability to...provide early identification and early intervention services for com-

munication disorders occurring at any time during the life span."

ASHA has produced several guidelines for audiologic screening of children, three of which are currently active. They include guidelines for screening high-risk newborns for hearing impairment (ASHA, 1989) and screening for hearing impairment and middle ear disorders in individuals from 3 to 40 years of age (ASHA, 1985, 1990). Of course, there are other documents that are relevant to screening hearing in the pediatric population, including Guidelines for Audiologic Assessment of Children from Birth Through 36 Months of Age (ASHA, 1991); Guidelines for Audiology Services in the Schools (ASHA, 1993); and Report on Audiologic Screening (ASHA, 1993). In addition, AAA has formed a task force to develop a position statement and guidelines related to screening for middle ear disease. The Joint Committee on Infant Hearing (JCIH), comprised of representatives from ASHA, AAA, and other interested associations has published position statements on infant hearing (JCIH, 1982, 1991, 1994). The ASHA (1993) Report on Audiologic Screening, which summarizes all of the ASHA guidelines for audiologic screening, identifies areas that need further study and makes suggestions for future development of guidelines.

Other resources are available as well. A collection of works regarding screening, based on an international symposium, was published by Bess and Hall (1992) and there was an issue of *Seminars in Hearing* (White and Behrens, 1993) devoted to one newborn screening program, the Rhode Island Hearing Assessment Project (RIHAP). In 1993, the National Institutes of Health sponsored a Consensus Conference on early identification of hearing impairment in infants and young children and published a consensus statement based on the conference (NIH, 1993).

## BASICS OF SCREENING

Screening is not the same as diagnosis. Screening is done to separate those who are at greatest risk of a target disease or condition from the general population. Diagnostic tests are those that are generally accepted by professionals to be the best determinants of the presence of a particular disease or condition. In general, the more similar the screening test is to the test used for diagnosis, the greater will be its validity. For example, a pure-tone hearing *screening* is very much like the pure-tone hearing *threshold test* that is done to *diagnose* hearing impairment, and so has a great deal of validity. On the other hand, screening can be done in ways that do not resemble the test that is used for diagnosis. For example, a questionnaire on communication difficulties might be used to screen for hearing impairment, but is not similar to pure-tone threshold audiometry and as such may have poorer validity than the pure-tone screening for identification of impairment.

## Principles of Screening

There are several principles of screening that apply to screening for any disease. It is important to understand that audiologic screening is not an exception and that the wisdom represented in these principles has been acquired over many years of study of identification and diagnosis of many diseases and disorders. It is important to understand and appreciate these basic principles before embarking on screening activities at any level. Different authors discuss these principles in slightly different ways. Some of the primary sources used in developing this summary of principles, which may be consulted for additional information, include articles by Cadman, Chambers, Feldman, and Sackett (1984); Feightner (1992); Frankenburg (1974); Griner, Mayewski, Mushlin, and Greenland (1981); and Thorner and Remein (1982).

### Purposes of Screening

The purposes of screening are to separate from among apparently healthy individuals those for whom there is a greater probability of having hearing impairment and then to refer them for appropriate diagnostic testing. That is, those screened are separated into a "pass" group and a "refer" group.

### Importance of the Disease or Disorder

Each disease or disorder has a cost to society; the greater the burden to society, the greater the reason to screen for the disease. Hearing impairment is associated with a fairly high morbidity, such as lost function or lost opportunities, that has personal, societal, and/or financial costs.

### Diagnostic Criteria

For a screening program to be successful, there must be a clear and measurable definition of what one is attempting to identify through screening. There must be a test that is accepted as a standard for diagnosis (e.g., such as the pure-tone threshold test or audiogram).

### Treatment

Before a screening program is implemented, it is necessary to demonstrate that treatments are available, effective, and shown to alter the natural history of the disorders. Intervention in the pre-symptomatic stage should result in a better outcome than intervention after symptoms appear, such as delayed speech and language development in the case of hearing impairment.

### The Program Must Reach
### Those Who May Benefit

It is important that screening programs be administered so that those who would probably benefit from early identification are easily included. Mechanisms for outreach to the targeted population should be in place. Education and public policy can influence how well screening programs succeed in reaching those they should reach.

### Availability of Resources and Compliance
### of Those Identified

Diagnostic and treatment resources appropriate for the population being served must be available before a screening program can be managed successfully. Following identification, those identified must comply with follow-up components of the screening program.

## Appropriateness of the Test

In general, a screening test that is easy to administer, comfortable for the patient, short in duration, and inexpensive will be well received by those being screened and by those responsible for its administration. The test must also meet performance criteria. It must be sensitive, specific, precise, and accurate. There must be an acceptably low over-referral rate so to minimize the number of those without the disorder who are referred.

## Screening Program Evaluation

Screening programs can and must be evaluated. Protocols should be based on data that demonstrate that individuals identified through screening have better outcomes than those not screened. Program costs can be estimated (Turner, 1991, 1992a, 1992b; Turner and Cone-Wesson, 1992). There are direct monetary costs of screening that can be computed. There are also costs associated with the level of risk involved in the screening test itself. There is a cost to the patient and family that is associated with assigning a label (such as "deaf" or "hearing impaired") to an individual. There are costs associated with false positives and the false negatives of a screening program.

## Importance of Screening within a Program

Screening for hearing impairment, or any disease, cannot be accomplished with a single test used in isolation. A screening test is used within a program that adheres to the principles of screening. Screening performance is dependent not only on the performance of the test, but on many other factors, some of which were mentioned in the previous section.

For example, the definition of the disease or disorder to be identified by the screening can affect the performance of the screening test as well as the screening program. In some cases, there are differences of opinion over what is to be screened or what criteria must be met for a positive finding. Treatment availability as well as population characteristics also may affect the program. Of course, the test criterion that is used for discriminating

among those with the disorder and those without the disorder must be established. For example, how hearing impairment is defined will affect the selection of the test and will have an effect on the outcome of the program. What frequencies should be screened? What hearing level is chosen for screening? Is the screening only for bilateral hearing impairment or is it to identify unilateral losses as well? What test should be used? Such questions are not always answered in the same way by screening program administrators because they must be answered in the context of a number of other factors related to specific circumstances and according to the accepted principles of screening.

## Deciding on Test Criteria

Choosing a test for screening depends, in part, on the test's performance in separating those with from those without the target condition. Whatever test is chosen for evaluation in the context of screening, some value, the test criterion, must be chosen. A test criterion is needed because most screening tests are imperfect. Tests usually produce scores over a range along a continuum (e.g., hearing thresholds vary along the dB hearing level scale, peak compensated admittance varies along the millimho scale, tympanometric width (TW) varies along the dekapascal scale, etc.) and often there is a region of possible scores for which a proportion of those with the disorder overlap with a proportion of those without the disorder (Griner et al., 1981). That is, rarely is a screening test able to identify correctly all of those with the target condition (e.g., hearing impairment or middle ear disease) and all of those without the target condition.

It is not possible to understand screening without understanding how performance of a screening test is estimated and how the different variables involved interact. The concepts of overlapping distributions and their relationship to sensitivity and specificity, prevalence, predictive values and over referral and under referral must be understood if a screening program is to succeed.

## Sensitivity and Specificity

Sensitivity and specificity of a test relate to the ability of the test to identify correctly both those with the disorder (sensitivity) and those without the disorder (specificity). Sensitivity is the ratio of the number with the disorder who are positive on the screening test (numerator) to the number of all those with the disorder (denominator). In other words, sensitivity represents the percentage labeled "positive" on the screening test of all those who truly have the target condition. Specificity is the ratio of the number of those without the disorder who are negative on the screening test (numerator) to the number of all those without the disorder (denominator). In other words, specificity is the percentage labeled "negative" on the screening test of all those who truly are free of the target condition. To determine sensitivity and specificity, controlled clinical trials must be done, in which the screening test is followed by a diagnostic test for verification of the patient's true status.

Figure 5.1 is an illustration of overlapping distributions. The data are from a study of tympanometry in ears with and without middle ear effusion (MEE) in a group of children undergoing surgery for placement of tympanotomy tubes (Nozza, Bluestone, Kardatzke, and Bachman, 1994). The diagnoses of MEE were made by surgeons. The tympanometric variable used in the example is TW (tympanogram width), which is the width of the tympanogram at one-half the peak admittance (Koebsell and Margolis, 1986). It is a simple means of quantifying the slope, or gradient, of the tympanogram. The distributions show the percentage of ears with each TW value for each group. Notice that the distribution of TW values for ears with no MEE overlaps with the distribution of ears with MEE. This is typical of distributions of many conditions for many test variables that might be used for identification. In screening, a single point along the continuum would be chosen as the criterion to separate positive from negative findings. For example, the vertical dotted line at TW 200 daPa is a possible criterion, with TW > 200 being a positive (refer)

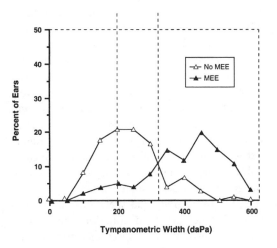

**FIGURE 5.1** Distributions of tympanometric width (TW) for ears without and for ears with middle ear effusion (MEE) from children undergoing surgery for placement of tympanotomy tubes. The data exemplify how distributions for those with a disease and those without the disease will overlap along a test continuum. The vertical lines at TW = 200 and TW = 325 represent two of many possible test cutoffs for use as criteria for diagnosis or screening. In the example, the percent of ears from each distribution to the right of the chosen criterion are those declared positive for MEE and the percent of ears from each distribution to the left of the chosen criterion are those declared negative. With the cutoff TW > 200, most of those with MEE are to the right of the cutoff, but a large proportion of those without MEE are also to the right. That is, sensitivity is high (89 percent), but specificity is low (47 percent). However, if we use a cutoff TW > 325, sensitivity and specificity (70 percent and 88 percent, respectively) change markedly. Data taken from Nozza, R. J., Bluestone, C. D., Kardatzke, D., and Bachman, R. N. (1994). Identification of middle ear effusion by aural acoustic admittance and otoscopy. *Ear and Hearing* 15:310–323.

test and TW ≤ 200 a negative (pass) test. If all ears with TW greater than 200 daPa were positive, then sensitivity would be 89 percent, which is determined by totaling the percentage of ears from the MEE distribution with TW greater than 200 daPa. From the distribution of ears with no MEE, the total percent of ears less than or equal to the TW cutoff value of 200 daPa, 47 percent, represents the specificity.

By moving the cutoff to the right to a TW of 325 daPa, the sensitivity and specificity values change to 70 percent and 88 percent, respectively. Notice that sensitivity and specificity change with a change in the cutoff value such that as one increases, the other decreases. More importantly, because of the overlapping distributions, no cutoff value can be chosen that will separate completely the group with MEE from the group with no MEE (i.e., yield sensitivity and specificity of 100 percent). By knowing the distributions, one can determine sensitivity and specificity for different cutoffs so that an informed choice of the test criterion can be made.

The overlapping distributions, and the resulting sensitivity and specificity, also provide other information. In the tympanometry example, because all those with middle ear disease are not correctly identified, some must be incorrectly identified. That is, some individuals without middle ear disease would be referred for either a retest or for diagnosis and follow-up (i.e., false positive identifications) and some individuals with middle ear disease would not be referred (i.e., false negative identifications). The false positive rate $(1 -$ specificity) and the false negative rate $(1 -$ sensitivity) depend on the degree of overlap of the two distributions on the continuum of test scores as well as on the specific test criterion (i.e., cutoff) that is used. For example, referring again to Figure 5.1, with a cutoff of TW > 200 daPa yielding 89 percent sensitivity, 11 percent (100 percent − 89 percent) of the ears *with* MEE will be to the left of the cutoff and not referred. Likewise, with 47 percent specificity, 53 percent of the ears with no MEE will be to the right of the cutoff and referred.

## Predictive Values

The test performance (sensitivity and specificity) together with the percentage of the population with the disorder (disorder prevalence), determine predictive values and the rates of over and under referral for diagnosis. Positive and negative predictive values are ratios also. Positive predictive value (PPV) is the ratio of the number of those scoring positive on the test who truly have the disorder (numerator) to the number of all those who scored positive on the test (denominator). Negative predictive value (NPV) is the ratio of the number of those scoring negative who truly do not have the disorder (numerator) to the number of all those scoring negative on the test (denominator). They are functions of sensitivity and specificity as well as of the proportion of those tested who truly have the disorder, otherwise known as the prevalence. The test administrator must know the probabilities that an individual will (or will not) have the condition given a positive (or negative) test outcome. Predictive ability is the information the practitioner needs because in the screening situation, it is the test outcome that is known rather than the true state of the individual such as must be known to determine sensitivity and specificity of the test.

Predictive values determine overreferral and underreferral rates. The overreferral rate is the proportion of those referred who do not have the disorder $(1 - \text{PPV})$ and the underreferral rate is the proportion of those not referred who do have the disorder $(1 - \text{NPV})$. An unacceptably high overreferral rate can cause dissatisfaction among those being screened as well as to those whom the referrals are sent, thereby reducing the effectiveness of the program. A high underreferral rate, whereby those with hearing impairment or middle ear disease are not identified, is also problematic and often results in delayed diagnosis and related consequences.

Figure 5.2 is an illustration of the difference in predictive ability and the over- and underreferral rates when prevalence of a target condition increases. The two-by-two matrix is a useful way to illustrate the outcomes of a test. The abscissa is for the true status of the disorder, present or absent, and the ordinate is for the test outcome, positive or negative. The combination results in four

**PREVALENCE = 1%**

**Disorder**

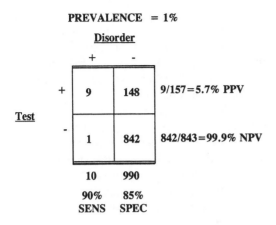

**PREVALENCE = 10%**

**Disorder**

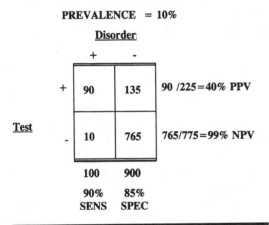

**FIGURE 5.2** Two-by-two matrices of hypothetical data illustrating the effects of disease prevalence on test performance. In both cases, the test has sensitivity (SENS) of 90 percent and specificity (SPEC) of 85 percent. However, positive predictive value (PPV) changes considerably with increase in prevalence of the disease. NPV = negative predictive value.

possible outcomes; the individual can have the disorder (first column) or not have the disorder (second column), and the test can be positive (first row) or negative (second row). For a given test cutoff (which determines sensitivity and specifici-

ty) and the prevalence of disease, we can determine predictive values and over- and underreferral rates easily from the matrix.

With sensitivity and specificity constant, the example shows that for 1000 screening tests done in the low (1 percent) prevalence group, there would be 148 false identifications (overreferred) while obtaining 9 correct identifications out of 10 with the targeted condition. In a group with a prevalence of 10 percent, 1000 screening tests would yield fewer false identifications (135) while obtaining 90 correct identifications out of 100 with the targeted condition. In the former case, the overreferral rate (1-PPV) is over 94 percent while for the latter case the over referral rate is only 60 percent. In screening for conditions with low prevalence, which is common, even a test with high sensitivity and specificity still produces a large number of over referrals. Underreferral rates (1-NPV) are .1 percent and 1 percent for the low and the high prevalence rates, respectively, in the example.

One mechanism for avoiding the problem of a high overreferral rate is to increase the prevalence of disorder in the population screened. This is done by identifying a subgroup within the population that is at greater risk for having the target condition than the larger general population. For example, use of a high-risk register for selecting newborns for hearing screening, or screening for middle ear disease only in preschool or young elementary grades, are practices based on the knowledge that risk is greater in those subpopulations than in the whole population. Identification of a high-risk group can reduce an otherwise unmanageable over referral rate to manageable proportions. Of course, there is a cost to such a maneuver. By selecting a high-risk subgroup for screening, those in the unscreened group who truly have the condition will be missed.

## AUDIOLOGIC SCREENING

Audiologic screening can cover different domains (e.g., impairment, hearing disability, middle ear disorders, central auditory processing disorders, etc.) over a wide range of ages. Even within the category covered by pediatric audiologists, there are many different things that one can screen for and different age groups that may be involved. The importance of screening for a given disorder may vary with age, and the ability to use and interpret certain screening test measures may be age dependent.

## Newborn Hearing Screening

Early identification of hearing impairment in the newborn child has been of interest to professionals in audiology, pediatrics, and otolaryngology for many years. In 1982, the Joint Committee on Infant Hearing (JCIH) recommended that screening for hearing impairment in newborns be done by identifying those at greatest risk and then performing an auditory screening test on them. Subsequently, an updated position statement (JCIH, 1991) expanded the criteria used to identify at-risk infants and recommended that auditory brain stem response (ABR) screening be used with them. Although screening can be done using behavioral observation techniques, high false positive rates associated with such techniques make them less desirable than objective measures for newborns. Even prior to the 1991 JCIH position statement, most newborn hearing screening programs were focusing on the ABR in favor of tests such as behavioral observation of reflexive responses, the Crib-o-gram (Simmons and Russ, 1974) and the auditory response cradle (Bennett, 1979). The ASHA (1989) guidelines for the audiologic screening of newborn infants who are at risk for hearing impairment suggested use of the high-risk criteria provided in the 1982 JCIH position statement. The ASHA guidelines have not been updated to reflect updated criteria (JCIH, 1991; 1994), but most programs use the current high-risk indicators, or some similar set of criteria, for selecting newborns for ABR screening. The updated high-risk indicators published in the JCIH 1994 Position Statement are provided in Table 5.1.

Newborn hearing screening programs that use the ABR vary in the application of the test

(Hall, 1992). Some programs use a diagnostic ABR test system and test infants who meet high-risk criteria. The ASHA guidelines recommend that a repeatable ABR to a click stimulus at a level no higher than 40 dB nHL be used as a screening criterion. Many programs use 35 dB nHL, a more strict criterion. Some programs also will test using a higher level (60 to 70 dB nHL) to provide information that helps the interpretation of poor or delayed responses at the lower level and to provide information about the integrity of the neural transmission through the brain stem. The test has been shown to have high sensitivity and specificity with the high-risk population. In such programs, a skilled and experienced audiologist typically reads the ABR and makes the decision on disposition (pass or refer) of the newborns. In some cases, if the infant does not meet criteria for passing the screening, a search for threshold will be done at that time. This is an advantage of using a diagnostic ABR system for screening; further testing can be done while the infant is prepared, thereby eliminating the need for a second ABR, at a later time, that is designed to estimate peripheral sensitivity (Galambos, Wilson, and Silva, 1994).

Alternatives to the use of a diagnostic ABR test system are automated ABR systems such as the Natus (i.e., the ALGO-II) by Natus Medical and the Smart Screener by Intelligent Hearing Systems (IHS). The Natus is a closed screening system in the sense that the operator has little flexibility in the application of the test. Once electrodes and the earphone (which is encased in a disposable, adhesive pad for placement over the infant's ear) are in place, the instrument is started and runs independent of operator control. The system will provide click stimuli and collect ABR data for as long as necessary (up to 15,000 sweeps) to detect with a certain degree of confidence that an ABR is present. In the standard application of the Natus screener, the ABR waveform is not readily available to the operator, although it can be obtained. The instrument has a sophisticated built-in algorithm that constantly analyzes the response until criteria for accepting the response are met or the maximum number of

**TABLE 5.1**    Indicators Associated with Sensorineural and/or Conductive Hearing Loss as Provided in the Joint Committee on Infant Hearing 1994 Position Statement

| A. For use with neonates (birth–28 days) when universal screening is not available. | B. For use with infants (29 days–2 years) when certain health conditions develop that require rescreening. | C. For use with infants (29 days–3 years) who require periodic monitoring of hearing. |
|---|---|---|
| 1. Family history of hereditary childhood sensorineural hearing loss.<br>2. In utero infection, such as cytomegalovirus, rubella, syphilis, herpes, and toxoplasmosis.<br>3. Craniofacial anomalies, including those with morphological abnormalities of the pinna and ear canal.<br>4. Birth weight less than 1500 grams (3.3 lbs.)<br>5. Hyperbilirubinemia at a serum level requiring exchange transfusion.<br>6. Ototoxic medications including but not limited to the aminoglycosides used in multiple courses or in combination with loop diuretics.<br>7. Bacterial meningitis.<br>8. Apgar scores of 0–4 at one minute or 0–6 at five minutes.<br>9. Mechanical ventilation lasting 5 days or longer.<br>10. Stigmata or other findings associated with a syndrome known to include a sensorineural and/or a conductive hearing loss. | 1. Parent/caregiver concern regarding hearing, speech, language, and/or developmental delay.<br>2. Bacterial meningitis and other infections associated with sensorineural hearing loss.<br>3. Head trauma associated with loss of consciousness or skull fracture.<br>4. Stigmata or other findings associated with a syndrome known to include a sensorineural and/or conductive hearing loss.<br>5. Ototoxic medications including but not limited to chemotherapeutic agents or aminoglycosides used in multiple courses or in combination with loop diuretics.<br>6. Recurrent or persistent otitis media with effusion for at least 3 months. | Some newborns and infants may pass initial hearing screening but will require periodic monitoring of hearing to detect delayed onset sensorineural and/or conductive hearing loss. Infants with these indicators require hearing evaluation at least every 6 months until age 3 years, and at appropriate intervals thereafter.<br><br>Indicators associated with delayed onset sensorineural hearing loss include:<br><br>1. Family history of hereditary childhood hearing loss.<br>2. In utero infection, such as cytomegalovirus, rubella, syphilis, herpes, or toxoplasmosis.<br>3. Neurofibromatosis Type II and neurodegenerative disorders.<br>4. Persistent pulmonary hypertension in the newborn period.<br><br>Indicators associated with conductive hearing loss include:<br><br>1. Recurrent or persistent otitis media with effusion.<br>2. Anatomic deformities and other disorders that affect eustachian tube function.<br>3. Neurodegenerative disorders. |

From Joint Committee on Infant Hearing (1994). Joint Committee on Infant Hearing 1994 Position Statement *Audiology Today, (6),* 6–9.

averaging sweeps is reached. At the end of the test, it simply reports "PASS" or "REFER." The Natus has also been shown to have high sensitivity and specificity and is increasing in popularity because of the ability of trained technicians to operate it (Hall, 1992).

The Smart Screener is a computer-based system that is also small and portable. In addition to an algorithm that recognizes the ABR and determines its presence or absence, it also has an automatic threshold-seeking algorithm, and waveforms are displayed for examination by the audiologist.

This system combines the advantage of an automated screener with the capabilities of a diagnostic ABR system.

The idea of combining the acoustic reflex with ABR to make newborn screening with the ABR more efficient was suggested by Hirsch, Margolis, and Rykken (1992). Among a small sample of newborns, they found that performance of the combined protocol was as good as ABR alone and was much less time intensive. This approach is worthy of further study.

More recently, otoacoustic emissions (OAEs) have been suggested for newborn screening (Bonfils, Dumont, Marie, Francois, and Narcy, 1990; Kemp and Ryan, 1991, 1993; Martin, Whitehead, and Lonsbury-Martin, 1990; Norton, 1994; Zwicker and Schorn, 1990). The test is simple, quick, and objective. Like the ABR, OAEs are present in newborns, even those born at risk and/ or prematurely. In fact, evoked OAEs in a normal-hearing newborn are quite robust. Although much of the data available are based on transient evoked otoacoustic emissions (TEOAEs), distortion product otoacoustic emissions (DPOAEs) also have potential for use in newborn screening and are under investigation for that application now. It is important to point out that OAEs are generated at the level of the outer hair cells in the cochlea, so the OAE test does not assess the integrity of the auditory system beyond that point.

A complete overview of the different OAE tests and ABR can be found in Chapter 7. It should be clear that whatever test is used, the primary objective will be to select a criterion that has good performance characteristics, that is, good sensitivity, specificity, and predictive values. For example, to maximize performance of TEOAEs as a screening test, it has been recommended that evidence of an emission, such as reproducibility above 50 percent or signal-to-noise ratio (S/N) greater than 3 dB, be present in octave bands centered at 1, 2, and 4 kHz (Norton, 1994).

Both ABR and OAE procedures have characteristics that make them good screening tests, especially with the development of automated systems. The tests meet criteria for ease of application, comfort for the patient, time efficiency, and performance. The ABR requires the attachment of electrodes, which may cost slight additional time relative to the OAE tests and may cause slight irritation to the skin. Both tests are vulnerable to the noise and electrical interference that is common in environments in which newborn hearing screening is typically done. Although current practice is to test infants born at risk (JCIH, 1991), which results in most infants coming from the neonatal intensive care unit (NICU), testing is typically not done until the infants reach a transition unit to avoid the high noise levels and electrical "noise" coming from the many complex instruments used in the NICU. The ABR is susceptible to both acoustic and electric noise related to the instruments and activities in the neonatal units, and the OAE tests are susceptible to acoustic interference.

### Universal versus High-Risk Screening

One major drawback to actively screening the hearing of newborns only if they meet the high-risk criteria of JCIH (1991, 1994) is that many newborns with permanent hearing loss will not be tested. As discussed in Chapter 2, a large proportion of infants who are born with permanent hearing loss have auditory impairment due to a recessive genetic trait that is not known to the families or is related to other factors not included in the risk categories. Consequently, the infants are not on the high-risk register and are not tested. It is estimated that 50 percent of newborns with permanent hearing impairment do not meet the high-risk criteria and are missed by the screening protocol. The poor sensitivity of the recommended protocol (ASHA, 1989) has led many professionals to advocate universal newborn hearing screening (AAA, 1988; NIH, 1993). Because prevalence is low, even a test with good specificity will have a large number of false positive outcomes, which is the problem that originally motivated use of the high-risk criteria. With test time, equipment and personnel costs to consider, universal newborn screening could be a costly endeavor and is an issue of concern among those who would administer such programs.

A number of events have occurred and documents produced that address the issue of universal early identification of hearing impairment in young infants (Mauk and Behrens, 1993). In 1993, the NIH consensus conference on universal newborn screening recommended that universal newborn hearing screening be implemented nationwide. Legislation proposed in the United States and the report Healthy People 2000: National Health Promotion and Disease Prevention Objectives (DHHS, 1990) both have supported the same concept. At the same time, the JCIH struggled with the concept of universal newborn screening in developing the 1994 position statement. However, the 1994 JCIH Position Statement, in using an outcome-based approach, does advocate universal detection of infants with hearing impairment.

Besides the fact that current screening practices fail to identify many newborns with hearing impairment, another impetus for screening all infants is the notion that the OAE test will provide an inexpensive and time-efficient means of screening newborns. Much of the attention received by OAEs in the context of universal newborn screening is attributable to the Rhode Island Hearing Assessment Project (RIHAP) (White, Vohr, and Behrens, 1993; White, Vohr, Maxon, Behrens, McPherson, and Mauk, 1994). The RIHAP is a study of the sensitivity, specificity, and practicality, of using TEOAEs for screening all newborns. The project was started in 1990 and has provided very encouraging data on the value of TEOAEs as a tool for universal newborn screening.

The RIHAP program is not without skeptics. That the OAE test is better and more cost-effective than ABR, including the automated ABR, for newborn hearing screening, has not been determined to everyone's satisfaction. One drawback to the OAE test in the context of universal newborn screening is that most of the infants are well babies who will be discharged from newborn nurseries shortly after birth. Because measurement of OAEs is affected by outer and middle ear disorders and because newborns sometimes have material in the outer ear, such as vernix caseous, a fatty substance that covers the skin of the fetus and often collects in creases and cavities, the OAE test has a false positive rate that is relatively high when administered within 24 hours of birth (Vohr, White, Maxon, and Johnson, 1993; Norton, 1994). This has raised concern that there will be an unacceptably high overreferral rate for universal screening programs that use the OAE test. Studies currently underway will clarify this issue over time.

## Older Infants and Young Children

Once infants leave the newborn nurseries, access to them for mass screening programs is limited. The JCIH (1990, 1994) position statements include suggestions for early identification of hearing impairment in infants up to 24 months of age. The high-risk indicators offered in the JCIH (1994) position statement for the older infants also are listed in Table 5.1. Unfortunately, neither ASHA nor AAA have specific guidelines for screening in this age group, but some reviews are available in the literature to help guide the practicing audiologist (e.g., Diefendorf, 1992; Mahoney, 1992). Although methods such as the ABR, OAEs, behavioral observation audiometry (BOA), and visual reinforcement audiometry (VRA) are available for screening in this age group, goals of the screening program and circumstances that are specific to each situation must be considered before choosing a screening test. A discussion of BOA and VRA, along with other behavioral methods for evaluation of hearing in infants and children, is provided in Chapter 6 on behavioral testing.

With techniques such as BOA, it is usually possible to rule out bilateral severe hearing loss. However, BOA is not good at identifying hearing impairments of mild to moderate degree and is not done with earphones, precluding ear-specific information. Also, although BOA-type techniques seem simple, false positive and false negative findings are common. We often advocate that primary care practitioners (nurses, pediatricians, family practice physicians, etc.) be a part of our early identification efforts, but office hearing screening techniques can be flawed. Most include some form of noise maker and the observation of responses, so they technically come under the category of BOA. However, under conditions in which there is noise in the background, uncalibrated stimuli, potential for inadvertent cues due to poor test technique and so on, there is great danger for errors to be made. Especially problematic is the false negative, whereby a truly impaired youngster passes the screening, thereby delaying identification and referral. Audiologists should be aware of the techniques used in their community for hearing screening and should serve as a resource to those involved in early identification of hearing impairment. All screening tests should be done as part of a program so that children who are screened positive receive appropriate management of their hearing loss.

For infants who are 6 months developmental age or more, VRA can be used successfully and works well with earphones. In particular, insert-type earphones seem to work better than the headsets with traditional MX41/AR cushions that are clumsy on infants. Due to the limits on the number of responses one might expect in a single session using VRA, decisions must be made by screening program administrators on the test protocol. A test in sound field will work well, but does not provide ear-specific information. Testing each ear with earphones often takes more time for familiarization and doubles the number of responses that are required. Trade-offs include the number of stimuli used and the number of responses required before acceptance as a "true" response. With VRA, some institutions will use a sound field presentation and two or three stimuli to cover the speech range, including high frequencies. The level of presentation is based on normative data collected in the same setting. The

objective in such cases is to rule out hearing impairment that may cause significant communicative difficulties and, as such, is not aimed at identifying unilateral losses. Other programs might choose to determine status of each ear individually, which would require a different protocol.

A computer-based VRA system (IVRA by Intelligent Hearing Systems) has an algorithm (CAST: Classification of Audiograms by Sequential Testing) for quickly screening infants behaviorally through either loudspeakers or earphones (Eilers, Ozdamar, and Steffens, 1993).

Of course, ABR and OAE tests are available for this age group as well. Typically, after infants reach about 6 months of age, they are unable to relax for sufficient periods of time to complete a successful ABR test. In such cases, sedation is usually recommended, but is a limitation that must be considered carefully by screening program administrators and directors. OAEs are also susceptible to the noise generated by an infant or toddler who is unable to relax. However, we have had success with TEOAEs in infants between 12 and 24 months when testing them on a parent's lap or in a crib. If they do not sleep, even a minute or two of quiet sitting is sufficient to get a TEOAE screening test completed. Our experiences with DPOAEs are more limited in this age group, but may also provide a means of screening without the need for medication. Our experience clearly suggests that when using OAEs in this age group, a sound-treated room will be very helpful in keeping background noise to appropriate levels.

Middle ear disorders are also a factor in this age group. Otitis media with effusion reaches its peak prevalence during the first two years of life, with the period between 6 and 12 months having particularly high incidence rates (Bluestone and Klein, 1988). Information from a hearing screening should be combined with information on status of the middle ear as determined using acoustic immittance tests as well. Immittance norms for this age group are scarce and there are fewer data on abnormal ears, which would be needed to determine a test criterion (overlapping distribution effect). Holte, Margolis, and Cavanaugh (1991) have published some data on normal infants up to about 4 months of age that can provide helpful information. In spite of the lack of data in infants up to 24 months, it is clear that middle ear immittance changes developmentally during early childhood, and it is not recommended that screening criteria for this age group be based on data from older children such as are provided in the next section. ASHA (1990) guidelines for screening for middle ear disorders are intended for children over three years of age, and thus are are not appropriate for this younger group.

In general, infants under 2 years of age produce tympanograms that have lower peak admittance and greater TW than those of older children. More data are needed from various clinics and laboratories so that a reasonable estimate of the normal range for infants under 2 years of age can be made and incorporated into screening criteria. It is important to repeat that to determine the performance of a tympanometric criterion in this age group, a clinical trial is required in which infants with and without middle ear disease are tested and in which the diagnosis of middle ear disease is made by qualified clinicians using specific diagnostic criteria.

Identification of middle ear disorders is a controversial issue in audiology and medicine. As discussed further in Chapter 3, the question of long-term developmental consequences of chronic or recurrent otitis media is still not answered to the satisfaction of many. Some believe that identifying asymptomatic middle ear effusion is not necessary because many of the cases resolve on their own without need of intervention. Over referral rates have been high in programs designed to identify asymptomatic otitis media with effusion, so strategies are used to try to identify only those with chronic middle ear effusion. For a review of the issues, the article by Bluestone and colleagues (Bluestone, Fria, Arjona, Casselbrant, Schwartz, et al., 1986) should be consulted. In spite of the fact that the debate continues, identification of the child with persistent middle ear

disease, especially when accompanied by hearing impairment, should be a goal of audiologic screening programs in this age group. However, especially in this context, careful monitoring of immittance test performance is critical so that the tenets of screening are met. That is, the false positive rate, which affects the number of overreferrals, must be monitored carefully, and communication between the screening program and those making diagnoses (usually pediatricians or family practice physicians in this case) must be constant. Early attempts at immittance screening were not successful because high overreferral rates caused problems for managing physicians and burdened families with "unnecessary" doctor visits and concern (Lous, 1983; Roush and Tait, 1985). Cooperation of the professionals to whom screening positives are referred and the population being screened is essential if the screening program is to succeed.

The JCIH (1990, 1994) places special emphasis on the value of parental/caregiver reports of abnormal auditory behavior and/or delayed development of speech and language with regard to the infant and toddler groups. Primary care physicians need to be sensitive to the concerns of parents and need to be aware themselves of signs of delayed auditory development (Matkin, 1984). After the newborn period, most infants and children with hearing impairment are first identified by a parent or caregiver. Unfortunately, the concerns of parents sometimes are minimized by primary care practitioners, largely because of the wide range of variability in normal development, a belief that hearing cannot be assessed adequately in the very young, or concerns over the cost of assessments. The consequences of delayed assessment of suspected hearing loss is delayed intervention; not only for the affected child but for the family as a whole (Bailey, 1992). The impact on the family presented by a child with a disability such as hearing impairment is great. This is complicated tremendously when parents are treated as overconcerned or are put off for many months by uninformed professionals. Parents are reliable reporters of their infants' development, and their concerns should be taken seriously.

## Screening Preschool and School-Age Children

There is a wealth of information on screening preschool and school-age children in the book *Screening Children for Auditory Function* (Bess and Hall, 1992), including considerable detail on test methods and strategies. Because preschool and school-age children can typically perform behavioral audiometric tasks, such as play audiometry or conventional audiometry, pure-tone hearing screening rather than methods such as OAEs or ABR are usually used. ASHA (1990) guidelines for screening for hearing impairment and middle ear disorders (Table 5.2, part III) recommend that for children 3 years of age and above, pure-tone hearing screening be done at 20 dB HL at test frequencies .5, 1, 2 and 4 kHz in each ear using behavioral test methods. A screening failure occurs when a child fails to respond to any frequency in either ear. As with all audiometric tests, noise in the test environment can artificially elevate thresholds, so screening done outside of sound-treated rooms must be done with an understanding of the potential pitfalls associated with poor environmental noise conditions. Pure-tone screening at 500 Hz is optional when using acoustic immittance screening for middle ear disorders. The rationale is that there will be many false positive findings at 500 Hz in poor acoustical environments and that most of the few children who will fail only at 500 Hz will fail due to middle ear disorders that will be identified using acoustic immittance testing. The risk in this approach is missing the rare child with a sensorineural hearing impairment that includes 500 Hz but no higher frequencies.

The ASHA guidelines (ASHA, 1990) also provide a suggested protocol for screening for middle ear disease (Table 5.2, part IV). The protocol has several components, including recent otologic history, visual inspection of the external auditory meatus and tympanic membrane, and acoustic immittance test along with the pure tone

**TABLE 5.2** Recommended Protocol of Referral for Hearing Impairment and Middle Ear Disorders as Presented by ASHA Guidelines

| REFERRAL CRITERIA |
|---|
| I. History |
|   A. Otalgia |
|   B. Otorrhea |
| II. Visual Inspection of the Ear |
|   A. Structural defect of the ear, head, or neck |
|   B. Ear canal abnormalities |
|     1. Blood or effusion |
|     2. Occlusion |
|     3. Inflammation |
|     4. Excessive cerumen, tumor, foreign material |
|   C. Eardrum abnormalities |
|     1. Abnormal color |
|     2. Bulging eardrum |
|     3. Fluid line or bubbles |
|     4. Perforation |
|     5. Retraction |
| III. Identification Audiometry—Fail air conduction screening at 20 dB HL at 1, 2, or 4 kHz in either ear (ASHA, 1985; these criteria may require alteration for various clinical settings and populations). |
| IV. Tympanometry |
|   A. Flat typanogram and equivalent ear canal volume (Vec) outside normal range unless PE tubes are known to be in place. |
|   B. Low static admittance (Peak Y) on two successive occurrences in a 4–6-week interval |
|   C. Abnormally wide tympanometric width (TW) on two successive occurrences in a 4–6-week interval |

From: American Speech-Language-Hearing Association. (1990). Guidelines for screening for hearing impairment and middle ear disorders. *Asha, 32*(Suppl. 2), 17–24.

hearing screening. The history is designed to learn, either from a parent/caregiver or the child, if there is any recent ear pain, drainage, or other related conditions that would signal need for immediate medical referral. The visual inspection using an otoscope is designed to identify gross obstructions or defects in the external auditory meatus or gross abnormalities of the tympanic membrane that require immediate medical referral. The visual inspection is *not* intended to be used for diagnosis of middle ear disease.

The acoustic immittance battery is designed primarily to identify ears that are at risk for MEE. However, one component is designed to determine if, in the presence of a flat tympanogram, the ear canal volume is abnormally large. In that case, an opening in the tympanic membrane is suspected and, unless the child is known to have PE tubes in place, warrants medical referral. With respect to identification of middle ear effusion, the need for the immittance test relates to the poor sensitivity of the pure-tone hearing screening for that purpose. Many children with middle ear effusion will have hearing thresholds that are at or below (i.e., better than) the screening fence of 20 dB HL and, as a result, would not be identified using a hearing screening alone.

The recommended acoustic immittance screening protocol (ASHA, 1990) is to use normative data from an appropriate group of children, similar in age and other characteristics to those to be screened, to determine the values for peak compensated acoustic admittance and for TW that are outside the normal range. The protocol suggests that peak compensated acoustic admittance values that are below the fifth percentile and TW values that are above the ninety-fifth percentile for the normative group should be positive on the screening. Because the protocol is designed to identify those with long-term or chronic middle ear disease, and because the natural history of middle ear disease is such that many ears will have transient episodes, the screening protocol requires that a child be positive on two immittance tests, separated by 4 to 6 weeks, to be referred for medical examination.

The guidelines (ASHA, 1990) provide in an appendix some interim norms, based on ears of preschool children (Margolis and Heller, 1987), that suggest the screening cutoff should be a peak compensated acoustic admittance less than 0.2 mmho or TW greater than 150 daPa. Data from Nozza and colleagues, (1992, 1994) suggest that different criteria might have better performance in the general school-age (i.e., older than preschool age) population (Table 5.3). In the latter studies, a number of possible screening criteria were analyzed and presented in table as well as in graphic form. For example, as shown in Table 5.3, specificity was higher for TW of 200 daPa rather than 150 daPa for ears in the school-age group (Nozza et al., 1994). Figure 5.3 illustrates some of the variability in test performance based on different test criteria using data, analyzed by child rather than by ear, from the same study. With the criterion changing from TW > 150 to TW > 200 to TW > 250, and counting as positive also those children for whom tympanometry could not be completed on both ears, PPV changes from 36 percent to 53 percent to 62 percent. However, there is no consensus on the best immittance screening protocol for identification of middle ear disease. Some (e.g., Silman, Silverman, and Arick, 1992) feel that the acoustic reflex test has a role in screening for middle ear disease. However, we (Nozza et al., 1992, 1994) have found that the acoustic reflex has a high false positive rate when screening for middle ear disease and that there are some children who will provide valid tympanograms but who will not sit still long enough to obtain a valid test of the acoustic reflex. For those children, the acoustic reflex is useless in a screening protocol. Also, because the acoustic reflex depends on more than middle ear function, other disorders, particularly sensorineural hearing impairment, will preclude use of the acoustic reflex for screening for middle ear disease in some special populations.

We have also demonstrated that the population tested could have a great effect on test performance. The criterion of TW > 150, as shown in Figure 5.4, has sensitivity of 89 percent and specificity of 93 percent using the ear as the unit of analysis. However, the same criterion, when applied to ears of children with chronic or recurrent otitis media and who were scheduled to undergo myringotomy with tube placement, produced sen-

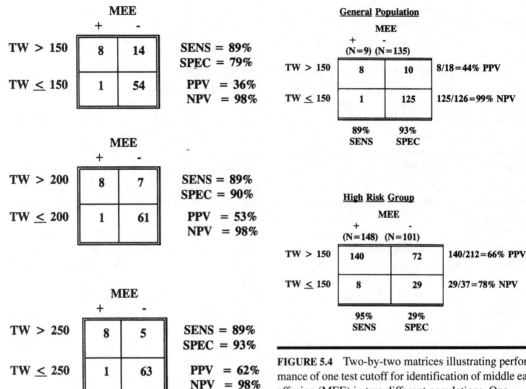

FIGURE 5.3    Two-by-two matrices to illustrate how changing a test criterion will affect test performance. The data are based on tympanometric measurements in school age children examined by a nurse/otoscopist for middle ear disease (Nozza et al., 1994). As the test cut-off (TW) increases, the specificity (SPEC) and the positive predictive value (PPV) change. MEE = middle ear effusion; + = present; – = absent; SENS = sensitivity; NPV = negative predictive value.

FIGURE 5.4    Two-by-two matrices illustrating performance of one test cutoff for identification of middle ear effusion (MEE) in two different populations. One group, the general population, was represented by children selected randomly from a hospital allergy outpatient clinic and the second, high-risk group was represented by children about to undergo surgery for placement of tympanotomy tubes because of chronic or recurrent middle ear disease. Notice especially the effect on specificity (SPEC) and predictive values as a function of the change in population and change in disease prevalence. TW=tympanometric width; + = present; – = absent; SENS = sensitivity; PPV = positive predictive value; NPV=negative predictive value. Data taken from Nozza, R. J., Bluestone, C. D., Kardatzke, D., and Bachman, R. N. (1994). Identification of middle ear effusion by oral aconstic admittance and otoscopy. *Ear and Hearing* 15, 310–323.

sitivity of 95 percent and specificity of only 29 percent. Others have investigated the performance of the recommended ASHA (1990) protocol in different settings with different age groups (Karzon, 1991; Roush, Drake, and Sexton, 1992) and have had some variation in results. The lack of consensus on the best method or the best test criterion relates to the effects of factors such as the definition and prevalence of the disease, population characteristics, test instrument settings, and others that may affect the outcome of a screening test or program (Nozza, 1995).

As mentioned earlier, interest in OAEs for screening newborns is at a peak. Nozza and Sabo (1992) investigated the potential role of TEOAEs

**TABLE 5.3** Performance of Selected Typanometric Criteria in Screening for Middle Ear Effusion

| | | GENERAL POPULATION | | | |
|---|---|---|---|---|---|
| Variables | Criterion | SENS (%) (N = 9) | SPEC (%) (N = 135) | PPV (%) | NPV (%) |
| TW | > 150 | 89 | 93 | 44 | 99 |
| | > 200 | 78 | 99 | 78 | 99 |
| | > 250 | 78 | 100 | 100 | 99 |
| TW or $Y_{tm}$ | TW > 150 or $Y_{tm} < .2*$ | 89 | 93 | 44 | 99 |
| | TW > 200 or $Y_{tm} < .3$ | 78 | 98 | 70 | 99 |
| | TW > 250 or $Y_{tm} < .3$ | 78 | 99 | 88 | 99 |

*Interim norms (ASHA, 1990).

From Nozza, R. J., Bluestone, C. D., Kadatzke, D., and Bachman, R. N. (1994). Identification of middle ear effusion by aural acoustic admittance and otoscopy. *Ear and Hearing, 15,* 310–323.

for screening for hearing impairment and middle ear disease in the school-age population. Because OAEs are sensitive to both hearing impairment and middle ear disease, it seems an ideal measure for screening school age children. The rationale is that OAEs may, with a single, brief, and simple measurement, separate those at risk for either hearing impairment, middle ear disease, or both, from the general population, which is in contrast to the present protocol that requires a pure-tone hearing screening and an acoustic immittance test. The data of Nozza and Sabo (1992) suggest that specificity of the OAE test would be at least as good as the current ASHA-recommended protocol (ASHA, 1990) and probably would be less time-consuming. Those passing an OAE test could be considered to have normal middle ear function and normal peripheral hearing. Those failing an OAE test could then be screened using immittance and/or pure tone hearing screening techniques. Whatever method is chosen for the stage following a positive outcome on the OAE test, it is clear that fewer tests would have to be given overall using the OAE test at the first stage. Research into optimal protocols for such a screening program is warranted.

### Other Issues in Screening

There are other dimensions of screening in pediatric audiology that cannot be covered in detail in this chapter. For example, as specified in the JCIH Position Statements (1990; 1994), screening should be done if children are at risk for hearing loss due to ototoxic medications. Also, many children participate in activities that may expose them to hazardous levels of noise especially as they get older. Periodic monitoring of children receiving medications that are known to be ototoxic or children who are being exposed to noise should be carried out using the most appropriate screening test, taking age, physical condition, and potential consequences into consideration.

Also, some children are believed to be at risk for central auditory processing disorders (CAPDs). There is a screening test available for children who exhibit behaviors that are consistent with such problems as we understand them (Keith, 1986). It should be noted that Stach (1992) does not recommend universal screening of school-age children for CAPDs. Further discussion on the somewhat controversial topic of CAPD is provided in Chapter 8.

### SUMMARY

Early identification and management of hearing impairment and middle ear disorders is important for children of all ages. Methods for screening infants, toddlers, and school-age children are available. It is important that audiologic screening of children takes place in the context of a program that meets all of the basic principles of screening so there is a well-thought-out and organized sequence of events and available resources for the follow-up of those identified. Screening programs designed for identification of hearing impairment should be directed by audiologists who have a good understanding of the principles of screening, including how to estimate performance of a test and how factors other than the test itself can affect program performance. Screening is only a part of the early identification program. The involvement of the community, the families, the schools, and the professionals to whom referrals will be made is essential.

The issue of screening for middle ear disorders is a controversial one. The belief that mild and/or fluctuating hearing impairment associated with otitis media with effusion can cause a disability is not universally accepted, so strong rationale should be given when attempting to screen for middle ear disease. As Downs (as cited in Bluestone et al., 1986) has stated, in spite of arguments over the methodological limitations of some of the research in this area, it is still clear that otitis media early in life can cause audiologic and other developmental consequences.

The best way to make a strong case for the early identification of hearing impairment is to learn more about the consequences of hearing impairment on the development and education of children of all ages as discussed in Chapter 1. Research is necessary that will help us learn how infants and children with normal hearing use auditory input in those processes and how abnormal auditory input affects those processes. Until we understand the effects of all types of hearing impairment, including the mild and/or fluctuating hearing impairment that often accompanies otitis media with effusion, and convey that understanding to others, we will be forced to continue to accept delayed identification and delayed intervention resulting in academic or social failure for some of our children.

## REFERENCES

American Academy of Audiology. (1988). Position statement of early identification of hearing loss in infants and children. *Audiology Today*, 8–9.

American Speech-Language-Hearing Association. (1993). Report on audiologic screening. Ad Hoc Committee on Screening for Hearing Impairment, Handicap, and Middle Ear Disorders. Rockville, MD: ASHA.

American Speech-Language-Hearing Association. (1993). Guidelines for audiology services in the schools. *ASHA, 35* (Suppl. 10), 24–32.

American Speech-Language-Hearing Association. (1991). Guidelines for the audiologic assessment of children from birth through 36 months of age. *ASHA,* (Suppl. 5), 37–43.

American Speech-Language-Hearing Association. (1990). Guidelines for screening for hearing impairment and middle ear disorders. *ASHA, 32*(Suppl. 2), 17–24.

American Speech-Language-Hearing Association. (1989). Guidelines for audiometric screening of newborn infants who are at risk for hearing impairment. *ASHA, 31*(3), 89–92.

American Speech-Language-Hearing Association. (1988). Position statement: Prevention of communication disorders. *ASHA,* 90.

American Speech-Language-Hearing Association. (1985, May). Guidelines for identification audiometry. *ASHA, 27,* 49–52.

Bailey, D. B., Jr. (1992). Current issues in early intervention. In F. H. Bess and J. W. Hall (eds.), *Screening Children for Auditory Function* (pp. 385–398). Nashville: Bill Wilkerson Center Press.

Bennett, M. J. (1979). Trials with the auditory response cradle I: Neonatal responses to auditory stimuli. *British Journal of Audiology, 13,* 125–134.

Bess, F. H., and Hall, J. W. (eds.) (1992). *Screening Children for Auditory Function.* Nashville: Bill Wilkerson Center Press.

Bluestone, C. D., and Klein, J. O. (1988). *Otitis Media in Infants and Children.* Philadelphia: W. B. Saunders Company.

Bluestone, C. D., Fria, T. J., Arjona, S. K., Casselbrant, M. L., Schwartz, D. M., et al. (1986). Controversies in screening for middle ear disease and hearing loss in children. *Pediatrics, 77,* 57–70.

Bonfils, P., Dumont, A., Marie, P., Francois, M., and Narcy, P. (1990). Evoked otoacoustic emissions in newborn hearing screening. *Laryngoscope, 100,* 186–189.

Cadman, D., Chambers, L., Feldman, W., and Sackett, D. (1984). Assessing the effectiveness of community screening programs. *Journal of the American Medical Association, 252,* 1580–1585.

Davidson, J., Hyde, M. L., and Alberti, P. W. (1989). Epidemiologic patterns in childhood hearing loss: A review. *International Journal of Pediatric Otorhinolaryngology, 17,* 239–266.

Department of Health and Human Services, Public Health Service. (1990). *Healthy People 2000: National Health Promotion and Disease Prevention Objectives.* Washington, DC: US Government Printing Office.

Diefendorf, A. O. (1992). Screening for hearing loss: Behavioral options. In F. H. Bess and J. W. Hall (eds.), *Screening Children for Auditory Function* (pp. 243–260). Nashville: Bill Wilkerson Press.

Eilers, R. E., Ozdamar, O., and Steffens, M. L. (1993). Classification of audiograms by sequential testing: Reliability and validity of an automated behavioral hearing screening algorithm. *Journal of American Academy of Audiology, 4,* 172–181.

Feightner, J. W. (1992). Screening in the 1990's: Some principles and guidelines. In F. H. Bess and J. W. Hall (eds.), *Screening Children for Auditory Function* (pp. 1–16). Nashville: Bill Wilkerson Center Press.

Frankenburg, W. K. (1974). Selection of diseases and tests in pediatric screening. *Pediatrics, 54,* 612–616.

Galambos, R., Wilson, M. J., and Silva, P. D. (1994). Identifying hearing loss in the intensive care nursery: A 20-year summary. *Journal of the American Academy of Audiology, 5,* 151–162.

Griner, P. F., Mayewski, R. J., Mushlin, A. I., and Greenland, P. (1981). Selection and interpretation of diagnostic tests and procedures. *Annals of Internal Medicine, 92,* 557–570.

Hall, J. W. (1992). Newborn auditory screening. *Handbook of Auditory Evoked Responses,* pp 475–508. Needham Heights, MA: Allyn and Bacon.

Hirsch, J. E., Margolis, R. H., and Rykken, J. R. (1992). A comparison of acoustic reflex and auditory brain stem response screening of high-risk infants. *Ear and Hearing, 13,* 181–186.

Holte, L., Margolis, R. H., and Cavanaugh, R. M., Jr. (1991). Developmental changes in multifrequency tympanograms. *Audiology, 30,* 1–24.

Joint Committee on Infant Hearing. (1982). Position Statement. *ASHA, 24*(12), 1017–1018.

Joint Committee on Infant Hearing. (1991). 1990 Position Statement. *ASHA, 33* (Suppl. 5), 3–6.

Joint Committee on Infant Hearing. (1994). Joint Committee on Infant Hearing 1994 Position Statement. *Audiology Today, 6*(6), 6–9.

Karzon, R. G. (1991). Validity and reliability of tympanometric measures for pediatric patients. *Journal of Speech and Hearing Research, 34,* 386–390.

Keith, R. W. (1986). SCAN: *A Screening Test for Auditory Processing Disorders.* San Antonio, TX: The Psychological Corporation/Harcourt Brace Jovanovich.

Kemp, D. T., and Ryan, S. M. (1993). The use of transient evoked otoacoustic emissions in neonatal hearing screening programs. *Seminars in Hearing, 14,* 30–45.

Kemp, D. T., and Ryan, S. (1991). OAE tests in neonatal screening programs. *Acta Otolaryngology* (Suppl. 482), 73–84.

Koebsell, K. A., and Margolis, R. H. (1986). Tympanic gradient measured from normal preschool children. *Audiology, 25,* 149–157.

Lous, J. (1983). Three impedance screening programs on a cohort of seven-year-old children. *Scandinavian Audiology* (Suppl. 17) 60–64.

Mahoney, T. (1992). Screening the preschool-age child. In F. H. Bess and J. W. Hall (eds.), *Screening Children for Auditory Function* (pp. 272–286). Nashville: Bill Wilkerson Press.

Margolis, R. H., and Heller, J. W. (1987). Screening typanometry: Criteria for medical referral. *Audiology, 26,* 197–208.

Martin, G. K., Whitehead, M. L., and Lonsbury-Martin, B. L. (1990). Potential of evoked otoacoustic emissions for infant hearing screening. *Seminars in Hearing, 11,* 186–203.

Matkin, N. E. (1984). Early recognition and referral of hearing-impaired children. *Pediatrics in Review, 6,* 151–155.

Mauk, G. W., and Behrens, T. R. (1993). Historical, political, and technological context associated with early identification of hearing loss. *Seminars in Hearing, 14,* 1–17.

National Institutes of Health (1993). Early identification of hearing impairment in infants and young children. *NIH Consensus Statement, 11*(1).

Norton, S. J., (1994). Emerging role of evoked otoacoustic emissions in neonatal hearing screening. *American Journal of Otology, 15*(Suppl. 1), 4–12.

Nozza, R. J. (1995). Critical issues in acoustic immittance screening for middle-ear effusion. *Seminars in Hearing, 16*(1), 86–98.

Nozza, R. J., Bluestone, C. D., Kardatzke, D., and Bachman, R. N. (1992). Towards the validation of aural acoustic immittance measures for diagnosis of middle ear effusion in children. *Ear and Hearing, 13,* 442–453.

Nozza, R. J., Bluestone, C. D., Kardatzke, D., and Bachman, R. N. (1994). Identification of middle ear effusion by aural acoustic admittance and otoscopy. *Ear and Hearing, 15,* 310-323.

Nozza, R. J., and Sabo, D. L. (1992). Transiently evoked OAE for screening school-age children. *The Hearing Journal, 45*(11), 29–31.

Roush, J., Drake A., and Sexton, J. E. (1992). Identification of middle ear dysfunction in young children: A comparison of tympanometric screening procedures. *Ear and Hearing, 13,* 63–69.

Roush, J., and Tait, C. (1985). Pure-tone and acoustic immittance screening for preschool-aged children: An examination of referral criteria. *Ear and Hearing, 6,* 245–250.

Silman, S., Silverman, C. A., and Arick, D. S. (1992). Acoustic-immittance screening for detection of middle-ear effusion in children. *Journal of the American Academy of Audiology,3,* 262–268.

Simmons, F. B., and Russ, F. (1974). Automated newborn hearing screening: Crib-o-gram. *Archives of Otolaryngology, 100,* 1–7.

Stach, B. A. (1992). Controversies in the screening of central auditory processing disorders. In F. H. Bess and J.W. Hall (eds.), *Screening Children for Auditory Function* (pp. 61–78). Nashville: Bill Wilkerson Press.

Thorner, R. M., and Remein, Q. R. (1982). Principles and procedures in the evaluation of screening for disease. In J. B. Chaiklin, I. M. Ventry, and R. F. Dixon (eds.), *Hearing Measurement: A Book of Readings* (2nd ed., pp. 408–421). Reading, MA: Addison-Wesley.

Turner, R. G. (1991). Modeling the cost and performance of early identification protocols. *Journal of the American Academy of Audiology, 2,* 195–205.

Turner, R. G. (1992a). Comparison of four hearing screening protocols. *Journal of the American Academy of Audiology, 3,* 200–207.

Turner, R. G. (1992b). Factors that determine the cost and performance of early identification protocols. *Journal of the American Academy of Audiology, 3,* 233–241.

Turner, R. G., and Cone-Wesson, B. K. (1992). Prevalence rates and cost-effectiveness of risk factors. In F. H. Bess and J. W. Hall (eds.), *Screening Children for Auditory Function* (pp. 79–104). Nashville: Bill Wilkerson Press.

Vohr, B. R., White, K. R., Maxon, A. B., and Johnson, M. J. (1993). Factors affecting the interpretation of transient evoked otoacoustic emission results in neonatal hearing screening. *Seminars in Hearing, 14,* 57–72.

White, K. R., and Behrens, T. R. (eds.). (1993). The Rhode Island Hearing Assessment Project: Implications for universal newborn hearing screening. *Seminars in Hearing, 14.*

White, K. R., Vohr, B. R., and Behrens, T. R. (1993). Universal newborn hearing screening using transient evoked otoacoustic emissions: Results of the Rhode Island Hearing Assessment Project. *Seminars in Hearing, 14,* 18–29.

White, K. R., Vohr, B. R., Maxon, A. B., Behrens, R. T., McPherson, M. G., and Mauk, G. W. (1994). Screening of all newborns for hearing loss using transient evoked otoacoustic emissions. *International Journal of Pediatric Otorhinolaryngology, 29,* 203–217.

Zwicker, E., and Schorn, K. (1990). Delayed evoked otoacoustic emissions—An ideal screening test for excluding hearing impairment in infants. *Audiology, 29,* 241–251.

# CHAPTER 6

# BEHAVIORAL HEARING TESTS WITH CHILDREN

*FREDERICK N. MARTIN AND JOHN GREER CLARK*

## INTRODUCTION

Performing voluntary or behavioral hearing tests with infants and children is both an art and a science, interest in which may be waning. A series of surveys (most recently Martin, Armstrong, and Champlin, 1994) suggest that as the use of electrophysiologic tests with less than fully cooperative patients increases in prominence, audiologists appear to relegate behavioral procedures to secondary importance. Perhaps the glamour of the newer procedures has something to do with this, although their usefulness is undeniable.

Although other procedures for determining the hearing status of children described in this book, such as auditory evoked potentials and otoacoustic emissions, are extremely useful, no diagnosis is complete until the results of voluntary hearing tests are obtained. It is often said that it is not hearing *per se* that we measure, but rather a series of responses to acoustic stimuli. This is true whether these responses are made voluntarily, as by a hand signal, or involuntarily, through the measurement of some change in physiologic state. In situations in which responses are difficult to obtain both approaches should be used in concert to obtain initial diagnoses. Acoustic immittance measures (Chapter 7) are an integral part of the audiologic assessment of children and are invaluable as a cross check of the validity of measured behavioral responses.

Before hearing tests on children are performed, experienced audiologists will usually have a plan of action. These clinicians know that testing must begin as soon as possible after the child and caregiver arrive in the clinic and that when testing is delayed it may become impossible due to fatigue or distraction. The result is the loss of valuable time, thereby obviating complete, or even partial, results. Such game plans are often called "age-appropriate," but a child's age has less to do with what will be attempted in testing than does maturity, self-discipline, and a desire to cooperate. Even very small children have been known to take adult-like tests, and we feel it is advisable to strive for the highest level of tests that the child is capable of taking.

Voluntary hearing tests may be separated into categories such as formal versus informal, those that seek to find auditory threshold versus an approximation of the degree of hearing loss, and ear-specific tests (using earphones) versus sound-field tests. Although a complete hearing test is often not obtained on the first attempt, even the most difficult-to-test children will afford some insights into their auditory status. It is important that parents/caregivers are apprised of these facts from the outset. To permit them to sit through a full session with their child and the audiologist expecting to receive habilitative recommendations at the conclusion of the test is unfair. Parents/caregivers need to know what to expect and that a full audiologic diagnosis may not be forthcoming at the conclusion of the first test.

The importance of careful measurement of behavioral thresholds in children cannot be overstated. The decisions made on the basis of these tests can reverberate through the entire life of a small child and impact, in the most dramatic ways, on the family. To assist in the administration and interpretation of informal hearing tests audiologists need to be familiar with the development of auditory skills in children.

## AUDITORY DEVELOPMENT AND MATURATION

Before audiologists can appreciate and interpret the responses children make to informal hearing tests, they must understand how the child's auditory development and maturation will affect the observed responses. The development of auditory skills proceeds through the same stages, albeit at different rates, for children with normal hearing and children with impaired hearing, provided that the latter receive appropriate amplification and aggressive auditory-based habilitation from an early age. If left unidentified, the auditory development of the child with hearing loss will become arrested. Through the first several months of life, however, the development of audition for these two groups of children may run parallel, thereby hampering the goals of early identification. This is one of the reasons that universal newborn hearing screening, as discussed in Chapter 5, is so very important.

Infant and childhood development is highly individual and varies greatly from child to child. Some children will excel in particular areas of skill development and lag behind their peers in other areas, while their developmental prowess continues to fall within accepted ranges of developmental guidelines. It is for this reason that pediatricians and other health-care providers may admonish parents not to compare one sibling's developmental patterns with another. While such comparisons are indeed often invalid and should be discouraged, prompt investigation is always warranted when parental concerns in the areas of delayed speech and language development are coupled with concerns about a child's hearing abilities. Toward this end, audiologists should be familiar with the developmental checklists detailed in Appendices 1 and 2 so they may be able to help identify a child not maturing as expected.

The auropalpebral reflex (APR) yields the familiar eye blink response to a sudden sound. This reflex is not only a very reliable response in neonates (Froding, 1960), its resistance to extinction provides a response that continues even after repeated presentation of stimuli (Eisenberg, Coursin, and Rupp, 1966). As with many reflexive and behavioral responses to sound, responses are more overt and occur at lower intensities as signal complexity increases. Within a quiet room an involuntary movement of the eyes toward the sound source (the cochleo-oculogyric response) can be reliably elicited to broadband signals and speech signals at 60 to 75 dB SPL (40 to 55 dB HL). Louder sounds may elicit a moro reflex, a rather gross response in which the knees and arms are drawn into the body. Less overt startle responses are often observable in infants in response to speech signals above approximately 65 dB HL. Elicitation of such responses can be good indicators that hearing is within or near normal limits for at least a portion of the frequency range of interest. However, relying on such measures alone, as may be done during a gross screening at a physician's office, will fail to identify significantly handicapping high frequency hearing loss. Similarly, startle responses to louder signals may be a sign of recruitment in the presence of hearing loss rather than an expected response from a child with normal hearing.

Other responses to sound, such as changes in respiration or sucking behaviors, may be observed when ambient noise levels are low. Bench (1970) observed that infant responses to sound tend to have an inverse relation to the prestimulus activity level of the child. The quieter the child before stimulus onset the more active the child will become. In contrast, if the child is more active the observer will see a general decrease in activity level with stimulus onset.

Before observing any response to sound, the audiologist should make note of the activity state of the child. The activity state of an infant is generally classified as deep sleep, light sleep, awake and quiet, or awake and active. A child in deep sleep will be quite still except for sporadic star-tling, little or no eye movement, and a rhythmic respiration pattern. When in light sleep, body and eye movements increase considerably and respira-tion is less rhythmic. When children are awake and quiet they appear quite peaceful and at ease with their eyes open, while the awake and active child is more vocal and squirmy.

Deep sleep and light sleep are most easily differentiated by observing a child's response to a light touch or stroking of the eyelid. While the child in deep sleep will not respond to such stimu-lation, in the lightly sleeping child this will elicit movement of the eyes and some slight squirming. Very young children are most easily tested for startle and APR responses when they are in light

sleep or when awake and quiet (Eisenberg, Grif-fin, Coursin, and Hunter, 1964).

As babies get older, the development of cer-tain motor patterns occur with the development of audition, which readily lend themselves to clinical observation when assessing hearing. The cochleo-oculogyric reflex gives rise to an infant's eye movement toward a sound source and with matu-ration is coupled to a head-turning response, first indirectly toward the sound and then more direct-ly (Figure 6.1). While localization behaviors be-gin to develop fairly early, neuromuscular control of the neck is not sufficiently established for clear assessment of hearing through localization re-sponses until 4 to 6 months. The utility of local-ization responses for hearing testing is reduced for

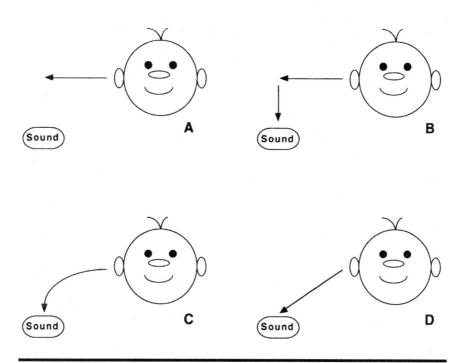

**FIGURE 6.1**    Development of auditory localization in infants. (*A*) At 3 months the head moves unsteadily along the horizontal plane toward the sound source. (*B*) At 5 months local-ization is in straight lines, first horizontally and then vertically. (*C*) At 6 months the head and eyes move in an arc toward the sound source. (*D*) At 8 months the head and eyes move directly toward the sound source.

children with motor retardation or in those in whom hearing loss has reduced the child's auditory experience (Hodgson, 1987).

## INFORMAL HEARING TESTS

Informal hearing tests are generally performed on children whose chronological or mental ages preclude the use of earphones, or who, for some other reason, will not tolerate them. Different kinds of stimuli may be used in these procedures but the audiologist should always strive for the use of the most frequency-specific signals possible.

One reason children do not like to wear earphones for testing, in addition to their threatening size and discomfort, is the fact that the cords restrict their movement and get entangled. We believe it is only a matter of time before some aggressive audiometer manufacturer produces cordless earphones that are light in weight and would allow active children to move about unencumbered and still take reliable hearing tests. This kind of innovation would be eagerly accepted by many pediatric audiologists.

Since ultimately all children must be tested using some kind of earphone, and many children refuse them, there are steps that can be taken to encourage acceptance. Most audiology clinics have old, broken, or otherwise unusable earphones and headbands lying about. These can be loaned to families to take home. The parents or older siblings can wear these around the house for short periods of time, and many small children will be enticed and indicate that they want to wear them as well. This can be "tolerated" for short periods of time at home, which in turn makes putting them on the child much easier the next time the child is seen by the audiologist.

### Noisemakers

As alluded to earlier, it has been recognized for some time that the more narrow the frequency range of an acoustic signal the less interesting it is for most children. The inverse is, of course, also true. Therefore, a pure tone is least likely to catch the attention of a child while a signal like a buzzer is most apt to do this. The former can more easily be controlled and responses interpreted in terms of hearing sensitivity at different frequencies. The latter lacks this specificity but may be chosen by default. The use of nonfrequency specific stimuli, however, must be used with caution. When using noisemakers it is likely that children will respond to the portion of the acoustic spectrum in which their hearing sensitivity is best. Children with severe high-frequency hearing losses, for example, have been known to turn to a moderately loud sound, such as the clapping of hands or the calling of their names, resulting in a diagnosis of normal hearing. It may later be learned that the child responded only to the low-frequency portion of the spectrum—the time lost before this is discovered may be critical to early intervention and education.

Despite the disadvantages stated, the use of noisemakers does have a place in testing some young or developmentally delayed children. When noisemakers are to be used they should be calibrated, at least in terms of their spectrum, and audiologists must practice using them until they can replicate, with reasonable accuracy, the intensity of the sound produced at a given distance from a child's ear. This can be accomplished by making tape recordings of the sounds and determining the results on a spectrum analyzer. Subjective impressions can be very misleading and a sound that appears to be primarily high-pitched (such as a whistle) may contain considerable energy in the mid- or low-frequency range. Noisemakers can include, among others, bells, clickers, buzzers, whistles, and crinkled cellophane.

### Behavioral Observation Audiometry

The use of noisemakers for behavioral observation audiometry (BOA) usually takes two clinicians, although the exigencies of routine clinical practice often require that an adult accompanying the child be pressed into service as an assistant. This may or may not prove useful. One clinician should be placed in front of the child, who may be seated on the floor of the examining room or held by a parent/caregiver. This clinician's responsibility is to watch for responses. The other clinician selects from a set of noisemakers that have been laid out in advance and placed out of the child's line of vision. While the child's attention is diverted by the first clinician, who works as silently as possible using puppets or other visually engaging devices, the second clinician activates the noisemaker behind and to the side of the child. The midline of the head should not be used since localization is difficult or impossible from this point.

BOA responses to noisemakers may be seen in searching behavior, such as turning the head or moving the eyes. Sounds should not be very loud initially and may be increased in volume when responses are not observed. Responses to loud sounds may occur as overall startle responses, searching behavior, APRs, or cochleo-oculogyric responses, as discussed earlier. With many children only one or two observations can be made before any semblance of cooperation disappears.

We usually look for the onset of a response from a controlled, calm activity state but this is not always the case. Some children may be engaged in play and will stop when they hear a sound. Many children with mild to moderate hearing impairments appear very interested in sounds once they exceed their thresholds, but children with profound losses, who have not heard sounds, may show no interest in them at all.

Although, as stated above, a parent's lap or the floor are the usual placements for babies and small children, we have experienced some difficulties with these arrangements. When a loud sound is presented parents with normal hearing will almost certainly convey *their* response to the child by tensing or tightening their hold, resulting in the child's response to a parent's response. We find that in many cases a high chair is ideal for testing.

There are several reasons why we recommend high chairs when examining small children. Most children are accustomed to sitting in these chairs at home and accept them readily. The myri-

ad distractions available on the floor are removed, as is the distorted, fish-eye appearance adults present to children as they hover above them, causing them to become frightened. We also find, when parents approve, that children enjoy eating small crackers from the high chair tray. It often takes a long time for children to eat these crackers and some reactions to sound can often be seen long before they are sated. Since we want a child's attention centered forward and down the tray is an ideal focus point (Figure 6.2).

When a series of responses can be seen to noisemakers this can be quite comforting to clinician and caregiver alike. However, the caveat that must always be remembered is that the test is incomplete until an audiogram is obtained. This is true whether responses have or have not been observed. As BOA does not incorporate a reinforce-

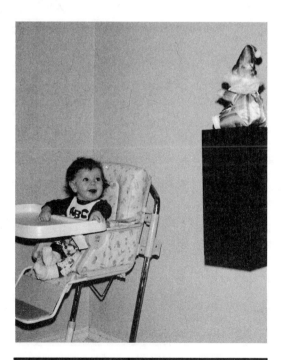

**FIGURE 6.2** A high chair provides ideal positioning for BOA, VRA, or COR testing with children. (Photo courtesy of HearCare, Inc.)

ment to the child for elicited responses, response habituation may be rapid. In addition, these techniques may be confounded by false positive responses, nonspecific responses, and observer bias.

## FORMAL HEARING TESTS

### Sound-field Audiometry

Sound-field setups in many audiology centers include at least two loudspeakers that are fed by an audiometer (Figure 6.3). The room should be cleared of any distracting objects or those that might cause injury to an inquisitive child. While some audiologists decorate the walls of their pediatric test suites with colorful pictures and interesting objects, we find this often to be highly distracting to some children.

Naturally, it is imperative that the system be properly calibrated and care given to avoiding interference patterns and standing waves. It is common to use frequency modulated tones, which are said to "warble." This warble is usually expressed as a percentage of the frequency of the pure tone tested, that is, a 1000 Hz tone warbled at 5 percent would change over time from 950 to 1050 Hz. The child may be seated on an adult's lap, on the floor, in a small chair, or in a high chair. Signals are directed from the right or left of the child. Stimuli may include pure tones, narrow noise bands, speech, recorded music, or sounds from the child's

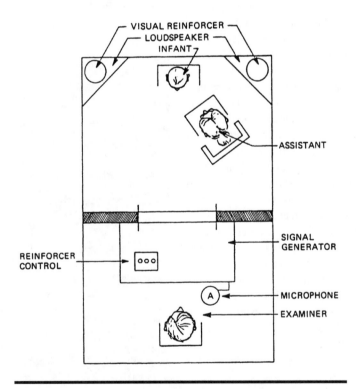

**FIGURE 6.3** Usual arrangement of a two-room sound suite for testing children. (From W. R. Hodgson, (1987). Tests of hearing: Birth through one year. In F. N. Martin (ed.). *Hearing Disorders in Children* (p. 201). Reprinted by permission of Prentice Hall, Englewood Cliffs, NJ)

daily activities such as a spoon in a cup. This test is more intensity specific than the use of hand-held noisemakers, but the sensation level at which the child elects to respond cannot be known. For this reason, when results are recorded, they should be specified as minimum response levels (MRLs) rather than thresholds. The number of decibels above threshold for a child's MRL cannot be known. However, Table 6.1 provides guidelines for the interpretation of MRLs in children.

Theoretically, although MRLs obtained to pure tones and narrow bands of noise surrounding that same frequency should be the same, this is only true when critical bands are used. The narrow noise bands used on audiometers for masking may be rather wide, containing considerable side-band energy, to which the child might respond rather than to the frequency in the center of the band. When narrow bands of noise are used in testing children, which is a common practice, results should be considered preliminary and the procedure a part of the child's training to take a pure-tone test.

## Visual Reinforcement Audiometry

Visual reinforcement audiometry (VRA) is any procedure by which a child reacts to sound, as presented through a loud speaker, and is visually reinforced for that response. During VRA the audiologist sits at the audiometer in the control room while an assistant sits with, distracts, and observes the child in the patient room. As mentioned in Chapter 9, it is advisable for at least one parent or

caregiver to observe the test to ease the flow of diagnostic information at the conclusion of testing. A child who is otherwise occupied is not likely to respond to a sound close to threshold; rather the sound will have to be loud enough catch the child's attention. An exception to this, of course, is the child with loudness recruitment, who may perceive a sound slightly above threshold as quite loud.

Many children are fitted with hearing aids before completely accurate test results are obtained. We believe this is appropriate if the audiologist has sufficient audiometric data to allow the fittings to approximate the child's hearing needs and the instruments are versatile enough for readjustment. As always, testing is an ongoing process with children who are hearing impaired. If the children are wearing hearing aids they can be tested with and without them, the difference, in decibels, being the wearable gain. This is true even if precise thresholds are not obtained. Sound-field gain measures must be used with caution, however, and only when probe-microphone measures cannot be obtained, given their many shortcomings, as discussed in Chapter 11.

One form of VRA that has become very popular is the conditioned orientation reflex (COR) described by Suzuki and Ogiba (1961). As discussed earlier, localization responses are fairly well established by 5–6 months of age permitting assessment of very young children with COR. For COR testing the child sits between two loudspeakers upon which are devices that light up and

**TABLE 6.1**  Typical Sound-Field Minimum Response Levels from Infants

| AGE (MONTHS) | NOISEMAKERS (dB HL) | PURE TONES (dB HL) | SPEECH (dB HL) |
|---|---|---|---|
| 0–4 | 40 | 70 | 45 |
| 4–6 | 45 | 50 | 25 |
| 6–8 | 25 | 45 | 20 |
| 8–10 | 20 | 35 | 10 |
| 10–14 | 20 | 30 | 10 |
| 14–20 | 20 | 25 | 10 |
| 20–24 | 15 | 25 | 10 |

produce some activity, such as the movement of a doll, when activated. This pleasurable viewing by the child follows the presentation of a tone from the loudspeaker. The child is expected to look in the direction of the speaker producing the sound and be rewarded by the visual activity. Ear-specific information is, of course, lacking since the child's better hearing ear is always the one to respond if there is a significant difference in hearing sensitivity between ears. If, however, clear and accurate localizations are observed, a statement of presumed balanced hearing can be made. A child with a severe hearing loss who has not had the advantage of wearing hearing aids may never have learned to localize sound, a fact that can mislead the audiologist when sounds above threshold appear to go unheard. It is only positive responses that are meaningful with children, for a lack of response means only that no response was observed and not necessarily that the child did not hear the signal.

A new system for performing COR tests requires no assistance and allows the audiologist to examine a child when they are both within the same room. The child is placed between the small loudspeakers that support the dolls (an elephant and a teddy bear) that provide the reinforcement. The audiologist holds what looks like a ping-pong paddle that has a distracting fuzzy animal to maintain the child's attention on one side and the controls to the COR system on the others. Signals that can be used are recorded on an audiocassette and include some warbled tones, a 3000 Hz narrow-noise band, a music box, and a baby's cry. Many clinicians find this device quite useful in obtaining preliminary information on the status of a young child's hearing.

We find high chairs are also useful when looking for localization responses from children. If the child will wear earphones, COR tests can be used to obtain individual ear information as the child localizes to the right or left for reinforcement. If earphones will not be worn, individual ear responses can be estimated by attaching the earphones to the high chair. The earphones from an audiometer can be easily mounted and re-moved from the seatback using Velcro strips that allow them to be moved up or down depending on the child's size. The proximity of the earphone to the child's ear often results in greater interest than and localization to a sound of identical intensity entering the external auditory canal from a loudspeaker. Appropriate calibration factors must, of course, be applied.

Any procedure involving sound localization can be contaminated by a number of factors. These include unilateral or markedly asymmetrical hearing losses and children with some central auditory disorders. Localization is a process that is often not developed until children are about 6 months of age. By the time children are 2 to 2½ years old they tend to tire quickly of visual reinforcers. This can be a difficult age to get accurate, frequency-specific information for more than a few frequencies during a single session as these children are also too young to condition to play audiometry.

**Play Audiometry**

A number of play procedures have been used with children who are capable of participating in some form of game. We have used methods that range from dropping a block in a bucket or placing a bead on a string each time a tone is heard, to moving a tiny horse in a simulated race, to making a move in a game of checkers. When a child moves a block from one bucket to another, many audiologists have learned to surreptitiously add blocks to the bucket from which the child selects the block to throw when a signal is heard. To some children an empty bucket signifies the end of the game. There are some very young or small children who will simply raise their hands when they hear a tone, and some older or larger ones who appear incapable of concentrating unless there is some strong motivation. The procedure itself is less important than the reinforcement for a correct response, which usually takes the form of a social reward like smiling or hand clapping. Clinicians must do whatever it takes to let children know that what they did in response to a signal is wanted and appreciated. Typically children are able to be conditioned to respond for play audiometry between 3 and 4 years of age.

A procedure that often works with small children is to draw a small "happy face" on the top of one index finger, fold the finger up and ask the child to look for the "happy face" by popping the finger up whenever the sound comes on, reinforcing this response when it occurs. Similarly, a small figure can be drawn on the inside of the child's hand, which is then rolled into a fist to be opened when a sound is heard, followed by obvious approval from the adult with the child. When using the ear-choice technique, in which the child is to indicate which ear heard the signal, a figure can be drawn on both hands and the child asked to hold each hand next to the corresponding ear and open it when the sound is heard on that side. A figure on the child's hand also works well when doing the Weber test.

Although signal buttons are usually rejected when testing children, they can be useful. Even some very young children play computer games at home and can be told to listen for the signal and "zap it" whenever it comes on. This sometimes works very well and children enjoy the game. Social reinforcement should always be used. Changes in response consistency and latency often signal satiation. The prudent audiologist will be prepared with a variety of play activities so that a change can be made when the child begins to tire of one activity.

When a child cannot be conditioned to respond to a test tone, the clinician may attempt to condition a response to flashing the room lights on and off. A profound hearing loss may quickly be suspected if the child conditions to light but not to sound. Similarly, the audiologist might assess whether the child conditions to the vibrations of a bone-conduction oscillator when held in the hand and a low-frequency tone is presented.

## Operant Conditioning Audiometry

For many children the kind of intangible reinforcement described above is not sufficiently motivating to keep their attention and thus result in a valid hearing test. The principles of operant conditioning, as described by B. F. Skinner, may be used with excellent results. Lloyd, Spradlin, and Reid (1968) describe a procedure called tangible reinforced operant conditioning audiometry (TROCA), which encourages the child to press a button each time a tone is heard, followed immediately by mechanical delivery of a tangible reinforcer such as a token or edible treat. Since the device is automated the reinforcer can be delivered with almost no delay, thereby facilitating conditioning. Whether the test is done in an operant paradigm or by using some form of social reinforcement, the principle is the same:

STIMULUS → RESPONSE → REINFORCEMENT
(e.g., a pure    (push-button,    (tangible or
tone)         hand raise)    intangible)

In general it is safe to say that tangible reinforcement yields better hearing test results than most forms of social reinforcement. Many audiologists may agree with this but run into problems deciding just what reinforcer to use, food being a popular choice. When food is used approval must first be obtained from the child's parent/caregiver for there may be some good reasons (or maybe not such good reasons according to the clinician) for not feeding a given child. Caregiver decisions in this matter, as in all matters, cannot be ignored. In most cases true operant conditioning cannot be carried out because the Skinnerian approach dictates that the subject (the child in this case) must select the reinforcer, something that almost never happens in the world of pediatric audiology. As with sound-field testing or more informal measures, the same cautions apply to signals that lack frequency specificity.

## Mechanical Devices

A number of mechanical devices have been developed through the years to encourage children to participate in hearing tests. These include the peep show (Dix and Hallpike, 1947), a device that encourages the child to press a button when a sound is emitted from a small loudspeaker. The response button is wired in series with a switch that turns on a series of pictures. The objective, of course, is to use the sight of the picture as a reinforcer for the appropriate response, eliminating false positives by not reinforcing inappropriate responses. This paradigm can easily incorporate earphones as well.

Other devices include the pediacouameter (Guilford and Haug, 1952), which uses small puppets popping out of a box as reinforcers. The pediacouameter has an advantage over the original design of the peep show in that the child does wear earphones, allowing for threshold measurements in each ear. There is reason to believe that the child may lose interest after all eight puppets have been viewed.

Several computer-driven instruments have been developed that work on operant principles but reward the child for a proper response with visual graphics that appear on a monitor. These can include cartoon animals or other colorful objects. Each of these devices has its own appeal but our feeling is that in many situations their efficacy is more logical than real. We seem to have better luck with less expensive procedures such as play audiometry or operant conditioning audiometry.

## PURE–TONE AUDIOMETRY

As stated earlier, the test that must be completed before a diagnosis can be made is the pure-tone audiogram. Many audiologists feel insecure if this cannot be carried out during the first visit the child makes to the clinic but it sometimes takes considerable training before it can be completed. Some children can be told or shown simply to raise one hand or finger when they hear a tone or to give a verbal response (which we often prefer) such as "Now" or "I hear it." As in all hearing tests the objective is to obtain the auditory threshold so that once a pattern of responses is developed the clinician can lower the intensity of the tone until responses cease, increase intensity until they reappear, and so forth. Because of the rigidity of some pure-tone procedures, such as described by ASHA (1978), they are not always appropriate for small children.

ASHA recommends that testing begin at 1000 Hz in what appears to be the better-hearing ear, then ascending in frequency, returning to 1000 Hz as a reliability check, and then descending in frequency. The seasoned audiologist realizes that every response obtained from a child may be the last one for the day. It seems to us, therefore, that the most critical information should be obtained first. For example, if the child appears to have good hearing it might be wise to begin at 2000 or even 3000 Hz, testing one ear and then the other. A low frequency, such as 500 Hz, should then be selected and each ear tested separately again. If the child discontinues the test—and certainly it is the child who has the power to do this—before a complete audiogram is obtained, at least some insight into degree of loss and audiometric configuration has been garnered. It may be desirable to test a couple of frequencies by air conduction and then switch to bone conduction.

False positive responses can cause clinicians more irritation than false negatives. When the child consistently claims to hear a pure tone that is either obviously below threshold, or not present at all, the process must necessarily slow down, which creates problems of its own. In addition, there are times when it appears that no measures at all can correct the false positives. Extreme patience is required when dealing with these cases.

## CASE REPORT—FALSE POSITIVE RESPONSES

*We once visited with a colleague and watched as he struggled with a 12-year-old boy who consistently gave false positives. He would simply raise his hand every few seconds whether a tone was or was not presented and continued to do this despite numerous attempts to correct this behavior.*

*Our colleague was at the end of his patience. While we sat in the control room he walked around to the patient room where the child was seated and admonished him for his behavior. He said words like, "We will finish this test if it takes all day. You must not raise your hand until you really hear a tone. Do you understand this?" The child said, "Okay." While the audiologist returned to the control room and out of the patient's view we heard the child say through the talkback system, "I hate you, I hate you, I hate you." So much for discipline.*

*Test results did improve with this child but we believe that a less threatening posture might have resulted in the same outcome.*

If acoustic immittance measures are carried out before audiometry they may dictate whether bone-conduction testing is needed. For example, children with normal tympanograms, including normal gradients and points of maximum compliance, along with normal acoustic reflexes, almost certainly do not have conductive components to their hearing losses. Before any child is finished with hearing testing we believe that bone-conduction tests should be completed, but given a situation such as described above, they can be delayed until all the more important data are collected.

We have noticed that many children present with small air-bone gaps, suggesting some conductive hearing impairment, when this is not extant. Of course, whenever an air-bone gap is seen masking must be applied to the nontest ear to eliminate its possible contribution to test results. Since bone-conduction tests almost always follow air-conduction tests many children get more proficient at test taking as the test proceeds and thus give responses closer to threshold. The thinking clinician will often try by retesting to close the air-bone gap by air conduction before pursuing the more arduous task of masking for bone conduction, in hopes that the air-conduction thresholds will be lower.

Clinical masking often cannot be carried out on nonverbal children, although there are surely exceptions to this statement. Many children can just be told, as their adult counterparts are, to ignore the loud noise in one ear and listen for the soft tone in the other. Many others cannot. In every situation the audiologist is a time manager, determining which procedure will be most efficacious for a particular child at a particular time.

The way in which children, especially nonverbal children, are approached with the transducers needed for testing can be all-important. It is possible to decorate earphones so that they are more appealing, or even to mount an audiometer earphone inside a telephone, which children are accustomed to seeing (Figure 6.4). As discussed in Chapter 3, ear canal collapse from the pressure of supra-aural earphones is more prevalent among young children than in the general population. We recommend placing a thin wedge of foam rubber behind the pinna before putting on the earphones when pinna inspection indicates the possibility of such collapse, or, just as a routine precaution. A thin sheet of foam, such as is sent as packing material with hearing aids and other paraphernalia, can be cut into many small wedges using a behind-the-ear hearing aid as a template.

We prefer the forehead as the testing site for bone conduction and have found that a feather placed in the headband can look like fun to a child. The forehead strap has the additional advantage of being much easier to position on small heads than the steel headband used for mastoid testing. Testing from either the forehead or the mastoid yield the possibility that a child's responses may be to stimuli that are felt rather than heard. This usually occurs at frequencies below 2000 Hz near the output limit of most audiometers (about 40 dB HL for 250 Hz, 60 dB HL for 500 Hz, 70 dB HL above 500 Hz). Clinicians can only guess whether what looks on the audiogram to be a profound mixed hearing loss may be the result of vibrotactile responses.

Insert earphones have a variety of advantages over the supra-aural type that accompany most audiometers. Because they are lighter and less frightening, they are often quite useful with children. Children who have been wearing hearing aids will be accustomed to devices placed in their ears and may offer less resistance than they would to standard earphones. That clinical masking will be required less often when insert earphones are used is motivation enough to use them whenever possible. Insert earphones also avoid the need for

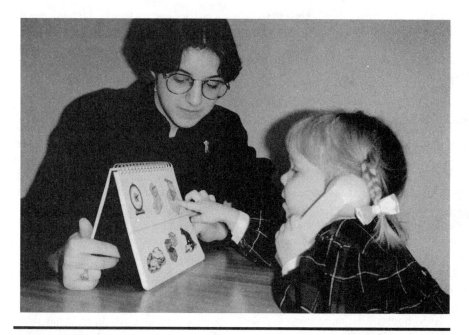

**FIGURE 6.4**   An audiometer earphone mounted in a telephone receiver helps this apprehensive 30-month-old child to continue with testing. (Photo courtesy of Hear Care.)

a foam pad placed onto a small child's head to occupy the space between the head and the headband and keep the headset from sliding off and possibly upsetting the child. It is likely, since insert phones use soft foam in the external ear canal instead of a hard rubber cushion over the pinna, that testing with inserts can minimize the likelihood that air-conduction thresholds will result from tactile stimulation.

Test instructions may be given verbally or pantomimed. One major mistake is to ask, "Would you like to put these earphones on?" or "How would you like to come with me and play a game?" This is fine if children answer positively but if they say "No" the audiologist cannot respond with "Well, put them on anyway" or "Well, we are going." It is better to use direct statements such as, "Let's see if these earphones fit you," or "Come with me and I'll show you the games I have." The less the child controls the procedure the better the chances that it will work. Audiolo-

gists need to be flexible and willing to abandon clinician-centered tests for child-centered tests as things progress, but children quickly learn when they control the situation and may assume that control whenever possible. And although audiologists must attempt to be pleasant and friendly, many children can sense insincerity and are turned off by adults who fawn over them.

## SPEECH AUDIOMETRY

Speech is an abstract concept in that it is only symbolic of objects and actions in the real world. In many ways, however, speech is far more concrete than other audiometric stimuli, like pure tones, because it exists in the child's environment. Hearing tests using speech stimuli should be carried out on children whenever possible. This statement applies to patients of any age, of course, but the corroboration needed for other tests, such as those using pure tones, is essential to make them believable. Speech audiometry provides this confirmation.

As with adults, speech audiometry with children consists of measurements of threshold, levels of comfort and discomfort, and the ability to discriminate among speech sounds, now called word recognition. This chapter is concerned primarily with threshold and word recognition scores. As with pure tones, children should be tested with earphones whenever possible, failing which, sound-field procedures may be used.

## Speech Detection Threshold

The speech detection threshold (SDT) is often called the speech awareness threshold and is generally defined as the lowest level at which speech can be heard and recognized as speech. This definition obviously excludes discrimination among the different speech sounds. The SDT is a popular test with children, often because it is the only measurement that can be made on many difficult-to-test patients.

Properly done, the SDT is carried out using a fairly lengthy selection of prerecorded materials like cold running speech, which the patient listens to and directs the audiologist to increase and decrease the intensity until the criteria for "just barely hearing" are met. This is not a test that children can take. Instead, in most cases, some form of brief live-voice speech signal is used, usually via the sound-field system of the audiometer, and the child is watched for a reaction. Often the child's name is used as a stimulus. Sometimes nothing short of "Would you like to go home now?" will evoke a response, at which time children may grab their mother's hand or bolt for the door. It this phrase is used it should be saved until all else fails because usually there is no going back after this. Innovative clinicians can make hearing testing enjoyable for many children, but children are almost always ready to flee the audiology clinic as soon as possible.

It is obvious that most children whose attention is properly being diverted will not respond at threshold and there is no way of knowing what the

exact sensation level of the signal might be before a child attends to it. Table 6.1 provides guidelines for the interpretation of response levels for speech and other signals.

Additionally, as we said in the section on noisemakers, if the child has a hearing loss in which sensitivity is significantly better in a particular frequency region (both high-frequency and low-frequency hearing losses are common in children) the response is likely to come from that frequency range. Consider a child with normal hearing at 250 Hz, whose audiogram falls, on average, at a rate of 30 dB/octave (not an uncommon finding)—results of the SDT could easily lead to a diagnosis of normal hearing if the child looks for the sound source when it is presented at 20 or 30 dB HL.

The numbers of misdiagnoses and consequent mismanagement of children who have been tested only using SDTs because "that was the only test that produced a response" are incalculable. Those kinds of statistics do not appear in the literature. We do not have a problem with using SDTs with children when all else fails, as long as clinicians and families alike understand that this is merely a preliminary measurement, to be followed as quickly as possible with more definitive tests, such as the speech recognition threshold.

## Speech Recognition Threshold

The speech recognition threshold (SRT), formerly called the speech reception threshold, is a measurement of the intensity at which a patient can barely discriminate about 50 percent of speech materials presented. The usual stimuli are spondaic words, and their use is recommended, although Martin and Mussell (1981) found that for children, SRTs using trochaic stress are quite close to those using spondaic stress with children. SRTs require approximately 10 dB greater intensity for persons with normal hearing than do SDTs, but this difference may be greater in the patient who has a falling or rising hearing loss.

Although many clinicians hold the SRT to be the patient's hearing loss for speech in decibels, there are many times when this can be misleading. At times the SRT will correspond with the pure-tone average at 250 and 500 Hz in patients with steeply falling audiograms who learn the spondees quickly and use their residual hearing well. We are eager to find SRTs with children primarily because they match, in most cases, the pure-tone average using the lowest two thresholds among 500, 1000, and 2000 Hz. Agreement between these tests is a source of great comfort in assessing the reliability of both of them.

Children with good spoken language can often simply repeat spondees to the examiner, which are usually presented using monitored live voice. At times, based on the child's vocabulary, the list is abbreviated. It is a good idea to make a quick check with the accompanying adults to be certain that the test words are in the child's vocabulary. When the child lacks speech, has poor articulation, is too reticent to respond, or for some other reason cannot or will not respond orally, special approaches may be used.

Commonly used are pictures representing spondaic words to which the child points, followed by smiles from the clinician or other reinforcement. Pointing to body parts on the child or attending parent/caregiver can also be useful. If desired, objects may be used instead of pictures or body parts. More than six pictures or objects can slow down testing, even with cooperative children as they search on the table or floor before them for the correct picture. Since most children who are difficult to test are seen for more than one diagnostic session we recommend that the parent or caregiver be asked to bring pictures or objects from home that they know the child can recognize. Whenever possible, stimuli should come from the child's activities of daily living.

Once the child has learned to point to the picture that represents the word that was presented, the intensity is lowered until about half a short list of four to six words is missed. Holding out for a precise 50 percent criterion is impractical for most children and so we recommend a working definition of SRT that calls for the lowest hearing level

at which *at least* 50 percent of the words can be identified. SRTs can often be obtained by clever clinicians in a very few minutes and can be extremely useful.

As with pure-tone tests, social reinforcement when measuring SRTs often does not work well with some children. Martin and Coombes (1976) developed a system for testing SRTs with children using a brightly colored clown. The child is instructed to push the portion of the clown (hand, eye, foot, etc.) when the name of that body part is heard. Microswitches behind each body part are wired in series with a programmer so the child is never reinforced for pressing a body part that was not named. The reward is a small piece of candy-coated chocolate that falls into a cup in the clown's hand. This procedure has been used successfully with very young children as well as with those who are mentally challenged (Weaver, Wardell and Martin, 1979). Variable ratio or variable frequency reinforcement schedules seem to work best.

Modern computer technology holds forth great possibilities for speech testing with children. We envision a video monitor that shows a set of four to six pictures representing words in a child's vocabulary (preferably, but not necessarily spondees) using a touch-screen procedure. The child would hear the word and be encouraged to touch the picture it represents. This would be followed by a short display of pictures and graphics exciting to the child. An incorrect response, of course, would not be reinforced. We are certain that these kinds of devices are merely waiting in the wings and will be available before long to be used in testing young children.

Many children can cooperate sufficiently to yield a reliable SRT, even when pure-tone results are not available. As a matter of fact, there are children who offer very accurate SRTs who give either no or spurious responses to pure tones. This being the case it is often useful when a conductive hearing loss is suspected or when bone-conduction thresholds are near the limit of the equipment (making it difficult to discern auditory from vibrotactile responses) to obtain SRTs by bone conduction in addition to air conduction.

If the SRT and pure-tone average do not agree it must be concluded that one or both of these measurements is incorrect, unless there is some explanation based on such findings as sharply falling audiograms. Although we are never certain that we are correct when we measure hearing in children we can feel more secure when two tests that use two different kinds of stimuli agree.

## Word Recognition Tests

Tests of word recognition are considered part of the basic audiometric examination of adults and have been a part of the basic test battery since audiology got its start in the 1940s. Unfortunately, many professionals and nonprofessionals believe that word recognition scores represent the actual percentage of speech that is discriminated by an individual in normal listening situations. For this reason there is danger in telling people their scores unless the audiologist is certain that this fact is understood.

Furthermore, we have observed that a significant number of people perceive their word recognition scores to be their percentage of hearing impairment, a concept we believe should not be conveyed to parents. Word recognition tests are clinical exercises that bear *some* resemblance to the degree to which patients discriminate speech in the real world. The variables are so manifold as to make these scores look far better or worse than the ways in which patients understand speech in different kinds of listening situations.

Despite this caveat, we continue to believe in the value of word recognition tests as a general guide to understanding a patient's auditory communication difficulties. While a number of tests are available for adults, the use of phonetically balanced (PB) word lists has historically been the most popular for clinical purposes (Martin et al., 1994). Adult PB word lists can frequently be used with children who simply respond to each word as it is presented at a comfortable sensation level (usually 30 to 40 dB above the SRT). This type of

test is called an open-message response test because the word said by the patient can be selected from any possibility.

For many children adult PB word lists are inappropriate because the words are not in their vocabularies. Haskins (1949) developed a set of word lists called PBKs, the "K" standing for kindergarten, that are appropriate for children of this age group. The test is performed and responded to as with adults, and the number of correctly repeated monosyllabic words is converted to a percentage to yield the word recognition score.

Open-message response tests are not appropriate for all children. This is true for some because they lack the ability to give oral responses, for others because they are unwilling or too shy, and for still others because their speech production is so poor that responses cannot be discriminated. For this reason, a number of closed-message response tests have been developed for children, including the Northwestern University Children's Perception of Speech (NU-CHIPS) test (Katz and Elliot, 1978), the Pediatric Speech Intelligibility test (Jerger and Jerger, 1982), the Discrimination by Identification of Pictures (DIP) test (Siegenthaler and Haspiel, 1966), the Auditory Numbers Test (ANT) test (Erber, 1980), and the Word Intelligibility by Picture Identification (WIPI) test (Ross and Lerman, 1970). The interested reader is encouraged to pursue the references cited above for more information on these procedures.

These tests are all similar in that they use a closed-response set with a picture-pointing paradigm. The word is delivered to the child, who searches a page containing colored pictures or line drawings whose labels rhyme (more or less), and then points to the picture. As stated earlier in the discussion of SRT tests, we envision a future test in which computers present the stimulus words along with their pictures, which are responded to on a touch screen. The computer can then advance to the next test word after storing a "correct" or "incorrect" in its memory.

The WIPI is the most popular test in use for children (Martin and Gravel, 1989). It requires two clinicians or a clinician and an assistant. Although there are tape-recorded versions of the WIPI that are commercially available[1] most clinicians prefer to use monitored live voice. The audiologist presents the words to the child, preferably through earphones, otherwise through the sound-field system. The carrier phrase "Show me ____" is used before each word. The assistant sits before the child with a book containing six pictures whose labels rhyme. The child is encouraged to point to the picture that corresponds to the word that was heard and notation is made of whether the response was correct or incorrect. Four of the six pictures on each page are test items, with the other two being foils to decrease the probability of a correct guess. The test is comprised of twenty-five picture sets so that each word has a value of 4 percent. Keeping track of the incorrect responses that were selected can further help to identify auditory confusion.

For children with no ability to recognize speech, clinicians can use the Sound Effects Recognition test (SERT) (Finitzo-Hieber, Gerling, Cherow-Skalka, and Matkin, 1980), which is a recording of environmental sounds that the child is asked to recognize. This is far from the discrimination of speech sounds but is useful when nothing else is available for use with a child.

Word recognition scores should be obtained on children whenever possible. They are useful in a variety of ways and should be pursued on future examinations when children cannot complete them on initial testing. When children are enrolled in auditory-aural programs, continued hearing testing, including attempts at finding word recognition scores, should be an ongoing enterprise. As with all tests with children, word recognition scores require audiologists who use persistence, ingenuity, and kindness.

## PSEUDOHYPACUSIS

The literature lacks incidence figures on the numbers of children with pseudohypacusis who are

[1]Auditec of St. Louis

seen by audiologists. We believe that the numbers may be larger than one might suppose. Some of the reasons why children fabricate or exaggerate hearing losses are not difficult to understand. It is likely that a child who is disposed to feign any kind of physical disorder has had the opportunity to observe that this can be a self-serving behavior. Some children are siblings of children who are truly hearing impaired and may be jealous of the extra attention given them. Other children may have attention focused on their hearing by erroneous failure of a school hearing test that brings them extra attention or sympathy. Such secondary gains can be persuasive for the child who makes a conscious effort to pretend to have a hearing loss.

Detecting nonorganic hearing loss in children should not be difficult in most cases. Children lack the insights required of the sophisticated malingerer. Lying appears to be a skill we hone as we get older when we think it will get us our way. An initial tip-off to pseudohypacusis is often a discrepancy between the SRT and the pure-tone average at 500, 1000, and 2000 Hz. We have even seen children who give no responses to pure tones until near the limits of the equipment and a normal SRT. Other children are much better at deceiving the audiologist.

The reader is doubtless familiar with tests for pseudohypacusis that are used with adults, many of which can be modified for children. The Yes-No test of Frank (1976) is done by asking children to say "Yes" when they hear a pure tone and "No" when they do not. The child who malingers will often say "No" every time a tone is presented, even below the suprathreshold level the child selects. It often works amazingly well.

There are times when children can be more skillful than described in this case report. This situation, as in all situations encountered when dealing with children, takes skill and tact on the clinician's part. There may be times when children must be tested using one of the electrophysiologic procedures described in Chapter 7. The challenge is often more what to say to the parent/caregivers who may have taken time from work or other duties and gone through the trouble and expense of escorting the child to the audiologist. They may not be kindly disposed to learning that this all may have been a "trick" played on them by their child to meet a certain need.

Audiologists, in situations as the one described above, must first determine the true hearing levels of the child and then act as advocates for that child. Certainly if the child initially presents with a hearing loss suggestive of pseudohypacusis, and normal hearing can be demonstrated, the parents must learn the truth of the hearing status, but can be spared some of the details. Just as careful wording and cajoling can enlist the cooperation of children, so can it work with the accompanying adults, by telling them, in the child's presence, that the hearing was normal while sparing them the gory details of how that was determined. The child learns that the clever scheme that was hatched did not work, and the adults are relieved to learn that their child is OK.

Even when we have determined hearing to be within normal limits, a child may return for a retest after failing a subsequent test at school. When it becomes apparent that a child is not relinquishing the feigned hearing loss, the audiologist should suspect that something in the child's life is at the root of this attention-seeking behavior. Posttest questioning of the parents of one child we worked with revealed the parents were newly married. It became apparent through the ensuing discussion that the child had lost the "only child" status she had enjoyed while her mother was single. Raising the parents' consciousness of the impact of this lifestyle change resulted in greater attention to the child and some time alone with the mother during this transition. Once this happened, the child began to pass the school hearing tests.

## REPORTING TEST FINDINGS

Too often, audiologists report test findings with little regard for the needs of those who may receive the reports. As discussed by DeConde Johnson (1994), reports that only state audiometric findings provide little on the implications that a child's hearing loss may have on instructional

and listening situations. Recommendations on amplification, preferential seating, and the need for follow-up testing are far from enough.

Audiologic reports of behavioral hearing test findings must provide habilitation specialists and educators with specific implications of the hearing loss in concrete and functional terms. Discussions of such factors as the impact of background classroom noise, resultant fatigue from attempts at visual compensation for the hearing loss, and what high-frequency consonant sounds may still be missed even with amplification, are glaringly omitted from most reports. Suggestions for more useful report writing and for classroom teaching modifications to help compensate for the limitations of amplification are provided in Appendices 5 and 9.

## DEVELOPMENTALLY DELAYED CHILDREN

Hearing loss among children with developmental delays may go undetected as the child's behaviors of auditory inattention may be attributed to the more overtly visible handicap. While a high percentage of children with developmental disability may have cognitive impairments as well, many have normal or greater than normal intelligence. However, children with any congenital anomaly are more likely to have a second concomitant disorder, perhaps less obvious or severe, than someone who does not have the first disorder (Lloyd and Young, 1969).

Developmental disability, as defined in Public Laws 94-103 and 95-602, refers to those with severe or chronic disability secondary to mental or physical impairments resulting in substantial functional limitations to life activities. This may include such disorders as mental retardation, cerebral palsy, epilepsy, or autism, and hearing loss is frequently seen as a disability that coexists with any of these. Visual impairments are also a frequent second disability, not only among those with multiple handicaps, but also among children whose only disabling condition appears to be hearing loss. For this reason audiologists must seek assurance of normal visual functioning for all children with impaired hearing. The identification of co-existing visual impairment in a child with hearing loss may further help identify what often remains an elusive etiology. In addition to visual impairment or hearing loss, children with developmental disabilities may have neuromuscular disorders, seizure disorders, and stereotypy, which is a rhythmic and repetitive movement that lacks any apparent adaptive significance (Young, 1994). Physiologic measures of hearing as discussed in Chapter 7 provide a dimension to the evaluation of difficult-to-test patients that was not available in the past. However, whenever possible, these measures should be used as a crosscheck to the results of behavioral assessment and not as a substitute. The ambiguous results of physiologic measures of hearing unfortunately increase with increased central nervous system involvement, thereby increasing the value of any behavioral results that may be obtained.

Audiologists evaluating children with developmental disabilities through behavioral techniques must be continually ready to alter their test paradigm to accommodate the needs of a given child, just as with the child who exhibits normal development. The response sought from the child clearly must be appropriate for the child's cognitive and neuromuscular abilities. When testing profoundly disabled children, it may be necessary, as discussed earlier, to rely on the auditory reflexes, localization responses, and changes in the child's activity state. The audiologist is wise to seek advice from the parent or caregiver on what the child with a neuromuscular disorder is capable of and what position may be most conducive to voluntary control and hence an observable and interpretable response (Young, 1994). Certainly the adult in attendance should be asked if the child is subject to seizures arising from photic stimulation. Such cases clearly preclude the use of visual reinforcers with flickering lights.

Responses from children who are profoundly multidisabled appear more reflexive than representative of true attention behaviors (Flexer and

Gans, 1985). Responses obtained are best evaluated in the context of the child's developmental rather than chronological age. Hearing may be considered normal if the development of auditory responses is generally consistent with the age level of the child's other developmental behaviors.

This judgment becomes more difficult if the child's cognitive and developmental ages have not yet been determined. As with young children, positive response behaviors can indicate the level of a child's hearing, but the absence of response is not indicative of hearing impairment. As when testing any young child, when testing those with developmental disabilities the audiologist should proceed as if any response may be the last. Therefore, it is always important during behavioral evaluations to begin with that deemed most important. Because the frequency range centered around 2000 Hz is often viewed as most critical to speech recognition, we recommend starting here. Severe neurologic, motor, and sensory problems preclude a description of hearing thresholds across the frequency range in each ear. As Gans and Gans (1993) point out, the primary goal in testing children with profound multidisabilities is to rule out moderate to profound hearing impairment between 500 and 2000 Hz.

The autistic-like behaviors that lead some children to avoid eye contact and reject physical interactions with others yields a general disregard to all speech signals that may be employed during testing. If the child's hearing is normal, startle responses and APRs should be elicited at expected levels. Some of these children will also search for sounds presented in the sound field, although the sound that may be of interest is impossible to predict. Generally, the less frequency-specific the sound the greater the interest, which correspondingly decreases the usefulness of the response.

Children who present with self-stimulatory behaviors (head swaying, body rocking, finger flicking, etc.) present a true challenge to the audiologist as these children are typically unaware of their environments when preoccupied with their own repetitive movements, especially if these movements are accompanied by vocalizations (Young, 1994). Young notes that the audiologist may try to calm more disruptive stereotypic acts while not confining the lessor ones because restraint may result in an increase in such behavior upon release.

Any child with developmental disabilities whose handicap does not preclude the conditioning of a voluntary and consistent response to sound can generally be assessed with tests used in the evaluation of nonhandicapped children of similar mental age. Modification permitting greater reinforcement for the listening task can be quite helpful. For example, pairing the hand delivery of an edible response with the dropping of a block during play audiometry can greatly help to keep the mentally challenged on task during an evaluation. TROCA can be used successfully with many of these children as well.

Working with children who have developmental disabilities presents a unique challenge to any pediatric audiologist. Every effort should be made to obtain as much hearing test data as possible. As with all children, the greater the degree of information on the status of the auditory system, the more successful intervention planning becomes.

## SUMMARY

A number of different kinds of tests are described in this book, ranging from what appear to be crude attempts at distracting children with sounds to sophisticated electrophysiological procedures. Testing is never completed until a pure-tone audiogram has been accomplished along with, when possible, speech audiometric results. When these test results are not obtainable from a child, other procedures should be used that may approximate a child's hearing sensitivity but these are stopgap measures requiring future hearing tests. Any audiologist who works with small children has an obligation to take both testing and follow-up management very seriously—audiology offers no greater challenge and no greater responsibility.

## REFERENCES

American Speech-Language-Hearing Association. (1978). Guidelines for manual pure-tone audiometry. *Asha, 20:*297–301.

Bench, J. (1970). The law of initial value: A neglected source of variance in infant audiometry. *International Audiology, 9:*314–322.

DeConde Johnson, C. (1994). Educational consultation: Talking with parents and school personnel. In J. G. Clark and F. N. Martin (eds.), *Effective Counseling in Audiology: Perspectives and Practice* (pp. 184–209). Englewood Cliffs, NJ: Prentice Hall.

Dix, M. R., Hallpike, C. S., (1947). The peep show: A new technique for pure tone audiometry in young children. *British Medical Journal, 2,* 719–723.

Eisenberg, R., Coursin, D., and Rupp, N. (1966). Habituation of an acoustic pattern as an index of differences among human neonates. *Journal of Auditory Research, 6,* 239–248.

Eisenberg, R., Griffin, E., Coursin, D., and Hunter, M. (1964). Auditory behavior in the human neonate: A preliminary report. *Journal of Speech and Hearing Research, 7:* 245–269.

Erber, N. (1980). Use of the auditory numbers test to evaluate speech perception abilities of hearing-impaired children. *Journal of Speech and Hearing Disorders, 45,* 527–532.

Finitzo-Hieber, T., Gerling, I., Cherow-Skalka, E., and Matkin, N. (1980). A sound effects recognition test for the pediatric audiological evaluation. *Ear and Hearing, 1,* 271–276.

Flexer, C. and Gans, D. (1985). Comparative evaluation of the auditory responsiveness of normal infants and profoundly multihandicapped children. *Journal of Speech and Hearing Research, 28,* 163–168.

Frank, T. (1976). Yes-no test for nonorganic hearing loss. *Archives of Otolaryngology, 102,* 162–165.

Froding, C. (1960). Acoustic investigation of newborn infants. *Acta Otolaryngologica, 52,* 31–40.

Gans, D. and Gans, K. D. (1993). Development of a hearing test protocol for profoundly involved multi-handicapped children. *Ear & Hearing, 14:*2, 128–140.

Guilford, F. R., and Haug, C. O. (1952). Diagnosis of deafness in the very young child. *Archives of Otolaryngology, 55,* 101–106.

Haskins, H. (1949). *A Phonetically Balanced Test of Speech Discrimination for Children.* Unpublished master's thesis, Northwestern University.

Hodgson, W. R. (1987). Tests of hearing: The infant. In F. N. Martin (ed.). *Hearing Disorders in Children* (pp. 185–216). Austin: Pro-ED.

Jerger, S. and Jerger, J. (1982). Pediatric speech intelligibility test: Performance intensity characteristics. *Ear and Hearing, 3,* 325–334.

Katz, D., and Elliot, L. (1978). Development of a new children's speech discrimination test. Paper presented at American Speech and Hearing Association Convention, San Francisco, Ca.

Lloyd, L. L., Spradlin, J. E., and Reid, M. J. (1968). An operant audiometric procedure for difficult-to-test patients. *Journal of Speech and Hearing Disorders, 33,* 236–245.

Lloyd, L. L., and Young, C. E. (1969). Pure-tone audiometry. In R. T. Fulton and L. L. Lloyd, (eds.), *Audiometry for the Retarded with Implications for the Difficult to Test.* Baltimore: Williams & Wilkins, 1–31.

Martin, F. N., Armstrong, T. W., and Champlin, C. A. (1994). A survey of audiological practices in the United States. *American Journal of Audiology. 3,* 20–26.

Martin, F. N., and Coombes, L. (1976). A tangibly reinforced speech reception threshold procedure for use with small children. *Journal of Speech and Hearing Disorders, 41,* 333–338.

Martin, F. N., and Gravel, K. L. (1989). Pediatric audiological practices in the United States. *The Hearing Journal, 42,* 33–48.

Martin, F. N., and Mussell, S. A., (1981). The influence of syllabic stress on children's thresholds for speech. *Journal of Auditory Research, 21,* 105–108.

Ross, M., and Lerman, J. (1970). A picture identification test for hearing impaired children. *Journal of Speech and Hearing Research, 13,* 44–53.

Siegenthaler, B., and Haspiel, B. (1966). Development of two standardized measures of hearing for speech by children. Co-operative Research Program Project No. 2372, United States Office of Education, Washington, DC.

Suzuki, T., and Ogiba, Y. (1961). Conditioned orientation reflex audiometry. *Archives of Otolaryngology, 74,* 84–90.

Weaver, N. J., Wardell, F. N., and Martin, F. N. (1979). Comparison of tangibly reinforced speech-reception and pure-tone thresholds of mentally retarded children. *American Journal of Mental Deficiency, 83,* 512–517.

Young, C. V. (1994). Developmental disabilities. In J. Katz (ed.). *Handbook of Clinical Audiology* (4th ed., pp. 521–533) Baltimore: Williams & Wilkins.

# CHAPTER 7

# PHYSIOLOGIC MEASURES OF AUDITORY AND VESTIBULAR FUNCTION

*CRAIG A. CHAMPLIN*

## INTRODUCTION

The auditory system is like a railway. Beginning with the outer ear, the metaphorical train carries sonic passengers from station to station until they reach the brain. For one to hear properly, it is essential that the train remain on the track and run on time. If something untoward happens (e.g., a pathological condition, a traumatic accident, etc.), rail traffic may be partially or totally disrupted.

This chapter focuses on the assessment of auditory and vestibular function in children using acoustic immittance, otoacoustic emissions, auditory evoked potentials, and electronystagmography. The first three clinical methods were designed to evaluate that portion of the railway devoted to hearing. Specifically, immittance reveals the status of the middle ear station, otoacoustic emissions yield information about the inner ear (cochlear) station, and auditory evoked potentials indicate whether the various stations in the central nervous system are working normally. The fourth physiologic approach, electronystagmography, was developed to assess the railway branch line that deals with balance. The main point of this analogy is that because auditory information is transmitted serially, what happens at one station can have a significant impact on the activity at other stations up the line. For example, a problem at the middle ear station will affect the assessment of the inner ear station even though there may be nothing wrong with the inner-ear station per se. The four physiologic measures overlap somewhat, and this mutual dependence must be kept in mind when applying these tests.

The chapter is divided into four sections. Each section contains background material, a general overview of the technique, and a description of how that technique may be applied to the evaluation of children. Emphasis is placed on the *process* rather than on the nuances associated with specific cases. Thorough treatment of a particular technique can be found in the various review articles and chapters that are cited in each section.

## IMMITTANCE

### Background

Although the sensory cells of hearing are located in the inner ear, the structures of the outer and middle ear play a role in transmitting sound to the cochlea. The outer ear is accessible and its status can be directly determined via otoscopy. Conversely, the middle ear can only be evaluated indirectly because it is sealed off from the outside world by the tympanic membrane. Immittance measures include those tests designed to assess the status of the middle ear (Jerger, 1975; Feldman and Wilber, 1976). Because the middle ear is part of an important reflex system, immittance measures also provide information regarding the integrity of certain neural pathways in the brainstem (Silman, 1984; Northern and Gabbard, 1994).

Acoustic immittance refers to the application of sound to a mechanical system and then measuring how much sound energy is either absorbed (acoustic admittance) or reflected (acoustic impedance) (Popelka, 1984; Van Camp, Margolis,

Wilson, Creten, and Shanks, 1986). Acoustic admittance is the reciprocal of acoustic impedance; therefore, only one of these quantities is required to adequately describe a system's behavior. This section focuses on acoustic impedance because it is the most widely used clinical measure.

In mechanical systems, two vector quantities—resistance and reactance—determine the system's impedance. The resistive quantity consists of purely frictional forces and is not affected by the frequency of the sound source. The reactive quantity is made up of two opposing (additive) factors—mass and compliance. The relative contribution of mass or compliance to reactance depends on the frequency of the sound (e.g., Shanks, 1984). Specifically, the effect of mass increases with an increase in frequency, while the effect of compliance decreases with an increase in frequency. Resistance and reactance combine vectorally to determine a system's impedance.

The middle ear, bounded laterally by the tympanic membrane and medially by the oval window of the inner ear, consists of three small bones that are delicately suspended by ligaments and tendons. The middle ear is a mechanical system, and thus has an impedance. The frictional contribution to impedance comes primarily from the ossicles rubbing together and the resistance offered by the ligaments (Lilly, 1973). The mass of the tiny bones provides the mass contribution, while the compliance contribution comes mainly from the fluid load of the inner ear (Lilly, 1973). Remember that acoustic impedance depends on the stimulus frequency. For example, if a low-frequency tone (e.g., 226 Hz) is introduced, the acoustic impedance of the middle ear will be comprised of both resistive and reactive-*compliance* components. The effect of mass is not revealed because mass reactance is negligible at low frequencies. Conversely, a high-frequency tone (e.g., 2260 Hz) will reveal the effects of resistance and *mass* reactance. The compliance effect is minimal in this condition. Most clinical devices employ a single, low-frequency tone, thus the impedance measurements are said to be compliance-dominant.

To measure the acoustic impedance of the middle ear, a small probe is hermetically sealed in the external auditory canal. Contained within the probe are a miniature loudspeaker that serves as the sound source, a miniature microphone that monitors the sound-pressure level in the canal, and a manometer that is connected to a pump that applies a positive or negative air pressure to the canal. Sound-pressure level in the external ear canal is directly related to acoustic impedance. The impedance, and therefore the sound-pressure level in the canal, can be manipulated pneumatically using the pump or by causing the middle ear muscles to contract. The two clinical procedures associated with changing the impedance of the middle ear are known as tympanometry and acoustic reflex measures, respectively.

**Tympanometry**

In tympanometry, acoustic impedance is measured as the air pressure in the external auditory canal is varied. Sufficient positive or negative pressure effectively immobilizes the tympanic membrane at its maximum inward or outward position. The reduced mobility associated with either of these positions produces relatively high acoustic impedance. When the air pressure in the canal of a normal ear is equalized (i.e., returned to atmospheric pressure), the middle ear system moves easily and the acoustic impedance is lower. The graph in which acoustic impedance or compliance is plotted as a function of air pressure is known as the tympanogram. A tympanogram obtained from a normal ear is shown in Figure 7.1A. Use the scale on the left side of the graph for adults and the right side for infants. The apex or peak in the function indicates the point of least acoustic impedance or greatest compliance. Obtaining tympanograms from a group of healthy ears yields normative data as indicated by the solid lines.

The pressure peak appears in the tympanogram because the air pressure in the external ear canal has been balanced against the air pressure in the middle ear cavity. The air pressure in the cavity is controlled by the eustachian tube. This tube, which leads to the back of the throat, is normally closed. It opens briefly when a need to equalize the pressure in the middle ear is detected. If the eustachian tube is not allowed to open because the

surrounding tissues are inflamed, respiration of cells within the middle ear causes the pressure to decrease or become negative with respect to the ambient air pressure, which, in turn, causes the tympanic membrane to retract. The pressure peak

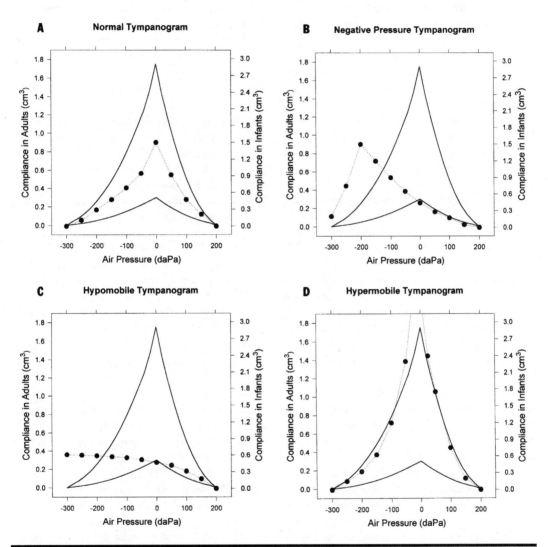

**FIGURE 7.1**   Sample tympanograms depicting (*A*) normal middle ear function; (*B*) negative middle ear pressure; (*C*) hypomobile (or flat) tympanogram suggesting the presence of middle ear fluid, and (*D*) hypermobile tympanogram consistent with a flaccid tympanic membrane or disarticulated ossicular chain. The left ordinate is used when testing adults or children older than 24 months of age, and right ordinate when testing infants who are 0 to 24 months old. Note that the ordinate scale depends on the type and brand of measurement device used. Solid lines indicate the boundaries of normal middle ear function.

in the tympanogram shifts in the direction of negative pressure. Negative pressure is of diagnostic significance because it often indicates the onset of otitis media. A tympanogram from an ear with negative pressure is plotted in Figure 7.1B.

It is possible to summarize the tympanogram as a single number. This value, known as static compliance, is obtained by subtracting the acoustic impedance measured when the tympanic membrane is "tight" (i.e., positive air pressure) from the acoustic impedance measured when the tympanic membrane is "loose" (i.e., at the point of maximum compliance). When the values from Figure 7.1 are referred to the right ordinate, this subject's static compliance is about 1.5 cm$^3$. Note that acoustic impedance and static compliance are inversely related.

Middle ear pathology causes the acoustic impedance to either increase or decrease relative to the normal system. Consider two illustrative cases, one toward each end of the impedance continuum. With otitis media, fluid produced by the epithelial cells lining the middle ear cavity accumulates. Impedance increases (compliance decreases) due to the added pressure exerted by the fluid, thus the tympanic membrane is *hypo*mobile. As shown in Figure 7.1C, a distinct peak in the tympanogram is not present and static compliance is less than normal. It is important to note that as the disease process associated with otitis media runs its course, the tympanogram has a series of distinct phases. At the onset of otitis media, the pressure peak is in a normal position. As the disease progresses, the pressure peak shifts in the negative direction, its amplitude decreases, and finally becomes indiscernible (hypomobile tympanogram). The sequence is reversed during recovery: no peak—negative pressure peak—normal peak.

With an ossicular disarticulation where the stapes has been completely fractured, impedance decreases (compliance increases) because the load of the cochlear fluids has been removed. Figure 7.1D reveals that the peak in the tympanogram is exaggerated and that static compliance is greater than normal. This condition results in a hypermobility, which is also seen in flaccid tympanic membranes.

For the most part, the two examples just discussed represent the range of abnormal tympanometric outcomes. However, in each of those cases, a low-frequency tone (226 Hz) was used. Low-frequency tympanometry provides useful diagnostic information about disorders of the tympanum (middle ear pressure or effusion), tympanic membrane (tympanosclerosis, scarring, perforation, retraction), and the eustachian tube (Lilly, 1984). However, low-frequency tympanometry is relatively insensitive in detecting lesions of the ossicular chain (otosclerosis, fracture or discontinuity, congenital malformation) (Lilly, 1984). To gain complete information on the status of the middle ear, measurements of both reactive components are necessary; therefore, multifrequency tympanometry is recommended.

## Acoustic Reflex Measurements

The stapedius muscle is connected by way of the stapedial tendon to the neck of the stapes. The acoustic reflex pathway consisting of the auditory nerve (cranial nerve VIII), the cochlear and superior olivary nuclei of the brain stem, and the facial nerve (cranial nerve VII) enables both stapedius muscles to contract when one or both ears are stimulated with an intense sound. The contraction causes the ossicular chain to stiffen, and acoustic impedance increases, or conversely, compliance decreases. The usual procedure for measuring the acoustic reflex involves stimulus presentation in steps of increasing intensity until the reflex is evoked. This intensity is known as the acoustic reflex threshold (ART), and in normal-hearing individuals the ART ranges from about 70 to 100 dB HL.

It is possible to measure the ART in the ear that receives the stimulus. The presence of the uncrossed or ipsilateral reflex suggests that the afferent and efferent neural pathways on the probe (i.e., measurement) side of the head are intact. Alternatively, the crossed or contralateral reflex is evaluated when one ear is stimulated and the ART is measured in the opposite ear. The presence of the crossed reflex indicates that the afferent pathways opposite the probe and the efferent pathways on the same side as the probe are intact. It is necessary to measure crossed and uncrossed reflexes in both ears to completely evaluate the integrity of the reflex pathways. Finally, when testing newborns, it is important to note that the probe tone must be greater than 800 Hz to observe the acoustic reflex (Bennett and Weatherby, 1982).

Reflex decay refers to the relaxation of the stapedius muscle over time. In normal ears, this effect is due to neural adaptation and occurs when the stimulus is continuous and contains frequencies above 1000 Hz (Borg, 1976). The rate of reflex decay is of diagnostic value. Specifically, an abnormally rapid rate of decay indicates a retrocochlear lesion.

A recent application of the acoustic reflex focuses on the detection of hearing impairment. This technique is based on two characteristics of the ART. First, in persons with normal hearing sensitivity, the ART for broadband noise is about 15 dB lower than the average ART obtained with tones at 500, 1000, and 2000 Hz (Popelka, Margolis, and Wiley, 1976). This difference is reduced or eliminated in persons with sensorineural hearing loss. Second, the ART is elevated relative to normal when a tone is presented in a frequency region of impaired hearing. When these characteristics are used together and the hearing loss exceeds 30 dB HL, it is possible to detect hearing losses in adults with a sensitivity and specificity greater than 90 percent (Margolis, 1993). (See Chapter 5 for further discussion of sensitivity and specificity of screening measures.) Although sufficient data have not been collected on children, preliminary results suggest that this technique may prove to be an efficient and accurate means for screening infant hearing.

### Neonates and Infants

The immittance results for infants less than approximately 1 month of age warrant special consideration. If immittance testing is performed

soon after birth, amniotic fluid may still be present in the baby's middle ear. In this case, tympanometry will reveal reduced compliance. The condition typically resolves spontaneously in a few days, and thus does not require medical intervention. However, it is likely that this baby will fail one of the newborn hearing screening techniques that is discussed later in this chapter and in greater detail in Chapter 5. Postponing the screening until after the middle ear has cleared is recommended.

Besides the flat tympanogram, another pattern often observed in neonates is the double-peak tympanogram. The peaks occur around –50 and +50 daPa (dekapascals) with a clear notch in between. The double-peak pattern is not due to the presence of fluid, but rather reflects the flaccidity of the newborn's tympanic membrane. This pattern is considered normal, and only appears when a low-frequency tone is used (Sprague, Wiley, and Goldstein, 1985).

The neonate's external ear canal is also very pliable. If the ear canal and/or the tympanic membrane are more compliant than more medial structures of the middle ear, a normal-looking tympanogram may be obtained even though a pathologic condition is present. This possibility has important diagnostic implications. For example, a normal tympanogram and absent acoustic reflexes could mean that the newborn has a middle ear problem that probably can be corrected or an inner ear or neural problem that cannot.

### Summary

Immittance (impedance or admittance) tests, including tympanometry and acoustic reflex measures, provide information on the status of the middle ear in children. This information is useful for three reasons. As discussed in Chapter 3, hearing loss associated with middle ear problems can interfere with the acquisition of normal communication skills and if left unattended, middle ear disease can lead to more serious and potentially life-threatening complications (e.g., meningitis). Finally, the interpretation of the tests described in subsequent sections requires that middle ear status be known.

# OTOACOUSTIC EMISSIONS

## Background

Otoacoustic emissions (OAEs) are low-level sounds that are generated in the cochlea, but can be recorded in the external ear canal using a sensitive microphone. Although the mechanisms underlying OAE production are not completely understood, they are believed to be manifestations of the motile response of the outer hair cells (OHCs) (Brownell, 1990). The function of the OHCs is to affect the mechanics of the cochlea in such a way that absolute sensitivity and frequency tuning are enhanced (Davis, 1983). This dependence on intact OHCs suggests that OAEs may provide an indirect means for evaluating cochlear status (Norton, 1993).

There are basically two classes of OAEs. Spontaneous otoacoustic emissions (SOAEs) are narrow-band signals that occur in the absence of external stimulation. They are usually inaudible, ranging in amplitude from –10 to 25 dB SPL (Zurek, 1981; Wier, Norton, and Kinkaid, 1984). SOAEs are present in neonates; therefore, it is unlikely that they are the consequence of pathological or traumatizing agents (Strickland, Burns, and Tubis, 1985). Because SOAEs are found in about half of normal human ears, their clinical usefulness is limited.

Evoked otoacoustic emissions (EOAEs) occur following acoustic stimulation. EOAEs are found in virtually all persons who have normal hearing sensitivity. The main types of EOAEs are transient and distortion-product. A third type, stimulus frequency emissions, has received relatively little attention due to the sophisticated equipment that is required to obtain them. This classification scheme merely reflects the properties of the stimulus; it is not known whether the EOAE types are generated by the same cochlear processes or independent ones.

## Transient Evoked Otoacoustic Emissions

Transient evoked otoacoustic emissions (TEOAEs) are typically elicited with brief acoustic pulses known as clicks, although short-duration tones are also used. The sound-pressure level of any resultant emission is recorded in the external ear canal for about 20 ms following each click. Time-domain averaging improves the signal-to-noise ratio of the recording. In order to separate the TEOAE from stimulus-related artifacts, a differential stimulus set is often used (Bray and Kemp, 1987). The stimulus set consists of four stimuli— three positive pulses that are equal in amplitude and a fourth negative pulse that is three times larger in amplitude. A subaverage consisting of responses to the four stimuli is formed, and because the stimulus polarity is inverted, the artifact is canceled. This technique, known as the "nonlinear" stimulus method, also reduces the amplitude of the TEOAE by a factor of two, but this small loss is rarely of practical significance (Kemp, Ryan, and Bray, 1990).

Two TEOAE waveforms obtained from a 4-year-old boy are shown in Figure 7.2. The clicks were presented at a peak sound pressure level of 80 dB using the nonlinear method. The first 2.5 ms have been zeroed out to remove the stimulus artifact. Although the waveform pattern varies considerably from person to person, it is very repeatable for a given individual. In fact, replicability is used as a criterion for detecting TEOAEs. Assume that a TEOAE has both signal (i.e., stimulus-related energy generated by the cochlea) and noise (i.e., random, non-stimulus dependent activity) components. Now consider the correlation coefficient derived from two hypothetical waveforms. A value of 1 would indicate a pure signal with no noise present while a value of 0 would indicate noise only, with no signal. The correlation is directly related to the signal-to-noise ratio. Kemp and colleagues (1990) recommend that the correlation coefficient exceed 0.50 before a TEOAE is considered present. The value obtained for the two waveforms in Figure 7.2 is 0.98, which suggests the presence of a strong

**Transient Otoacoustic Emission Waveform**

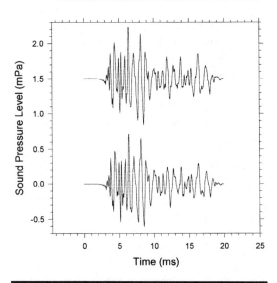

**FIGURE 7.2** Transient otoacoustic emission waveforms successively obtained under identical stimulus conditions from a 4-year-old male. The stimulus, an 80-microsecond click, was delivered at 80-dB peak SPL using a nonlinear mode of presentation. The first 2.5 ms were zeroed to remove stimulus artifacts. The top waveform has been displaced vertically by 1.5 mPa to show replicability.

emission and presumably a healthy cochlea (i.e., intact OHCs).

The correlation coefficient indicates the replicability of the entire waveform. Using digital filtering, the reproducibility of individual frequency bands also can be measured (Kemp and Ryan, 1993). The cochlea is systematically laid out according to frequency. Therefore, knowing whether a TEOAE is present, based on the correlation derived from the band-limited waveform, provides place-specific information on cochlear status. The TEOAE in Figure 7.2 was analyzed using bandpass filters centered at 1, 2, 3, 4, and 5 kHz; each band was 1000 Hz wide. The correlation coefficients are all greater than 0.95. Applying the presence-absence criterion of 0.50 reveals that, in this case, a TEOAE is present in each of the five

frequency regions. This type of analysis allows information to be gained on the slope of the hearing loss. For example, had a high-frequency sensorineural loss been present, the correlation associated with the high-frequency bands would have been lower.

The overall amplitude of the TEOAE in Figure 7.2 is 20.1 dB SPL. However, a number of factors are known to affect TEOAE amplitude. One factor is the intensity of the stimulus. Although TEOAE amplitude increases with intensity, the rate of growth is nonlinear (Norton and Stover, 1994). At low and moderate levels, TEOAE amplitude increases at a rate of about 0.5 dB/dB, while at high levels the growth rate is less, about 0.2 dB/dB (Kemp et al., 1990). Another factor that influences TEOAE amplitude is the status of the middle ear. Because OAEs are propagated from the cochlea via the ossicles to the ear canal, these structures must be working properly for an emission to be detectable. For example, the amplitude of the TEOAE will be reduced if there is fluid in the middle ear cavity. A third factor that affects TEOAE amplitude is the presence of a sensorineural hearing loss. Amplitude decreases as the amount of hearing loss increases up to 40 to 50 dB HL. Emissions are not typically observed if the loss exceeds this amount (e.g., Norton, 1993). A final factor that controls TEOAE amplitude is the age (or the ear canal size) of the patient. TEOAEs measured in infants are approximately 10 dB higher than those obtained from adults (Norton and Widen, 1990). This could be due to the fact that infants have smaller ear-canal volumes (infants = 0.7 $cm^3$ versus adults = 1.4 $cm^3$, or about a 6-dB effect). It is also possible that infants have more efficient middle ear systems or more powerful cochlear generators. Given that several factors influence TEOAE amplitude, it is not a particularly good predictor of absolute sensitivity.

TEOAE data have been analyzed using frequency-domain methods. One such technique is illustrated in Figure 7.3. The cross-power spectrum derived from the waveform is indicated by the solid line. The power spectrum of the noise, based on the difference of the two waveforms, is indicated by the dotted line. A TEOAE is considered present when the solid line exceeds the dotted line by 3 dB. In this example, although the amplitude does vary somewhat across frequency, the TEOAE is present from 500 Hz to 6000 Hz. A high-pass filter (cutoff frequency = 500 Hz) attenuated the low-frequency noise caused by blood flow, breathing, and slight movements by the patient. Although zeroing out the first 2.5 ms helped reduce the stimulus artifact, it also removed emission-related energy above 6000 Hz. The emission amplitude at a given frequency is believed to reflect the status of the cochlea at a particular place. Therefore, it is worth noting that had a high-frequency hearing loss been present, the energy in that frequency region would have been noticeably reduced.

## Distortion-Product Otoacoustic Emissions

Because the cochlea is essentially a nonlinear device, it has long been known that presenting two external tones (F1 and F2, where F2 is greater in frequency than F1) causes numerous additional tones to be generated in the inner ear. These supplemental tones are known as distortion products and when recorded in the ear canal they are called distortion-product OAEs (DPOAEs) (Kemp, 1979). The largest of the DPOAEs is the cubic difference tone (CDT). The frequency of the CDT is equal to two times F1 minus F2, and the frequency of F2 is typically 1.2 times that of F1 (Harris, Lonsbury-Martin, Stagner, Coats, and Martin, 1989). The two tones are presented continuously at equal levels. Time-domain averaging is performed, but relatively few (8–32) samples are required to obtain a detectable DPOAE. The DPOAE (i.e., the CDT) obtained from a 2-month-old girl is shown in Figure 7.4. The frequencies of F1 and F2 are 2000 Hz and 2400 Hz, respectively; therefore, the frequency of the CDT is 1600 Hz [(2000 × 2) – 2400]. The level of the primaries is 75 dB SPL, and the amplitude of the CDT is about 15 dB SPL.

It is believed that the CDT is generated at the cochlear place that corresponds to the geometric mean of the two primaries and then propagates apically (Brown and Kemp, 1984; Martin, Probst, Scheinin, Coats, and Lonsbury-Martin, 1987). Further, the amplitude of the CDT is assumed to reflect the cochlear status at the generator site (Smoorenburg, 1972). By changing the frequency of the primaries while maintaining a fixed frequency ratio and a constant primary level, it is possible to obtain CDTs from various regions in the cochlea. Figure 7.5 illustrates the "DPOAE audiogram" (Lonsbury-Martin, McCoy, Whitehead, and Martin, 1993). The circles connected by the solid line represent the amplitude of the CDT obtained at various frequencies. The dotted line shows the noise floor of the system. A number of factors contribute to the fact that the noise floor is not perfectly flat. These include head noise (low frequency), various ear resonances (mid-frequency), and microphone insensitivity (high frequency). A DPOAE is considered present at any frequency where the solid line exceeds the dotted line by at least 3 dB. Note that unlike TEOAEs, the ampli-

**Transient Otoacoustic Emission Spectrum**

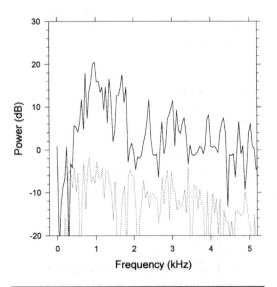

**FIGURE 7.3** Amplitude spectra of a transient otoacoustic emission (*solid line*) and accompanying noise (*dotted line*).

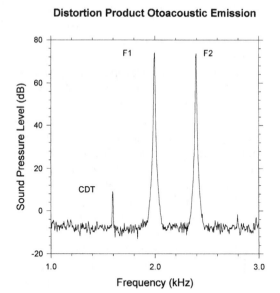

**Distortion Product Otoacoustic Emission**

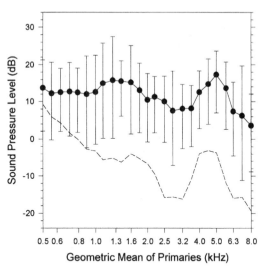

**DPOAE Audiogram**

**FIGURE 7.4**   A distortion product otoacoustic emission as revealed by the cubic difference tone (CDT). Also shown are the two primary tones, F1 and F2.

**FIGURE 7.5**   Audiogram of the distortion product otoacoustic emission (*solid circles, solid line*) and noise (*dotted line*) obtained from a 4-year-old male. Errors bars indicate the 95% confidence interval. The overall level of the primary tones was 75 dB SPL. The F2/F1 ratio was 1.2.

tudes of DPOAEs between infants and adults are not markedly different (e.g., Lonsbury-Martin et al., 1994). The infants', however, are generally noisier (Prieve, 1992). The average level of the noise floor measured in infants is about 5 dB higher than that of adults (Lonsbury-Martin et al., 1995).

It is also possible to compare an individual patient's results to normative data. The error bars in Figure 7.5 indicate the 95 percent confidence interval based on data obtained under similar stimulus conditions from a group of fifteen normal-hearing adults. Any point lying between the error bars is within two standard deviations of the mean, and normal cochlear function is predicted in that frequency region.

Rather than sweeping the primaries through a specified frequency range, it is also possible to fix the primary frequencies and vary their levels. The graph showing the change in CDT amplitude as a function of primary level is known as the input-output (I-O) function. A typical I-O function is indicated by the circles and the solid line in Figure

7.6. The frequencies of F1 and F2 were 1825 and 2195 Hz, respectively. The dotted line shows the noise floor. The error bars indicate the 95 percent confidence interval based on normative data. The variables of interest for the I-O function are the slope, dynamic range, and DPOAE detection "threshold" (Lonsbury-Martin et al., 1993).

At the present time, it is not known whether the DPOAE audiogram or the I-O function will ultimately be the most useful to the clinician. More than likely, each of these measures will provide helpful information, and it will be the evaluation context that dictates which one is measured.

## Applications of Otoacoustic Emissions in Children

A prerequisite of normal auditory function is an intact cochlea, and TEOAEs and DPOAEs both can be used to evaluate cochlear status. Other features of evoked emissions are that (1) active par-

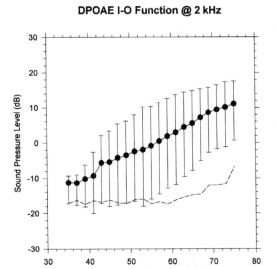

**DPOAE I-O Function @ 2 kHz**

**FIGURE 7.6** Input-output (I-O) function of the distortion product otoacoustic emission (*solid circles, solid line*) and noise (*dotted line*). Errors bars indicate the 95% confidence interval. The geometric mean of the primary tones was 2000 Hz. The F2/F1 ratio was 1.2.

ticipation by the patient is not required; (2) subject preparation is noninvasive and minimal; (3) measurement time is brief, about 5 minutes per ear; and (4) the data are reliable both within and across sessions. These characteristics make EOAEs a logical and attractive choice for assessing auditory function in children.

### Hearing Screening

The main goal of any hearing screening program is to identify children with hearing loss. There are several working definitions on what constitutes a "pass" or a "fail." In the Rhode Island Hearing Assessment Project (White, Vohr, and Behrens, 1993), 1850 infants were initially screened using the TEOAE technique described by Bray and Kemp (1987). The screening results were classified as pass, partial pass, or fail. A pass was assigned if the signal power exceeded the noise power by 3 dB in each of three frequency bands

(1–2, 2–3, and 3–4 kHz). A partial pass was given if a signal was present in one or two bands. A fail was assigned if no signal was present in any band. The partial passes and failures were subsequently grouped into a "refer" category. Using these categories, follow-up evaluation with evoked potential and behavioral tests revealed that the specificity and sensitivity of the TEOAE procedure were 81 percent and 100 percent, respectively (White et al., 1993). (See Chapter 5 for further discussion of sensitivity and specificity of screening measures.) These values are consistent with those reported by Stevens, Webb, Hutchinson, Connell, Smith, and Buffin (1990) whose criterion for passing was an interwave correlation of 0.50 or greater. To summarize the TEOAE screening performance, nearly one infant in five who failed the screening ultimately was found to have normal hearing. All infants whose hearing loss (conductive or sensorineural) was confirmed were successfully identified with TEOAEs.

Although comparatively few babies have been screened with DPOAEs, the DPOAE audiogram appears to be the measurement of choice for screening purposes. Lafreniere, Smurzynski, Jung, Leonard, and Kim (1993) have developed specific pass/fail criteria for the DPOAE test. Based on the data from the ears of thirty-one normal infants (ages 2–4 days), a failure was defined as three (or more) consecutive CDT amplitudes that fell below the tenth percentile of the normative group. Using this definition or others, it is anticipated that sensitivity and specificity data will soon be available for the DPOAE screening procedure.

Regardless of whether TEOAEs or DPOAEs are used, the ease and rapidity with which an emission screening is performed has lead to the suggestion that every baby should be tested. In the past, only those infants who were at risk for hearing loss were screened (for high-risk factors, see Table 5.1, page 103, this text). This strategy successfully identified most youngsters with hearing loss in the at-risk category. The problem was that the nonrisk infants were not screened, and a significant number (about 50 percent) of children with sensorineural loss was missed (White et al., 1993). While it remains to be determined whether universal screening is economically feasible, the fact is that high-risk registers are inadequate in their coverage of the pediatric population with potential hearing problems. Further discussion of universal screening of newborns is presented in Chapter 5.

*Monitoring Changes in Cochlear Status*
As mentioned previously, evoked emissions in normal ears are very stable over time. Certain kinds of medications, however, are toxic to sensory cells in the inner ear (see discussion in Chapter 4), and damage to these cells causes a reduction in the amplitude of the emission. The drugs that are potentially the most ototoxic include antimicrobials (aminoglycosides, e.g., mycin group drugs), analgesics (salicylates [e.g., aspirin]), loop diuretics (furosemides [e.g., Lasix]), and antiarrhythmics (quidinine sulfate [Quidinex]) (White and Regan, 1987). While these agents must be administered to control disease or other medical conditions, the side effect of permanent cochlear damage needs to be monitored. Obtaining EOAEs before drug therapy is initiated then again at regular intervals during the course of treatment can alert medical personnel that cochlear status and, therefore, hearing sensitivity, is changing. Given that EOAE tests require no patient cooperation, they are excellent measures for monitoring the early effects of ototoxic medications in children.

Intense sounds also can produce irreversible damage to structures in the cochlea. Another possible monitoring application would be to obtain EOAEs from relatively young children before they receive substantial noise exposure. For example, "baseline" EOAEs could be acquired from all kindergarten-age children. Measurements obtained in subsequent years could then be compared to the baseline. If a significant reduction in EOAE amplitude was noted, the child would be required to participate in a hearing conservation education program.

Because the basal end of the cochlea is predisposed to the effects of both ototoxicity and intense sounds, a reduction in the EOAE amplitude is usually first seen in the high-frequency components. Technical limitations associated with TEOAEs restrict their measurement to frequencies below 5 kHz (Kemp et al., 1990). Conversely DPOAEs are recordable to at least 8 kHz (Lonsbury-Martin et al., 1990). Therefore, it is entirely possible that monitoring applications will be better served by DPOAE measurement.

*Site-of-Lesion Testing*
Because otoacoustic emissions are generated by the OHCs, they are considered "sensory" responses. Evoked potentials, on the other hand, reflect the integrity of structures in the central nervous system; they are considered "neural" responses. In the past, a hearing loss associated with a lesion in the cochlea and/or central auditory pathways has been known as a sensorineural loss. Today, the potential exists to provide more specific site-of-lesion information. For example, the following combinations of test results and diagnostic classifications are possible: abnormal EOAE—"sensory" hearing loss; abnormal evoked potential (e.g., auditory brain stem response)—"neural" hearing loss; and, if both EOAE and evoked potential were abnormal—"sensorineural" hearing loss. The ability to separate sensory from neural losses in children, especially those with multiple disabilities, may lead to earlier and more effective medical intervention and habilitation.

*Evaluating Pseudohypacusis*
Occasionally, a child's auditory behavior is not consistent with the results of a standard hearing test. One explanation for the discrepancy is that auditory thresholds have been consciously (or unconsciously) exaggerated. Children may feign a hearing loss for a variety of reasons such as to gain attention, to provide a reason for poor school performance, or because a deeper psychological problem exists (Martin, 1994). Recall that EOAEs are not a measure of hearing per se. However,

they can be used to quickly rule out moderate to profound cochlear losses in youngsters who do not cooperate for behavioral tests.

### Assessing Middle Ear Function

As mentioned previously, the middle ear system must be functioning normally for an EOAE to be detectable. While I am not advocating that EOAEs be performed in lieu of immittance testing, emissions measurements may complement the traditional procedures for evaluating middle ear function (Prieve, 1992). In the section on immittance, it was noted that the neonate's ear canal and tympanic membrane are highly compliant. It is possible, therefore, to obtain a normal tympanogram even though fluid is present in the middle ear. Performing an EOAE (either TEOAE or DPOAE) test would be useful in this case because the presence of fluid would reduce (particularly in the low frequencies) or eliminate the EOAE.

Additionally, emissions could be used as an objective indicator of the transmission characteristics of the middle ear. This information would be particularly helpful when evaluating the success of medical treatment or a surgical procedure (Owens, McCoy, Lonsbury-Martin, and Martin, 1992).

Returning to the issue of hearing screening, it may not be absolutely necessary to do both immittance and EOAE tests on a given neonate. Because EOAEs are affected by the status of the middle ear, perhaps immittance testing would only need to be performed on those infants who failed the EOAE screen. Moreover, EOAEs appear to have the potential to identify babies who are at risk for middle ear diseases such as otitis media (Maxon, White, Vohr, and Behrens, 1993; Lonsbury-Martin, et al., 1995).

### Summary

Otoacoustic emissions provide information on the status of the cochlea, and the outer hair cells in particular. Transient and distortion-product OAEs are the most widely used types of OAEs because they can be obtained from virtually anyone who

has normal or near-normal absolute sensitivity. Likely applications of OAE measurements in children include hearing screening, monitoring cochlear status, site-of-lesion testing, evaluating pseudohypacusis, and corroborating tests of middle ear function.

## AUDITORY EVOKED POTENTIALS

### Background

Auditory evoked potentials (AEPs) are measurable neuroelectric responses that occur following the presentation of sounds (Davis, 1976; Hall, 1992). The AEP waveform represents auditory nervous system activity from the eighth cranial nerve to the cortex, and, therefore, can provide information on the function of the pathways within this system. In children, AEPs are mainly used to determine hearing status and to evaluate the functional integrity of auditory neural pathways.

To acquire the AEP, electrodes are attached to the head (e.g., scalp and ear lobes), and stimuli are presented via earphones or a bone vibrator. The typical stimulus is a click or brief tone burst. All electrical activity picked up by the electrodes is recorded for a specified time immediately after each stimulus presentation. The stimuli are repeated many times and the response to each stimulus is added to previously obtained responses to yield an averaged response. Averaging is essential in order to differentiate the small AEP from the background noise (i.e., ongoing electrical activity that is not time-locked to the stimulus). Supplemental techniques that are used to facilitate AEP detection include differential amplification, artifact rejection, and band-pass filtering. The child must remain still during the AEP recording. Children younger than 6 to 9 months of age will normally sleep if they have just been fed, have a fresh diaper, and are tired. Older children may require sedation (e.g., chloral hydrate) if there is not sufficient time to wait until they fall asleep naturally.

As many as fifteen individual components have been identified in the human AEP waveform. These "peaks" are traditionally classified on the basis of latency or the time when they appear relative to the onset (or offset) of the stimulus. Although there are several classification systems, I prefer the one described by Picton, Hillgard, Krausz, and Galambos (1974). According to their scheme, the early components have latencies of 10 ms or less and are collectively known as the auditory brain stem response (ABR). The middle components have latencies between 10 and 50 ms and are referred to as the middle-latency response (MLR). The components having latencies between 50 and 500 ms are known as the long-latency response (LLR). Because latency reflects the "travel time" through the auditory nervous system, each latency category is *loosely* associated with gross anatomical structures. Møller (1994) suggests that the ABR reflects neural activity in the eighth cranial nerve and brain stem, the MLR is generated in the midbrain and the cortex, and the LLR originates from various cortical sites.

Of the three AEPs, the ABR is by far the most widely used with children. There are two reasons for this. First, the ABR appears at an earlier age than either the MLR or the LLR. A general rule of neurologic development is that the peripheral structures mature more rapidly and become functional sooner than central ones. Because the ABR emanates from relatively peripheral loci, it is the first AEP to emerge in the infant. Second, unlike the MLR or the LLR, the ABR is not affected by the subject's state of consciousness. Satisfactory ABRs may be obtained regardless of whether the child is sleeping naturally, sedated, or awake and resting quietly. Although there are important applications for the MLR and LLR in the pediatric population, the popularity of the ABR suggests that I focus on it.

## Auditory Brain Stem Response

For the purpose of illustration, an ABR waveform obtained from a 6-year-old girl is plotted in Figure 7.7. The stimulus was an alternating polarity click that was presented at 70 dB nHL (nHL refers to the average hearing level for normal-hearing listeners). The seven positive peaks are identified

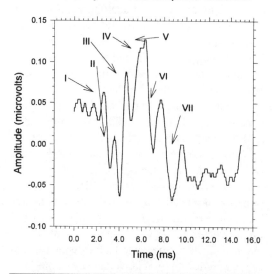

**Auditory Brainstem Response Waveform**

**FIGURE 7.7**   Auditory brain stem response from a 6-year-old female. Individual components are indicated with Roman numerals. An acoustic delay of 0.9 ms was introduced by the insert earphone. Absolute latency (in ms) for each positive peak are in parentheses: wave I (2.61), wave II (3.57), wave III (4.61), wave IV (5.88), wave V (6.31), wave VI (7.71), and wave VII (9.60). Relative latencies (in ms) are 2.00, 1.70, and 3.70 for interpeak intervals I-III, III-V, and I-V, respectively.

with Roman numerals (I–VII). Each peak has an absolute latency and amplitude. It is also possible to compare the absolute value of one peak to that of another. Such measures are known as either relative latency or relative amplitude. Normative data for both latency and amplitude are collected from groups of age-matched individuals of both sexes to establish criteria for clinically significant abnormality. Because latency is more stable than amplitude both within and between recording sessions, it is of greater diagnostic significance (Stockard, Stockard, Westmoreland, and Corfitts, 1979). Further, applications related to hearing status tend to focus on absolute latency, while those related to neurologic integrity typically emphasize relative latency.

In children, the ABR becomes essentially adult-like by two years of age (Gorga, Kaminski, Beauchine, Jesteadt, and Neely, 1989). The ABR waveform in infants differs from the adult pattern in that three peaks (I, III, and V) are usually discernible (Starr, Amlie, Martin, and Sanders, 1977), and the absolute latencies are longer (Schulman-Galambos and Galambos, 1975). The three or four additional peaks found in the adult ABR gradually appear as the brain stem structures develop. Although the absolute latencies decrease with increasing age, the rate of change is not the same for all components of the ABR. Over a given period of time, the latency of wave V decreases much more rapidly than does the latency of wave I (Gorga et al., 1989). One consequence of the differential change in absolute latency is that a concomitant reduction in relative latency occurs. The fact that the absolute latency in young children decreases as a function of age underscores the need to establish age-specific norms. It is recommended that normative data be collected by week during the preterm period, biweekly between term and 3 months, by months until 24 months, and by decades in children over 2 years of age (Jacobson and Hall, 1994).

Another factor that affects the ABR is the intensity of the stimulus. With decreasing intensity, all peaks in the ABR exhibit increases in absolute latency and decreases in absolute amplitude. It is useful to show these trends graphically, where the ordinate is absolute latency (or absolute amplitude) of a given ABR component (e.g., wave V) and the abscissa is stimulus intensity. Such a graph is known as an intensity-latency (or intensity-amplitude) function and will be described in more detail later.

## Evaluating Hearing Status

The ABR is not a measure of hearing per se, but it can provide useful information on hearing loss without active participation by the subject. From an audiologic perspective, the four factors needed to describe a hearing loss are the affected ear, type, magnitude, and slope of loss. Determining the affected ear requires that each ear be selectively stimulated. This is readily accomplished with standard or insert earphones. There are at least three advantages to using insert earphones when testing children (Berlin and Hood, 1987). One advantage is that insert earphones provide greater interaural attenuation than standard earphones. With insert earphones the acoustical energy is distributed over a relatively small area that effectively increases the isolation between the ears, thereby reducing the need for masking. A second advantage is that the opportunity for collapsing ear canals is minimized. Because the cartilaginous portions of the outer ear are extremely pliable in newborns and infants, pressure exerted by placing a standard earphone against the head can cause the external auditory canal to collapse temporarily and become occluded. Occluding the ear canal can lead to the erroneous diagnosis of conductive hearing loss. A third advantage of insert earphones is that the transducer can be positioned approximately 21 cm from the head. This distance imposes an acoustical delay of about 0.9 ms, which makes it easier to separate the stimulus artifact from the neural response.

The type and amount of hearing loss are obtained from the intensity-latency (I-L) function. Recall that as the intensity of the stimulus decreases, the latency of the ABR peaks increases. Figure 7.8 shows a normal I-L function and functions for two different hearing losses. The solid circles represent the I-L function from a 3-month-old infant with normal hearing sensitivity. The dotted line represents the average wave V latency based on a large group of normal subjects; the error bars indicate the 95 percent confidence interval (Gorga et al., 1989). There are two features of interest. The first one is the slope of the function. With a conductive or retrocochlear loss the I-L function parallels the normal one, but is shifted rightward by the amount of the loss (see the open circles). With a cochlear loss the function is steeper than normal, and may converge to within normal limits at high intensities (see the open triangles).

## Intensity-Latency Function

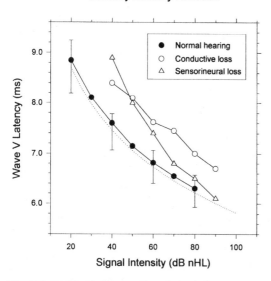

**FIGURE 7.8** Intensity-latency functions are shown for three children, each about 3 months of age—one with normal hearing (*solid circles, solid line*), one with a mild conductive loss (*open circles, solid line*), and one with a mild sensorineural loss (*open triangles, solid line*). The dotted line and the error bars represent the mean and two standard deviations, respectively based on normative data from Gorga, M. P., Kaminski, J. R., Beauchine, K. L., Jesteadt, W., and Neely, S. T. (1989), Auditory brainstem response from children three months to three years of age: II. Normal patterns of response. *Journal of Speech and Hearing Research, 32,* 281–288.

It is not always possible to determine the type of loss from the I-L function. For example, a high-frequency sensorineural loss often yields a function that parallels the normal one, and thus may be mistaken for a conductive loss. There are two ways to minimize this error—obtain immittance measures and stimulate via bone conduction (Schwartz, Larson, and DeChicchis, 1985). Performing immittance measures will indicate whether the outer and middle ear are operating normally. An important exception occurs in the neonate, whose highly compliant tympanic membrane may

hide a conductive loss and the presence of fluid in the middle ear. The relationship between the I-L function obtained via bone conduction and the one acquired via air conduction (i.e., using earphones) determines the type of hearing loss. The loss is likely conductive if the two functions do not overlap and sensorineural if they do. As an application note, the bone vibrator should be placed on the mastoid, rather than the forehead, when testing babies. Because the bones of the infant skull are not yet rigidly connected, the frontal (forehead) and temporal (inner ear) bones are decoupled, which results in less effective stimulation with forehead placement (Berlin and Hood, 1987).

The second feature of the I-L function is the "threshold" or lowest intensity at which a response is detected. When evaluating hearing status, ABRs are acquired in a series of decreasing intensity steps. The sensitivity of the ABR procedure typically will not tolerate a step size smaller than 10 dB; however, efficiency considerations may dictate the use of somewhat larger steps. The physiologic threshold is defined as that point midway between the lowest intensity at which a response is observed and the highest intensity at which a response is not detected. The physiological threshold then provides a rough approximation of the magnitude of the hearing loss. It should be noted that the physiologic threshold obtained with the ABR does not correspond exactly to the one that is measured behaviorally. Cooperative, well-trained subjects can detect the presence of a series of clicks at a lower intensity than is revealed by the physiologic technique. Specifically, the behavioral threshold for clicks is typically 10–20 dB lower than the ABR threshold (Coats and Martin, 1977). If hearing status is to be based on the behavioral threshold, it is necessary that the physiological threshold be "corrected" or adjusted in some way. Jerger and Mauldin (1978) have suggested multiplying the ABR threshold by 0.6 to estimate behavioral threshold.

The final piece of information needed for diagnostic audiologic purposes is the configuration or slope of the hearing loss. Although a click has a broad amplitude spectrum, it tends to produce a maximal response in the mid-frequency region of the cochlea (Ozdamar and Dallos, 1976). Consequently, ABRs obtained with transient stimuli reflect the hearing status of the 2- to 4-kHz region. To gain information about the slope of the loss, a low-frequency threshold is needed, too. The problem is that it is difficult to evoke an ABR with frequency-specific stimuli and low-frequency tones, in particular. For a stimulus to be frequency-specific, it must be both long in duration and with an abrupt onset. Such stimuli cause relatively few neurons to discharge synchronously and the quality of the ABR is poor. One solution is to use a brief ($\leq$ 10 ms) tone burst with a rapid ($\leq$ 2 ms) rise time. The target frequency is usually 500 Hz. To ensure that high-frequency regions are not contributing to the response, it is recommended that either a high-pass (Kileny, 1981) or a notch-noise (Stapells, 1989) masker be presented to the same ear as the tone burst. A moderate-level (70–80 dB SPL) masker is generally sufficient.

In summary, the ABR can be used to detect the presence of hearing loss in children. If a hearing loss is found, the ABR can show which ear is affected and the type, magnitude, and slope of the loss. Although not as sensitive as behavioral methods, this physiologic technique is a safe, noninvasive means of evaluating the hearing status of those who may otherwise be untestable.

## Hearing Screening

For nearly two decades, the ABR has been the tool of choice for screening neonatal hearing (Shimizu, Walters, Proctor, Kennedy, Allen, and Markowitz, 1990). Typically, only those newborns who exhibit one or more of the risk factors for hearing loss are screened. As discussed in Chapter 5, this level of coverage misses a significant number of babies with hearing loss. Therefore, the current trend is toward screening all babies residing in neonatal intensive care units or even more dramatic, screening all newborns.

As is the case with any screening procedure, the objective is to quickly and accurately deter-

mine whether the infant responds to sound. Consequently, the ABR is acquired at one stimulus level (e.g., 35 dB nHL) using a fairly rapid presentation rate (e.g., 38.3 clicks/s) (Weber and Jacobson, 1994). Anywhere from 1000 to 2000 responses are averaged, so a single run takes 30 to 60 seconds under optimal conditions. For replicability purposes, two runs are performed on each ear.

A number of pass-refer (or fail) criteria have been used. In the Rhode Island Hearing Assessment Project, a "pass" was defined as a replicable wave V, obtained at 30 dB nHL, with a latency that fell within one standard deviation of the nursery norms for the infant's conceptual age (White et al., 1993). Using this criterion, the sensitivity and specificity of the ABR procedure were 94 percent and 89 percent, respectively.

The sensitivity and specificity of ABR screening methods are comparable to those found with otoacoustic emissions. A logical question is, which one should I choose? Presently, there are not sufficient data to adequately answer this question. It may be instructive, however, to outline the advantages and disadvantages of each procedure. There are three advantages of the ABR method. First, it has been around longer, and, therefore, the procedural details are well understood. In fact, the ABR method has been automated sufficiently that it can be administered by trained volunteers. Second, an obvious advantage of using volunteers is that the screening cost is reduced. Third, the integrity of auditory neural pathways rostral to the cochlea is assessed. There are two main disadvantages of the ABR method. First, electrodes must be applied, which takes time and may disturb a baby who is already asleep. Second, the ABR is most affected by stimulus energy in the 1000 to 4000 Hz range, thus is relatively insensitive to low-frequency hearing loss. The advantages and disadvantages of the otoacoustic emissions procedure are essentially opposite those of the ABR method. Besides the similarity in sensitivity and specificity, equipment costs are about the same for both methods, and most importantly, neither one actually measures hearing. The fact that the ABR and the otoacoustic emissions have somewhat different strengths and weaknesses makes it unlikely that either one will "win out" over the other. Rather, complementary usage, where the positive aspects of both techniques are exploited, appears to be the most effective strategy.

## Evaluating Neurologic Status

Assuming that the individual peaks in the waveform are loosely correlated with anatomic structures, the ABR can provide information on the integrity of the neural pathways. In a simple sense, the absolute latency of particular components of the ABR reflects the neural travel time through the auditory nerve and brain stem. The effect of a lesion is to increase the travel time. Further, the more distal the lesion, the greater the number of ABR components affected. This is because it is not possible to make up lost time. For example, a lesion in the upper brain stem may just delay the latency of wave V. However, a lesion in the lower brain stem may result in increased latencies of both waves III and V, while a lesion of the auditory nerve may cause the latencies of waves I, III, and V to be prolonged. It is important to note that the ABR does not provide information about neurological structures above the brain stem and possibly midbrain levels.

Relative measures are comparisons, thus the minimum number of components required to obtain a relative latency is two. Said another way, measuring an interpeak latency (IPL) requires that there be at least two, but preferably three (waves I, III, and V), identifiable peaks in the ABR. Recall that the amplitude of the ABR components is affected by the sensation level of the stimulus. Therefore, to facilitate the detectability of individual peaks, the stimulus must be presented 60 to 70 dB above the patient's absolute threshold. The presence of a moderate (or greater) hearing loss coupled with the output limitations of the equipment may preclude testing at this level. In such situations, alternative procedures such as electrocochleography (ECoG) may need to be undertak-

en. Briefly, ECoG is an AEP technique specifically designed to obtain a measurable wave I (Ferraro and Ruth, 1994). If wave V is present in the ABR and wave I is identifiable via ECoG, then the I-V IPL can be calculated.

The neurologic applications of the ABR in children are essentially the same as for those in adults. However, depending on the age of the child, complete information on hearing status may not be available. Therefore, it is important that immittance and bone-conduction ABRs be performed prior to obtaining the neurologic ABR. Specific neurologic applications include identifying space-occupying lesions (e.g., tumors), evaluating demyelinating diseases, and monitoring coma and brain death (Hecox, Cone, and Blaw, 1981).

## Other Auditory Evoked Potentials

As mentioned at the outset, other AEPs, such as the middle-latency response (MLR) and the long-latency response (LLR), have not been widely used in children because the neural generators of these responses may not be fully developed. Further, both AEPs are affected by the patient's state of consciousness, which may be difficult to control, especially in infants and young children. In the case of the LLR, it is also necessary that children be able to understand and follow instructions (i.e., they must have acquired language). These limitations notwithstanding, the MLR and LLR are capable of providing information on the integrity of the auditory nervous system above the level of the brain stem. Additionally, the so-called cognitive components of the LLR (e.g., P300) may yield valuable insights into the mechanisms underlying the "central auditory processing disorders" that are observed in older, school-aged children (Jirsa and Clontz, 1990; Musiek and Bornstein, 1992).

## Summary

Auditory evoked potentials provide information regarding the status of the peripheral and central auditory pathways. The ABR is the most widely applied AEP because it can be recorded in very young children including neonates. There are two primary applications for AEPs. One is evaluating hearing. The four parameters of hearing loss—ear affected, type, magnitude, and configuration—can be specified via AEPs. The other application is assessing neurologic integrity, where the presence of a lesion can be confirmed physiologically.

## VESTIBULAR ASSESSMENT

### Background

Dizziness is a broad term used to collectively describe a range of conditions including vertigo, lightheadedness, ataxia of gait, loss of equilibrium, and motion sickness (Rubin and Brookler, 1991; Tusa, Saada, and Niparko, 1994). One manifestation of these disorders is the loss of balance. The overall balance system consists of sensory (vestibular, ocular, and proprioceptive) and motor subsystems plus various neural pathways and integrative centers in the brain stem, cerebellum, and cortex. The peripheral components are functional at birth while the structures in the central nervous system require several years to completely develop (Balkany and Finkel, 1986).

The vestibular subsystem refers to the inner ear, the muscles that move the eyes, the control centers in the brain stem and cerebellum, and associated neural pathways. The vestibular portion of the inner ear consists of the saccule, utricle, and three semicircular canals. Like the cochlea, the sensory cells in each of these structures are hair cells. The effective stimulus for these hair cells is motion, which may take the form of linear or angular (rotatory) acceleration. Either kind of acceleration causes the hair cells to bend, which affects the discharge rate in the afferent nerve fibers. Bending the hair cells in one direction causes the rate to increase (an excitatory effect), while bending in the opposite direction produces a decrease in rate (an inhibitory effect). Additionally, a given head movement evokes an excitatory response in one ear and an inhibitory response in the other. The brain uses the imbalance in neural activity be-

tween the two ears to determine the direction of the movement.

The vestibular branch of the auditory nerve (cranial nerve VIII) connects the inner ear to the vestibular nuclei in the brainstem. Cranial nerves III and VI are also connected to the vestibular nuclei. These latter two cranial nerves are part of the oculomotor system, which controls the rotation of the eyes. A reflex arc exists between the ears and eyes so that stimulating the inner ear causes the eyes to move and thus maintain the point of fixation. The function of this reflex, and therefore the vestibular system itself, is to help maintain the head in an upright position and to coordinate eye movement.

The eye movements brought about by vestibular stimulation are known as nystagmus. Nystagmic eye movements are repetitive and may be primarily in the vertical or horizontal direction. Each cycle or "beat" of the nystagmus consists of a smooth, slow phase and a rapid, snap-back phase. The slow phase is mediated by the peripheral system, while the fast phase is controlled by centers within the cerebellum and cortex. Because the eye is polarized (i.e., the cornea is positively charged and the retina is negatively charged), it is possible to record voltage changes associated with eye movement using surface-applied electrodes positioned near each eye. An example of a nystagmus waveform is schematically shown in Figure 7.9. The slope of the slow-phase segment points to the right, thus the nystagmus is classified as right-beating.

### Electronystagmography

The clinical procedure in which nystagmus is monitored electrically as the vestibular system is stimulated in various ways is known as electronystagmography (ENG). The ENG procedure is probably the most widely used means of assessing the dizzy patient. It must be emphasized, however, that the ENG evaluation is never performed in isolation (Dickins and Graham, 1986). A medical history is required, paying particular attention to details related to the dizziness (e.g., onset, dura-

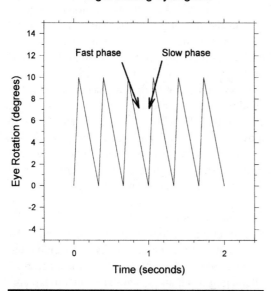

**Right-beating Nystagmus**

*Fast phase*    *Slow phase*

Eye Rotation (degrees)

Time (seconds)

**FIGURE 7.9**  Schematic nystagmus waveform. The slow and fast phases of one nystagmus cycle, or "beat," are shown. The nystagmus is right-beating.

tion, severity, etiologic factors, medications, traumatic incidents, presence of nystagmus, etc.). A physical examination is also necessary including otologic, head-neck, and neurologic examinations. An audiologic evaluation including the acquisition of auditory brain stem response should be performed. Various laboratory and radiographic tests also may be requested.

The ENG battery consists of a calibration followed by gaze, tracking, optokinetic, position, rotation, and caloric tests. Each test is designed to evaluate the function of a particular part of the vestibular system. The diagnostic questions that the ENG evaluation is capable of answering are the following: (1) Is there a lesion? (2) Is the lesion peripheral (i.e., inner ear and/or auditory nerve) or central? and (3) Is the lesion on the right or left side of the head? The adult ENG procedure can be successfully used with children over the age of 7 years. By this age children are cooperative and capable of understanding instructions.

Because complete descriptions of the ENG tests are provided elsewhere (e.g., Coats, 1986; Rubin and Brookler, 1991), only the essential details and special techniques used with children will be covered here.

Eye movements can be recorded using one channel (horizontal) or two channels (horizontal and vertical). A single channel will suffice for most pediatric cases. An advantage of the single-channel procedure is that it requires that only three electrodes be applied whereas the two-channel technique requires five electrodes. To record horizontal eye movements, a pair of small electrodes is placed just lateral to the outer canthus of each eye and a ground electrode is attached to the forehead. The voltage picked up by the electrodes is amplified, filtered, and directed to an output device (e.g., strip-chart recorder or computer system) for the purpose of plotting and analysis.

*Calibration or Saccade Test*

The variables of interest in ENG are the direction of nystagmus (e.g., left or right) and the magnitude (in degrees) of eye rotation. (The velocity of the eye movement may also be of interest and is defined as magnitude per unit time.) Obtaining accurate measurements requires that the equipment be calibrated. Calibrating the *direction* of eye rotation is accomplished by manipulating the input to the amplifier so that, for example, looking rightward produces an upward deflection at the output device. Calibrating the *magnitude* of eye movement involves adjusting the gain of the amplifier so that a specific amount of eye rotation corresponds to a given amount of deflection at the output device. This latter phase of calibration requires that the patient look back and forth between two fixation points that are subtended by an angle of known size (Coats, 1986).

Besides its implicit function, the calibration test is used to check the patient's ability to perform back-and-forth eye movements known as saccades (Stockwell, 1983). The waveform of normal saccades is essentially square or rectangular in appearance. (Filtering the wave may cause its corners to appear rounded.) Departures from this pattern include overshooting the target (hypermetric saccades), multi-step saccades, and one eye moving slowly while the other eye moves briskly. Abnormalities revealed during the calibration test are indicative of a central pathology of the brain stem or cerebellum.

### Gaze Test

In adults, the gaze test is an expanded version of the calibration test. The two tests differ in three ways: (1) The total amount of eye rotation is 2 to 3 times greater with the gaze test; (2) the gaze is maintained for 20 to 30 seconds; and (3) the patient must maintain a given gaze position with eyes open and with eyes closed. Additionally, the patient is requested to perform a mental task (e.g., counting forward or backward by two's) during the eyes-closed phase. The purpose of the eyes-closed-with-mental-task procedure is to prevent the suppression of nystagmus exerted by the control centers in the central nervous system.

Children may have difficulty both maintaining the gaze position and performing mental tasks. Consequently, the gaze test is often combined with the calibration test, and the eyes-closed phase is omitted. For example, Cyr (1980a) advocates using 20 degrees of eye rotation, rather than the more common value of 10 degrees, for calibration purposes.

At some point during the gaze test, the presence of spontaneous nystagmus is evaluated. Spontaneous nystagmus is defined as eye movements that are present in the absence of external stimulation. The patient is seated, looking straight ahead. A 20-second recording is obtained with eyes open and with eyes closed. If spontaneous nystagmus is suppressed by visual fixation (i.e., eyes open), it is likely the result of a peripheral vestibular lesion. Failure to suppress spontaneous nystagmus usually suggests a brain stem or cerebellar lesion. Congenital spontaneous nystagmus has a "spiky" appearance and may disappear or change directions with eyes closed.

### Tracking Test

The tracking test is a dynamic version of the gaze test. In the tracking test, the patient fixates on a small object, such as a tennis ball, as it is swung back and forth with a pendular motion. The extent of the excursions is 20 to 30 degrees. An alternative procedure for testing infants is to hold the child while gently rocking from side to side (Cyr, 1980a). In either case, the normal pattern of eye movement is smooth and sinusoidal. Step-like interruptions in the waveform are known as saccadic pursuits and suggest that a lesion exists in the central nervous system.

### Optokinetic Test

Optokinetic nystagmus is induced when a repetitive pattern is presented visually to an individual (Coats, 1986). The typical stimulus is a series of alternating black and white stripes that move unidirectionally across the visual field. The direction (right-to-left and left-to-right) and the speed (slow and fast) of the pattern are manipulated. Modifications for pediatric testing described by Cyr (1980b) include positioning the child's head inside a large, rotating drum that has vertical stripes on its inside wall. Alternatively, cartoon characters can be projected as a moving pattern on the wall of the room. Cyr (1980a) reports that it is possible to induce optokinetic nystagmus in infants younger than 4 months of age using these techniques.

In the normal patient, the nystagmus should change direction and remain symmetrical as the direction of the pattern is changed. Additionally, the frequency of the nystagmus (in beats per second) should increase with the speed of the stimulus. An abnormal optokinetic test suggests that a pathology exists in the central nervous system.

### Position Test

The purpose of the position test is to evoke nystagmus by changing the position of the head. The standard positions are sitting upright, supine, supine with right ear down, and supine with left ear down. Changing to a new position is undertaken in a slow, deliberate fashion so as to avoid the effects of movement. The presence of nystagmus during the position test is not normal. A peripheral lesion is likely if the nystagmus changes with changes in position; this result usually occurs when the patient's eyes are closed. A lesion in the central nervous system is probable if the nystagmus changes direction in a single position. The presence of nystagmus with eyes open also is indicative of a central lesion.

### Rotation Tests

Vestibular testing is also accomplished with children using the torsion-swing chair. The child sits alone or on an adult's lap. The chair rotates slowly in a 180-degree arc. Nystagmus is normally induced, and it changes direction as the chair swings back and forth. The number of nystagmus beats measured while rotating in one direction is compared to that obtained while swinging in the opposite direction. When the two directions are compared, a difference in the number of beats suggests the presence of a peripheral pathology, although it may be difficult to determine which side is affected (Cyr, 1980a).

A recent advance in rotational testing is slow harmonic acceleration (SHA) (Cyr and Beauchine, 1984). The chair is rotated sinusoidally at one of several different velocities (e.g., 0.01–0.64 Hz). The patient is in total darkness and is distracted by conversation or the performance of a mental task. The velocity of the eye movement is compared to the velocity of the head (Stockwell and Bojrab, 1993). A decrease in the relative velocity in one direction suggests a unilateral weakness while a decrease in both directions indicates a bilateral weakness. It is worth noting that SHA provides a more consistent stimulus than caloric irrigation, so responses are less variable (Stockwell and Bojrab, 1993). Further, SHA is more tolerable because, unlike caloric testing, it does not induce vertigo.

### Caloric Test

The purpose of the caloric test is to induce nystagmus by stimulating the lateral (horizontal) semicircular canal in one ear. Stimulation is brought about by irrigating the external auditory canal with water (air is also used) that is either slightly cooler or warmer than normal body temperature. The irrigation produces a localized temperature change in the affected ear, which causes the fluid in the semicircular canal to "flow." This flow bends the cilia of the hair cells, the neural discharge pattern is altered (increased with warm water, decreased with cool water), and the imbalance in neural activity is manifested as nystagmus.

An alternative to the water irrigation just described is the closed-loop system. With this method, a small balloon is positioned in the external auditory canal, and water is circulated through this water-tight system during irrigation. Compared to irrigating with water, the closed-loop system is neater and easier to control, and, therefore, better tolerated by children.

The complete caloric test requires that both ears are stimulated with warm (44° C) and cool (30° C) water, thus four irrigations are performed. The eyes are closed for the most part, although they are open for a brief period to determine whether the nystagmus can be suppressed. The nystagmus resulting from each irrigation is quantified, and two differences are calculated. The first difference is based on a comparison of the two ears after combining the temperature results. If the difference is sufficiently large (e.g., > 25 percent), a unilateral weakness is present. The presence of a significant unilateral weakness suggests that a lesion exists in the periphery on the weaker side. Finding that the responses from both ears are reduced relative to normative values indicates a bilateral weakness. The second difference is based on a comparison of the two temperatures after combining the results from the two ears. If this difference is significant (e.g., > 25 percent), a directional preponderance is present. A directional preponderance is nonlocalizing; that is, the lesion(s) could be in the peripheral or central parts of the vestibular system on the affected side.

Besides the blindfold and conversational distraction techniques that were previously mentioned for the positional tests, several alternative procedures have been developed for performing the caloric test on children. Balkany and Finkel (1986) suggest turning the infant over from stomach to back immediately following caloric stimulation. The normal response is for the nystagmus to reverse its direction with the change in position. Another technique is known as the simultaneous binaural bithermal caloric test (Brookler, 1976). With this test, both ears are irrigated at the same time with the same water temperature. No nystagmus or vertigo is induced if the two inner ears are equally responsive because a neural imbalance is not created (Cyr, 1980a). This situation is more tolerable to children than the dizziness that accompanies unilateral stimulation. It must be noted that a bilateral weakness cannot be detected with the simultaneous binaural caloric test.

## Postural Reflexes

Another approach to assessing vestibular function in children focuses on the evaluation of postural reflexes. As children mature, their gross motor capabilities become more sophisticated—progressing from rolling over, to sitting, to crawling, to standing, to walking, etc. Associated with each of these skills is a set of reflexive responses to postural change. Knowing when a given postural reflex is normally manifested allows the maturational level of the central vestibular system to be determined. It should be noted that although the observation of postural reflexes can provide useful information on vestibular function, the visual, proprioceptive, and vestibular systems are stimulated together. Thus, it may not be possible to partial out the relative contribution of each system and thereby localize the source of the balance disorder (Cyr and Beauchine, 1984). The evaluation of postural reflexes is generally the province of the occupational or physical therapist, and further discussion of the methodology is beyond the

scope of this chapter (for more information, see Eviatar and Eviatar, 1978).

## Causes of Dizziness in Children

Various factors can produce dizziness in children. The conditions that commonly result in an otologic and/or neurologic referral are categorized according to the site of lesion (i.e., peripheral or central) listed in Table 7.1. Complete descriptions of the symptoms and the management approaches associated with each condition can be found in Fried (1980), Balkany and Finkel (1986), and Tusa et al. (1994).

Two or more disorders may be simultaneously present, allowing for both peripheral and central manifestations. Further, dizziness may be classified as functional or psychosomatic when testing fails to reveal an organic source. Functional dizziness rarely occurs before school age (Balkany and Finkel, 1986). Finally, certain congenital conditions such as Joubert syndrome, Usher syndrome, Scheibe deformity, Mondini dysplasia, Arnold-Chiari malformation, Dandy-Walker cyst, and others may cause vestibular dysfunction and dizziness (Tusa et al., 1994).

**TABLE 7.1** Primary Causes of Dizziness in Children

**PERIPHERAL LESIONS**

Benign paroxysmal vertigo in children
Labyrinthitis
Labyrinthine fistula
Meniere disease
Otitis media
Ototoxic medications (e.g., streptomycin)
Traumatic incident
Vestibular neuritis

**CENTRAL LESIONS**

Brain stem—tumor or trauma
Cortex—tumor or trauma
Demyelinating disease
Meningitis
Migraine

## Summary

The balance system is complex, involving sensory, motor, and integrative components. Because of this complexity it is difficult to evaluate the entire system completely. The various tests in the ENG battery tap a portion of the overall system, and they are the most sensitive and reliable means for assessing balance disorders. Adaptations of the standard adult tests have been made so that even infants can be evaluated.

## OVERALL SUMMARY

The four physiologic methods described in this chapter allow a child's auditory and vestibular systems to be tested at various anatomic levels. Although each tool has certain limitations, these techniques generally do not require active participation by the patient, thus newborns and infants can be evaluated noninvasively. The primary implication of early auditory testing and diagnosis is that, if a problem is discovered, medical and/or nonmedical intervention can be provided sooner, which may help reduce the problem's impact on communication development and overall health. Early vestibular testing aids in the early diagnosis and subsequent management of balance disorders in children.

The four methods overlap somewhat in their scope of measurement. This is useful because it allows for cross-checking, that is, the findings from one test can be used to corroborate those from another. Further, each tool's diagnostic power is additive in the sense that two tests are better than one. These tools are meant to be used together rather than alone.

## REFERENCES

Balkany, T. J. and Finkel, R. S. (1986). The dizzy child. *Ear and Hearing, 7,* 138–142.

Bennett, M. J. and Weatherby, L. A. (1982). Newborn acoustic reflexes to noise and pure tone signals. *Journal of Speech and Hearing Research, 10,* 265–281.

Berlin, C. I. and Hood, L. J. (1987). Auditory brainstem response and middle ear assessment in children (Chap 5, pp. 151–184). In F. N. Martin (ed.), *Hearing Disorders in Children.* Austin: Pro-Ed.

Borg, E. (1976). Dynamic characteristics of the intra-aural muscle reflex (Chap. 11, pp. 236–299). In A. S. Feldman and L. A. Wilber (eds.), *Acoustic Impedance and Admittance: The Measurement of Middle Ear Function.* Baltimore: Williams & Wilkins.

Bray, P. and Kemp, D. T. (1987). An advanced cochlear echo technique suitable for infant screening. *British Journal of Audiology, 21,* 191–204.

Brookler, K. (1976). The simultaneous binaural bithermal: A caloric test utilizing electronystagmography. *Laryngoscope, 96,* 1241–1250.

Brown, A. M. and Kemp, D. T. (1984). Suppressibility of the 2f1-f2 stimulated emissions in gerbil and man. *Hearing Research, 13,* 29–37.

Brownell, W. E. (1990). Outer hair cell electromotility and otoacoustic emissions. *Ear and Hearing, 11,* 82–92.

Coats, A. C. (1986). ENG examination technique. *Ear and Hearing, 7,* 143–150.

Coats, A. C. and Martin, J. L. (1977). Human auditory nerve action potentials and brainstem evoked responses: Effect of audiogram shape and lesion location. *Archives of Otolaryngology, 103,* 605–622.

Cyr, D. G. (1980a). Vestibular testing in children. *Annals of Otology, Rhinology and Laryngology, 89,* Suppl. 74, 63–69.

Cyr, D. G. (1980b). Vestibular testing in children: Rationale, technique, and application. *Audiology: An Audio Journal for Continuing Education, 5,* 1–4.

Cyr, D. G. and Beauchine, K. A. (1984). The role of vestibular function in the development of communication (Chap. 7, pp. 127–138). In D. S. Beasley (ed.), *Audition in childhood: Methods of study.* San Diego: College-Hill Press.

Davis, H. (1976). Principles of electric response audiometry. *Annals of Otology, Rhinology and Laryngology, 85,* Suppl. 28, 4–96.

Davis, H. (1983). An active process in cochlear mechanics. *Hearing Research, 9,* 79–90.

Dickens, J. R. E. and Graham, S. S. (1986). Evaluation of the dizzy patient. *Ear and Hearing, 7,* 133–137.

Eviatar, L. and Eviatar, A. (1978). Neurovestibular examination of infants and children. *Advances in Otorhinolaryngology, 23,* 169–191.

Feldman, A. S. and Wilber, L. A. (1976). Introduction (Chap. 1, pp. 1–7). In A. S. Feldman and L. A. Wilber (eds.), *Acoustic Impedance and Admittance: The Measurement of Middle Ear Function.* Baltimore: Williams & Wilkins.

Ferraro, J. A. and Ruth, R. A. (1994). Electrocochleography (Chap. 5, pp. 101–122). In J. T. Jacobson (ed.), *Principles and Applications in Auditory Evoked Potentials.* Boston: Allyn and Bacon.

Fried, M. P. (1980). The evaluation of dizziness in children. *Laryngoscope, 90,* 1548–1560.

Gorga, M. P., Kaminski, J. R., Beauchine, K. L., Jesteadt, W., and Neely, S. T. (1989). Auditory brainstem responses from children three months to three years of age: II. Normal patterns of response. *Journal of Speech and Hearing Research, 32,* 281–288.

Hall, J. W. III. (1992). *Handbook of Auditory Evoked Responses.* Boston: Allyn and Bacon.

Harris, F. P., Lonsbury-Martin, B. L., Stagner, B. B., Coats, A. C., and Martin, G. K. (1989). Acoustic distortion products in humans: Systematic changes in amplitude as a function of f2/f1 ratio. *Journal of the Acoustical Society of America, 85,* 220–229.

Hecox, K., Cone, B., and Blaw, M. E. (1981). Brainstem auditory evoked responses in the diagnosis of pediatric neurological disease. *Neurology, 31,* 832–840.

Jacobson, J. T. and Hall, J. W. III. (1994). Newborn and infant auditory brainstem response applications (Chap. 13, pp. 313–344). In J. T. Jacobson (ed.), *Principles and Applications in Auditory Evoked Potentials.* Boston: Allyn and Bacon.

Jerger, J. (ed.). (1975). *Handbook of Clinical Impedance Audiometry.* Dobbs Ferry, NY: American Electromedics Corporation.

Jerger, J. F. and Mauldin, L. (1978). Prediction of sensorineural hearing level from the brainstem evoked response. *Archives of Otolaryngology, 104,* 456–461.

Jirsa, R. E. and Clontz, K. B. (1990). Long latency auditory event-related potentials from children with auditory processing disorders. *Ear and Hearing, 11,* 222–232.

Joint Committee on Infant Hearing (1991). 1990 Position Statement. *Audiology Today, 3,* 14–19.

Kemp, D. T. and Ryan, S. (1993). The use of transient evoked otoacoustic emissions in neonatal hearing screening programs. *Seminars in Hearing, 14,* 30–44.

Kemp, D. T., Ryan, S., and Bray, P. (1990). A guide to the effective use of otoacoustic emissions. *Ear and Hearing, 11,* 93–105.

Kileny, P. (1981). The frequency specificity of tone-pip evoked auditory brain stem responses. *Ear and Hearing, 2,* 270–275.

Lafreniere, D., Smurzynski, J., Jung, M., Leonard, G., and Kim, D. O. (1993). Otoacoustic emissions in full-term newborns at risk for hearing loss. *Laryngoscope, 103,* 1334–1341.

Lilly, D. J. (1973). Measurement of acoustic impedance at the tympanic membrane (Chap. 10, pp. 345–406). In J. Jerger (ed.), *Modern Developments in Audiology.* New York: Academic Press.

Lilly, D. J. (1984). Multiple frequency, multiple component tympanometry: New approaches to an old diagnostic problem, *Ear and Hearing, 5,* 300–308.

Lonsbury-Martin, B. L., Martin, G. K., McCoy, M. J., and Whitehead, M. L. (1995). New approaches to the evaluation of the auditory system and a current analysis of otoacoustic emissions. *Otolaryngology Head and Neck Surgery* 112: 50–63.

Lonsbury-Martin, B. L. McCoy, M. J., Whitehead, M. L., and Martin, G. K. (1993). Clinical testing of distortion-product otoacoustic emissions. *Ear and Hearing, 14,* 11–22.

Margolis, R. H. (1993). Detection of hearing impairment with the acoustic stapedius reflex, *Ear and Hearing, 14,* 3–10.

Martin, F. N. (1994). *Introduction to Audiology* (5th ed.). Englewood Cliffs, NJ: Prentice Hall.

Martin, G. K., Probst, R., Scheinin, S. A., Coats, A. C., and Lonsbury-Martin, B. L. (1987). Acoustic distortion products in rabbits. II. Sites of origin revealed by suppression and pure-tone exposures. *Hearing Research, 28,* 191–208.

Maxon, A. B., White, K. R., Vohr, B. R., and Behrens, T. R. (1993). Feasibility of identifying risk for conductive hearing loss in a newborn universal hearing screening program. *Seminars in Hearing, 14,* 73–86.

Møller, A. R. (1994). Neural generators of auditory evoked potentials (Chap. 2, pp. 23–46). In J. T. Jacobson (ed.), *Principles and Applications in Auditory Evoked Potentials.* Boston: Allyn and Bacon.

Musiek, F. and Bornstein, S. (1992). Auditory event-related potentials in central auditory disorders (Chap. 12, pp. 151–160). In J. Katz, N. A. Stecker, and D. Henderson (eds.), *Central Auditory Processing: A Transdisciplinary View.* St. Louis: Mosby-Year Book.

Northern, J. L. and Gabbard, S. A. (1994). The acoustic reflex (Chap. 21, pp. 300–316). In J. Katz (ed.),

*Handbook of Clinical Audiology.* Baltimore: Williams & Wilkins.

Norton, S. J. (1993). Application of transient evoked otoacoustic emissions to pediatric populations. *Ear and Hearing, 14,* 64–73.

Norton, S. J. and Stover, L. J. (1994). Otoacoustic emissions: An emerging clinical tool (Chap. 29, pp. 448–462). In J. Katz (ed.), *Handbook of Clinical Audiology.* Baltimore: Williams & Wilkins.

Norton, S. J. and Widen, J. E. (1990). Evoked otoacoustic emission in normal-hearing infants and children: Emerging data and issues. *Ear and Hearing, 11,* 121–127.

Owens, J. J., McCoy, M. J., Lonsbury-Martin, B. L., and Martin, G. K. (1991). Influence of otitis media on evoked otoacoustic emissions in children. *Seminars in Hearing, 13,* 53–65.

Ozdamar, O. and Dallos, P. (1976). Input-output functions of cochlear whole-nerve action potentials: Interpretation in terms of one population of neurons. *Journal of the Acoustical Society of America, 59,* 143–147.

Picton, T. W., Hillyard, S. A., Krausz, H. I., and Galambos, R. (1974). Human auditory evoked potentials: I. Evaluation of the components. *Electroencephalography and Clinical Neurophysiology, 36,* 179–190.

Popelka, G. R. (1984). Acoustic immittance measures: Terminology and instrumentation. *Ear and Hearing, 5,* 262–267.

Popelka, G. R., Margolis, R. H., and Wiley, T. L. (1976). Effect of activating signal bandwidth on acoustic-reflex thresholds. *Journal of the Acoustical Society of America, 59,* 153–159.

Prieve, B. A. (1992). Otoacoustic emissions in infants and children: Basic characteristics and clinical application. *Seminars in Hearing, 13,* 37–52.

Rubin, W. and Brookler, K. H., (1991). *Dizziness: Etiologic Approach to Management.* New York: Thieme Medical Publishers.

Schulman-Galambos, C. and Galambos, R. (1975). Brain stem auditory evoked responses in premature infants. *Journal of Speech and Hearing Research, 18,* 456–465.

Schwartz, D. M., Larson, V., and DeChicchis, A. R. (1985). Spectral characteristics of air and bone transducers used to record the auditory brainstem response. *Ear and Hearing, 6,* 274–277.

Shanks, J. E. (1984). Tympanometry. *Ear and Hearing, 5,* 268–280.

Shimizu, H., Walters, R. J., Proctor, L. R., Kennedy, D. W., Allen, M. C., and Markowitz, R. K. (1990). Identification of hearing impairment in the neonatal intensive care unit population: Outcome of a five-year project at the Johns Hopkins Hospital. *Seminars in Hearing, 11,* 150–160.

Silman, S. (ed.). (1984). *The Acoustic Reflex: Basic Principles and Clinical Application.* New York: Academic Press.

Smoorenburg, G. F. (1972). Combination tones and their origin. *Journal of the Acoustical Society of America, 52,* 615–632.

Sprague, B. H., Wiley, T. L., and Goldstein, R. (1985). Tympanometric and acoustic-reflex studies in neonates. *Journal of Speech and Hearing Research, 28,* 265–272.

Stapells, D. (1989). Auditory brainstem response assessment of infants. *Seminars in Hearing 10,* 252–261.

Starr, A., Amlie, R. N., Martin, W. H., and Sanders, S. (1977). Development of auditory function in newborn infants revealed by auditory brainstem potentials. *Pediatrics, 60,* 831–839.

Stevens, J. C., Webb, H. D., Hutchinson, J., Connell, J. Smith, M. F., and Buffin, J. T. (1990). Click evoked otoacoustic emissions in neonatal screening. *Ear and Hearing, 11,* 128–133.

Stockard, J. E., Stockard, J. J., Westmoreland, B. F., and Corfits, J. L. (1979). Brainstem auditory-evoked responses: Normal variation as a function of stimulus and subject characteristics. *Archives of Neurology, 36,* 823–831.

Stockwell, C. W. (1983). *ENG Workbook.* Austin: Pro-Ed.

Stockwell, C. W. and Bojrab, D. I. (1993). Background and technique of rotation testing (Chap. 10, pp. 237–258). In G. P. Jacobson, C. W. Newman and J. M. Kartush (eds.), *Handbook of Balance Function Testing.* St. Louis: Mosby-Year Book.

Strickland, E. A., Burns, E. M., and Tubis, A. (1985). Incidence of spontaneous otoacoustic emissions in children and infants. *Journal of the Acoustical Society of America, 78,* 931–935.

Tusa, R. J., Saada, A. A., Jr., Niparko, J. K. (1994). Dizziness in childhood. *Journal of Child Neurology* 9: 261–274.

Van Camp, K. J., Margolis, R. H., Wilson, R. H., Creten, W. L., and Shanks, J. E. (1986). *Principles of Tympanometry.* Rockville, MD: ASHA Press.

Weber, B. A. and Jacobson, C. A. (1994). Newborn hearing screening (Chap. 15, pp. 357–386). In

J. T. Jacobson (ed.), *Principles and Applications in Auditory Evoked Potentials.* Boston: Allyn and Bacon.

White, J. and Regan, M. (1987). Otologic considerations. In G. Mueller and V. Geoffrey (eds.), *Communication Disorders in Aging: Assessment and Management.* Washington, DC: Gallaudet University Press.

White, K. R., Vohr, B. R., and Behrens, T. R. (1993). Universal newborn hearing screening using transient evoked otoacoustic emissions: Results of the Rhode Island Hearing Assessment Project. *Seminars in Hearing, 14,* 18–29.

Wier, C. C., Norton, S. J., and Kincaid, G. E. (1984). Spontaneous narrow-band oto-acoustic signals emitted by human ears: A replication. *Journal of the Acoustical Society of America, 76,* 1248–1250.

Zurek, P. M. (1981). Spontaneous narrowband acoustic signals emitted by human ears. *Journal of the Acoustical Society of America, 69,* 514–523.

# CHAPTER 8

# CENTRAL AUDITORY PROCESSING DISORDERS IN CHILDREN: ARE WE LISTENING?

*DANIEL P. HARRIS*

## INTRODUCTION

The purpose of this chapter is to discuss substantial issues concerning the audiologist's role in the diagnosis and management of pediatric central auditory processing disorders (CAPDs). In the course of doing so, some suggestions are offered for improving professional education and CAPD evaluation methods. The chapter purposely does not provide a comprehensive review of the literature on CAPDs and does not focus on how to administer commercially available tests. This information is available elsewhere (Musiek, 1985; Musiek and Baran, 1987; Musiek and Chermak, 1994; Sloane, 1985, 1986; Willeford, 1985), and is secondary to the chapter's main intent of identifying methods and skills that can be improved to increase the competence of audiologists who work with children.

Regarding your professional work with children, please ask yourself what you are most qualified to do. Many audiologists will say that they are well trained to assess pediatric hearing. Now ask yourself as a professional, what you are less qualified to do? In my experience, many audiologists will report that they have little or no formal training and minimal experience in pediatric CAPDs. Indeed, the respondents of a recent nationwide survey of community speech and hearing clinic managers perceived on average that the preparedness of recent audiology graduates to assess central auditory processing is only "fair," ranking slightly above preparedness in deaf culture, cerumen management, aural rehabilitation, and vestibular assessment (Henri, 1994).

This perception is particularly unfortunate for the profession of audiology at this time, because the diagnoses of ADD (attention deficit disorder) and ADHD (attention deficit-hyperactivity disorder) are now common for preschool and elementary school children who demonstrate learning and/or behavior problems. Although precise incidence and prevalence figures are lacking, it is estimated that as many as 6 percent of American children from 4 to 16 years old meet the diagnostic criteria for attention deficit disorder (Barkley, 1990). Often, CAPDs are suspected to be among the causes or sequelae of ADD or ADHD in such children (Willeford, 1985), and other children may appear to demonstrate specific auditory processing problems without signs of ADD, ADHD, or more generalized learning disabilities (Sloane, 1980; Willeford, 1985). It is not surprising, then, that audiologists increasingly are being called upon to contribute to the diagnostic and remediative process, in what should be a team effort including the child, family, school, and medical community. However, due to insufficient expertise in pediatric CAPDs, the audiologist could end up being a weak team member, perhaps a benchwarmer capable only of marginal contributions (Henri, 1994).

Lack of knowledge about the specific causes and characteristics of pediatric CAPDs currently limits our ability to provide audiologists with optimal education and training experiences. Indeed, at present there is no single definition or set of terminology commonly used by professionals to define, diagnose, or describe childhood CAPDs. For the purposes of this chapter, a very general definition is employed so that a wide variety of topics can be considered: Pediatric CAPDs comprise sets of cognitive and behavioral deficits including reduced ability to attend selectively to the auditory environment, inaccuracy in decoding speech from the acoustic signal, and difficulty in incorporating auditory information into language, memory, and learning functions. These deficits may differ in severity and interrelatedness from child to child, and their etiology may be known or unknown. Given such an inclusive definition, the diagnostic pronouncement of "abnormal" for any particular child would be stated best in terms of developmental delay, auditory-linguistic dysfunction, and cognitive limitations, rather than in terms of neurologic deficits or possible sites of lesion. Although the audiologist may be well-intentioned in making direct pronouncements about neurologic status, such diagnostic terminology is more appropriately used by physicians.

It has been said that the road to hell is paved with good intentions. The audiologist sincerely may want to help the child suspected of having auditory processing problems and may believe that current methods of testing and remediation will suffice. Examples of such good intentions include accepting referrals without physician orders or supportive evidence from appropriate professionals, blindly following commercial test protocols, reporting only numerical scores (percentiles, standard deviations, age equivalents, grade equivalents, etc.), and recommending assistive listening devices and preferential classroom seating as panaceas. This sort of well-meaning behavior can earn the audiologist a place on the treatment team, but it ultimately fails to help the team members understand what, if anything, is actually wrong with the child's auditory processing. Also, if audiologists are not prepared through education and experience to improve current methods of testing and remediation, then children with CAPDs may continue to receive good intentions rather than the best possible professional services.

## AUDIOLOGY'S STEPCHILD

It is reasonable to ask why audiologists typically do not acquire as much formal training in pediatric CAPDs as in hearing evaluation, electrophysical

diagnostics, and other clinical methods commonly used with children. The analogy that the study of CAPDs presently holds the status of audiology's stepchild may help to answer this question as well as provide some direction for future professional development. To be good parents, we should have welcomed this stepchild into our professional family with open arms, but our adjustment to handling pediatric CAPDs has not been quite so easy. We have not given our family member the attention it deserves due to some natural, but regrettable doubts.

The first of these doubts may arise from the fact that we did not create this stepchild. Many early central auditory processing investigations were laboratory studies focused on the anatomy and physiology of the auditory nervous system. These studies often involved animal models and described neural activity and auditory behavior following carefully induced central nervous system lesions (Zimmerman, 1985). Other early investigations centered on auditory perceptual abnormalities in adults with known CNS lesions such as tumors and cerebrovascular accidents (Musiek, 1985). However, some of the experimental paradigms applied in these studies are widely used today by audiologists to test for CAPDs in children, many of whom do not have obvious CNS lesions. It is natural to have some reservations about adopting procedures from distant professional origins, with no clear idea of what is being tested and little indication of how the results should be used. With these reservations in mind, it is small wonder that many audiologists have not given the same time and energy to gaining expertise in pediatric CAPDs as they have to other more familiar offspring of our professional family.

A second source of doubt concerning our stepchild stems from the consideration that we have yet to define where our responsibilities begin or end in the management of pediatric CAPDs. Should we assume the role of a primary parent by setting professional standards, granting privileges for clinical practice, and specifying guidelines for the allocation of resources? Or is it more appropriate to take a less active role, assuming that audiologists function better as support personnel for other professionals?

Some of this doubt is due to the fact that we are uncertain about how we should relate to our stepchild's other professional families. Speech-language pathologists are said to be our closest relatives, but they speak in terms of phonology, morphology, syntax, semantics, and pragmatics. These terms might be only vaguely familiar to many audiologists. Educational psychologists may sound even less familiar when they use terms from psycholinguistics, learning and memory theories, and cognitive processing models to discuss pediatric CAPDs. Physicians, when called upon, can certainly present some challenging medical terminology from specialties such as pharmacology, neuroradiology, and electroencephalograpy. And finally, classroom teachers may sound alien to all when they ask everyone involved to drop the fancy terminology and give them a clear indication of exactly what is "wrong" with the child, and what practical strategies can be used to facilitate learning.

What can we do to resolve doubts about our stepchild, increase our willingness to give it appropriate attention, and improve our relationships with its other professional families? For all children, the best way to promote security and healthy development is to cultivate each child's unique and special qualities. At present, three general issues seem to be hindering many audiologists from giving such attention to pediatric CAPDs.

## Training of Audiologists

The finding that recent audiology graduates are perceived as being marginally prepared to deal with CAPDs (Henri, 1994) may be but a symptom of a more general problem in the way audiologists currently train and practice. Much of the education and experience audiologists devote to topics such as hearing evaluation, amplification, and evoked potentials will not translate directly into knowledge and skills optimal for the management of pediatric CAPDs. The capability to assess the relationships between neural maturation, speech, language, cognition, and memory appears to be critical, although the associations between these facets of child development and CAPDs are not well understood (Sloane, 1980, 1985, 1986; Willeford, 1985).

Also, familiarity with the basic principles of test construction, score standardization, and interpretation of results currently seems very important for two reasons. First, many central auditory processing tests commercially available today do not come with proven scoring criteria or objective guidelines for interpretation. Purchasers are often simply instructed to develop their own norms, without regard to their qualifications to do so. Of the commercial tests now available, the SCAN (Keith, 1986) probably has the most complete set of norms, but it is clearly designated as a screening instrument. Incredibly, tests with less comprehensive norms must therefore be considered among the approaches available to actually confirm a CAPD. Second, to design new assessments that may be more sensitive, specific, and descriptive for pediatric CAPDs, audiologists need to have a sound understanding of how effective and efficient tests may be developed and utilized. Given the fact that methods developed for laboratory and clinical studies of neural anatomy, physiology, and site of lesion still predominate test protocols for pediatric CAPDs, there may be room in the future for improving assessment procedures.

## Lack of Agreement on Terminology

Suppose that today the U.S. Department of Health, Education, and Welfare published a report with the following statement:

*There is an urgent need to improve the diagnostic procedures for disorders of auditory processing. The use of precise descriptive terms will help facilitate communication between disciplines. One of the basic steps that should be taken [is] to provide detailed and comprehensive descriptions of the behavioral responses to auditory stimuli, which are characteristic of peripheral and central deafness, mental retardation, emotional disturbance, apha-*

*sia, and disorders in the processing of auditory stimuli.*

Many professionals who currently work with pediatric CAPDs would probably agree with the statement and advocate that it should be acted upon as soon as possible. In fact, this statement has been published, some 25 years ago (Chalfant and Scheffelin, 1969). However, 25 years later there is still no general agreement on terminology appropriate for use by singular or multidisciplinary groups of professionals to describe normal or abnormal central auditory processing. For example, the authors of one study published in a journal devoted to public school services found that a "lack of concentration may be directly related to poor listening performances" observed by teachers of children labeled as having CAPDs (Smoski, Brunt, and Tannahill, 1992). Authors of a different study published in a journal dedicated to a wide range of research in audition found that one child's "difficulty appears specific to the extraction of acoustic features from noise when the signal is of brief duration" (Breedin, Martin, and Jerger, 1989). This is not to say that the authors of these two studies reached inaccurate, or even conflicting, conclusions. It could be said that they simply used different terms to convey the single conclusion that auditory attention and analysis are problematic for children with CAPDs.

## Lack of Agreement on Test Methods

If there is so little agreement on the appropriate terminology to describe pediatric CAPDs, then it is not hard to see why there is also some discrepancy over the methods that should be used in assessments. Opinions on this subject can be divided into two general groups: those who believe it is both possible and necessary to differentiate auditory processing from other sensory, linguistic, and cognitive processes, and those who believe it is not possible to do so. For example, Willeford (1985) makes a statement representative of the point of view that auditory processing can be differentially assessed:

*Children with central auditory deficits commonly have learning difficulties, and many learning-disabled children have central auditory disorders as a contributing cause of their problems.... Diagnosis in either case rests on confirmation of an auditory deficit through the use of appropriate measures of central auditory function. In the final analysis it is necessary to evaluate a given child's performance on auditory tests per se rather than on tests in which uncontrolled auditory stimuli theoretically play an integral part in the assessment of other skills such as oral, read, or written language.*

On the other hand, Sloane (1980) states that:

*The best means of evaluation and diagnosis is to assess the child with a variety of speech and language instruments that focus on different aspects of speech, language, and auditory function. In addition, it is important to make careful observations of the child's spontaneous behavior and a report of its history. It is more important to look at the qualitative aspects of the child's responses, than at any score per se. A score may have value as a reference for comparison later, but the immediate goal of evaluation is to understand how the child is processing the situation before him.*

In addition to this basic two-way divergence on the best approaches to use in assessing pediatric CAPDs, there is another body of research currently developing on the potential uses of physiologic measures of neural function, such as auditory event-related potentials, topographic brain mapping, and regional cerebral blood flow, to determine the possible relationships between physiologic and behavioral test results and to investigate the CNS correlates of auditory processing disorders (Hall and Harris, 1994; Harris and Hall, 1990; Jirsa, 1992; Jirsa and Clontz, 1990; Knopman, Rubens, Klassen, and Meyer, 1982; Kraus and McGee, 1994; Musiek and Baran, 1987). While these physiologic measures appear to be worthy of attention, at the present time they also add to the monumental challenge of determining which assessment methods may be the most sensitive and specific for CAPDs in any given child in any given situation.

## IMPROVING THE ASSESSMENT AND REMEDIATION OF PEDIATRIC CAPDs

If audiologists are to make any significant improvements in their current capacities to work with children with auditory processing problems, the four issues of specialization, training, terminology, and assessment methodology discussed above must be addressed in a timely and systematic manner. Until then, pediatric CAPDs could continue to be viewed as audiology's stepchild, deprived of essential attention due to professional doubts and lack of knowledge. Therefore, the following suggestions are offered to those willing to consider the need for improvement. In the course of discussing these suggestions, it is necessary to engage in constructive criticism of methods and materials presently in use. Any such criticism is intended to be positive in spirit and objective in nature. It is in no way intended to diminish the sizable contributions of many dedicated professionals who have spent a great deal of productive time and energy in developing current methodologies.

### Pediatric CAPDs as a Specialty

One of the first steps in the development of any particular personal or professional specialty is to identify and cultivate interests that define the area of specialization. In the case of pediatric CAPDs, it may sound simplistic to say that, first of all, one should be vitally interested in children. However, it seems very important to understand that neural maturation, cognitive processes, and behavioral limitations specific to children can dictate the need for assessment and remediative strategies that differ from those appropriate for adults. Also it would be beneficial to have an interest in family dynamics, cultural backgrounds, and socioeconomic forces as significant factors in the development of communication skills during childhood. Furthermore, the strengths and weaknesses of current educational systems, especially the ways in which school services are mandated and allocated for students with special needs, should be of keen interest to the professional considering specialization in pediatric CAPDs.

The desire to work in educational settings, rather than medical or commercial endeavors, represents the kind of commitment needed to promote the perception that audiologists can and should be specially prepared to assume a leadership role on the professional team for children with auditory processing problems. There is no better way for a professional specialty to gain visibility than to be recognized by other specialists interested in the same areas of practice. To that end it would be salutary for audiologists interested in pediatric CAPDs to undertake cooperative research projects with speech-language pathologists, educational psychologists, physicians, teachers, and other relevant personnel. The following research questions are suggested:

1. What are the causes of pediatric CAPDs?
2. Which diagnostic methods have the greatest sensitivity and specificity?
3. How do CAPDs affect the child's life, including life within the family?
4. What are the relationships between CAPDs and other childhood communication disorders?
5. What are the most effective methods of remediating pediatric CAPDs?
6. Are there residual effects of childhood auditory processing problems in adults?

Until such cooperative efforts are initiated, it is highly unlikely that the present lack of agreement on the terminology appropriate for describing childhood auditory processing problems can be resolved. Therefore, direct advice on the use of specific terms is not offered in this chapter. The terminology that is used herein reflects my own experiences and preferences.

### Educational Requirements for Competency in Pediatric CAPDs

Professional education in audiology is presently within a major transition. The present chapter is not intended to support any particular point of view on how the training of audiologists ought to proceed. The education and skills required for expertise in pediatric CAPDs should be addressed in any program dedicated to providing audiologists with opportunities for effective professional development. Regardless of the degree received upon graduation, the audiologist is better prepared to work with childhood auditory processing disorders if competencies are cultivated in the following areas.

### Anatomy and Physiology of the Central Nervous System

Knowledge of the anatomy, physiology, and development of the central nervous system is basic to understanding the perceptual and behavioral correlates of CAPDs. This learning should not be limited solely to the auditory pathways. It is also important to survey what is known about the neurobiology of awareness, perception, emotion, learning, and memory.

To present one small example of why such knowledge is important, there is some evidence that auditory event-related evoked potentials have neural generators in the limbic system of the brain (Smith, Stapleton, and Halgren, 1986). This finding may be relevant to the understanding of auditory processing disorders because the limbic system is also thought to be involved in the generation of emotions and the transfer of information into recent memory (Netter, 1975). Thus we have a neural system that is not often mentioned in discussions confined to the auditory pathways, even though it may play a significant role in determining responses and behaviors that affect auditory function.

### Child Psychology

Familiarity with behavior and learning theories, particularly as they are applied in the study of child psychology, may be helpful in designing remediative programs for children with CAPDs. Obviously, the main differences in learning capacities between children and adults can be attributed

to the cognitive developments that must occur during normal maturation. There is ample evidence that "the progressive changes in cognitive structure may vary in rate from person to person but they follow an invariant sequence, always moving in the same order, and the progressive changes in the way children organize information can be characterized as a sequence of stages" (Mayer, 1977).

Perhaps the best-known theory of stage-dependent cognitive development was proposed by Jean Piaget (Flavell, 1963). According to Piaget, children normally progress through four general stages that define and limit cognitive abilities (Flavell, 1963; Mayer, 1977):

1. Sensorimotor period (0–2 years)
2. Preoperational period (2–7 years)
3. Concrete operations period (7–11 years)
4. Formal operations period (11–adult)

Because these stages appear to be invariant in sequence, effective remediation for pediatric CAPDs may hinge on matching stimuli and tasks for therapy to the child's stage-dependent capabilities. For example, the preoperational period is characterized by "concreteness," in that the child performs best with concrete objects that are physically present. Furthermore, the preoperational child typically can attend to only one dimension of a situation at a time (Mayer, 1977). Appropriate strategies for remediating auditory processing in a preoperational child, then, would not include comparisons of shapes, sizes, or quantities in hypothetical situations. Thus, a task centered on identifying coins that would give a "small amount" of money may lead the preoperational child to specify dimes, rather than pennies, due to physical differences in the sizes of coins. As a result, the clinician could confuse poor task performance with the child's innate inability to understand the intent of the task.

### Speech and Language Development

In addition to familiarity with behavior and learning theories, an understanding of normal childhood speech and language acquisition and childhood communication disorders is essential in preparing to work with pediatric CAPDs. The sensitivity and specificity of assessments, as well as the effectiveness and efficiency of remediation depends on the ability to detect and describe deviations from normal communication development.

Some years ago, a well-known authority flatly stated: "There is no test for auditory processing disorders. There are many tests that present stimuli primarily through the auditory modality (receptive language tests, auditory language comprehension tests, speech sound discrimination tests, auditory retention tests), but none is comprehensive enough to provide a basis for differential diagnosis" (Sloane, 1980). This statement still seems accurate today, and will probably hold true in the future, because the aspects of auditory processing that are most relevant to the development of communication are often closely linked with linguistic functions.

The phenomenon of categorical discrimination (Lieberman, 1977) represents a very good example of the integration of auditory and linguistic functions, many of which seem to develop very early in childhood (Kuhl, 1980). In a typical categorical discrimination experiment, speech sounds created by computer are presented either singly for identification, or in pairs for discrimination between two sounds. Most often, syllables are used as stimuli, and varying frequency transitions are synthesized for the initial consonants. The results of such experiments consistently show that both the identification and discrimination of consonants depend on frequency "boundaries" between perceptual "categories" of sounds (Lieberman, 1977). In other words, listeners do not classify two speech sounds as being different, unless the difference in frequency transitions applied to them falls across a critical range representing a perceptual boundary.

Apparently these perceptual boundaries are shaped by linguistic influences during the first few months of childhood, so that the discrimination of speech sounds comes to depend on an infant's exposure to a specific language (Kuhl, 1980). It is easy to see, then, why anyone interested in designing central auditory assessments or interpreting auditory processing test results should be aware that stimulus construction could lead to some unanticipated effects of perceptual phenomena like categorical discrimination. Assessment approaches such as filtered speech, speech-in-noise, and dichotic speech create listening environments in which the interactions of acoustic, auditory, and linguistic variables are difficult to control. Therefore, responses that seem to be errors may actually be justified by the uncontrolled influences of particular stimuli upon any given child.

Categorical discrimination is only one of these possible influences. When other important dimensions of linguistic functioning, such as morphology, syntax, semantics, and pragmatics, are also considered, it becomes quite obvious that understanding normal and abnormal aspects of child language development is essential to competency in working with pediatric CAPDs. Additionally, proficiency in child language allows the audiologist to communicate more effectively with speech-language pathologists, educational psychologists, physicians, and teachers, thereby increasing professional recognition.

### Speech Science

If we accept that an understanding of language development is important to proficiency in managing childhood auditory processing problems, then we also can see that speech science laboratory training will provide the practical knowledge and skills necessary to put our understanding to work. Speech science training may incorporate overlapping topics such as the physics of sound, perception of sound, acoustics for speech and hearing, experimental phonetics, and psycholinguistics. However, our ultimate goal should be familiarity with the methods and results of speech perception experiments.

Classic studies, like those performed by Peterson and Barney (1952) and Miller and Nicely (1955), provide a wealth of information that directly applies to the construction of auditory processing tests and the interpretation of results. Overall, the results of these studies graphically demonstrate that central auditory test responses may be influenced by complex interactions between an individual's auditory and linguistic functioning and the nature of the stimuli and response modes used to sample auditory processing. The following examples illustrate this important point.

Peterson and Barney (1952) studied the perception of English vowels and found that the ease with which listeners classified various vowels varied greatly. To illustrate, the vowel /i/ was unanimously identified by 70 adult listeners in 143 out of 152 presentations. However, the same listeners unanimously identified /a/ in only 9 out of 152 presentations. In all cases, the vowels were presented in the single-syllable carrier /h/ + vowel + /d/. This finding is significant today for designers and users of central auditory processing tests because single syllable words are often used as stimuli, without direct attention being paid to inherent differences in discriminability associated with specific phonetic contexts.

Figure 8.1 shows the number of occurrences per vowel in the Competing Words Subtest of the SCAN Screening Test for Auditory Processing Disorders (Keith, 1986). It is evident that there is a wide range of vowel occurrence (1–18), which inherently contributes to uncontrolled variation in the sampling of phonetic contexts. Numerical scores, as derived for the Competing Words Subtest, do not give any hint of the specific effects of

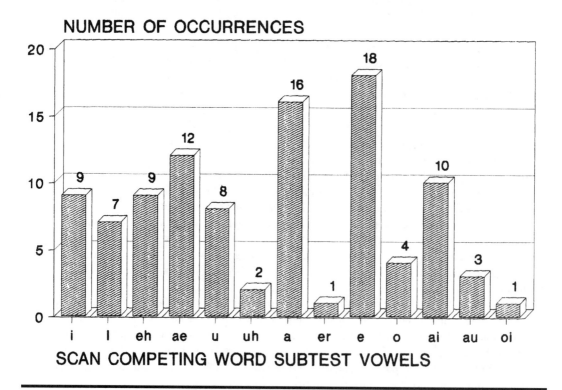

FIGURE 8.1  Occurrences per vowel in the Competing Words Subtest of the SCAN Screening Test for Auditory Processing Disorders.

this sort of variation. However, the results of speech perception research employing highly controlled auditory stimuli clearly indicate that phonetic context can greatly affect discrimination in normal listeners (Peterson and Barney, 1952). Anyone seeking to describe auditory processing beyond the level of numerical scores should be aware of this fact.

Figure 8.2 shows the percent of correct identification of single-syllable words (NU-6, List A or B) presented in three different filter conditions (500-Hz lowpass, 750-Hz lowpass, 300–3200 Hz band-reject binaural fusion) to a group of twenty-five college students with normal hearing with no history of auditory processing deficits (Harris Cannito, Descouzis, and Stiritz, 1990). Percentages are displayed according to the place of articulation for initial consonants of the stimulus words. It can be seen that word identification may be related to interactions between filter characteristics and the place of articulation. For example, identification of words with palatal initial consonants (/j/, /l/, /r/) was much worse for the 500-Hz lowpass condition than for 750-Hz lowpass filtering or binaural fusion, which involves both lowpass and highpass filters. On the other hand, identification of words with the glottal initial consonant /h/ appeared relatively easy in all three conditions.

In 1955, Miller and Nicely studied perceptual confusions among English consonants in normal listeners and found that specific confusions were related to the spectral properties of speech filters and experimentally generated noise, particularly as the filters or noise affected articulatory features including voicing, nasality, affrication, duration,

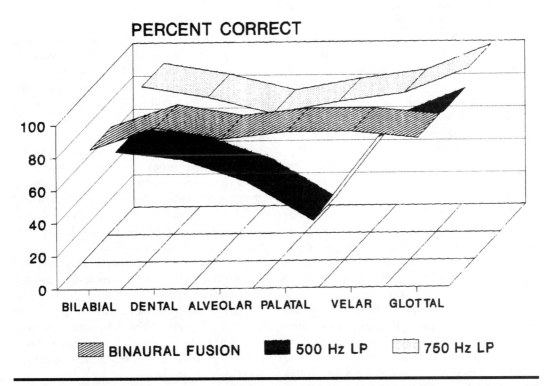

**FIGURE 8.2** Percent of correct identification of single-syllable words (NU-6, List A or B) presented in three different filter conditions (binaural fusion, 500-Hz lowpass [LP], 750-Hz lowpass [LP]).

and place of articulation. The results of more re-cent filtered speech tests of auditory processing, as described above (Harris et al., 1990), support the possibility that some "errors" in such tests may be due more to stimulus conditions (Miller and Nicely, 1955) than to inadequate auditory pro-cessing abilities in listeners. In light of these find-ings, it is evident that speech-science laboratory training can provide the audiologist with skills necessary to distinguish between the influences of stimulus conditions and perceptual limitations in the responses of children with CAPDs.

## Assessment Methods

Earlier in this chapter, I suggested that classroom teachers may sound alien to other professionals when they ask for a clear indication of exactly what is "wrong" with a particular child, and what practical strategies can be used to facilitate learn-ing. Although there is an element of jest in this statement, those who work with children with CAPDs will also recognize an element of truth. Specifically, the astute teacher wants to know at what functional level the child actually fails to handle auditory input well enough to perform acceptably in school, and what can be done about it. Others interested in the child, such as the par-ent, speech-language pathologist, educational diagnostician, and physician may pose their con-cerns in different (or more technical) terms, but they are all interested in this same fundamental question.

For the most part, the assessments currently used by audiologists to define and describe pedi-atric CAPDs fail to provide any direct answers as to the specific nature of auditory functions that may be problematic for any given child. Levels of dysfunction are typically expressed in numerical terms such as standard deviations, standard scores, percentiles, age equivalents, and the like. The audiologist who exclusively relies on these numerical representations really does not have much to offer other than an opinion as to whether a problem exists, and if one does exist, whether it is a small, medium, or large problem.

This sort of quantitative interpretation may be less than impressive to the parent, teacher, or oth-er concerned individual, because referral to an au-diologist never would have occurred unless a problem was already strongly suspected. Further-more, recommendations for improving auditory function based solely on numerical test scores can suggest only general strategies, such as control-ling environmental distractions, using assistive listening systems, and arranging preferential classroom seating. Although these strategies may facilitate better behavior and classroom perfor-mance in some children, they do not ensure that efforts to remediate auditory function have been maximized. To improve methods available to the audiologist for assessing pediatric CAPDs and contributing to effective remediation, issues of test construction and the reporting of results must be addressed.

### Test Construction

Today most audiologists test auditory processing by using speech or nonspeech stimuli presented in conditions that presumably make processing diffi-cult enough to cause more errors in children of a given age with CAPDs than in children of the same age without CAPDs. Filtered speech, speech-in-noise (figure ground), dichotic listening (competing speech), time-alteration (compres-sion, rapid alternation), and pitch patterns are fa-miliar examples of stimulus conditions currently employed in auditory processing tests for children (Willeford, 1985). The main strength of all these methods is that they attempt to provide consistent listening conditions through the use of sound rooms, audiometers, earphones, and prerecorded sets of stimuli. Their main weakness is that they all produce listening conditions that, to some de-gree, are unlike conditions children experience in daily living situations. This limits our capacity to draw direct conclusions about any given child's ability to process auditory information in the real world.

Also, each method of assessing auditory pro-cessing, and each test based upon a particular method, has limitations that result from complex interactions between the child's auditory and linguistic functioning and the nature of the stimuli used to sample auditory processing. Some of these limitations were touched upon in the previous section on speech science training for audiologists, but further discussion may be helpful if improvements are to be made.

Responses from tests employing speech stimuli with any type of filtering, background noise, or competing stimuli may be influenced by acoustic and phonetic contexts. The top half of Figure 8.3 shows a spectrogram of the stimulus word "vine" from a tape-recorded (NU-6, A) list of phonetically balanced words. The bottom half of Figure 8.3 shows a spectrogram of the same word "vine" filtered at 300-Hz lowpass and 3200-Hz highpass for a binaural fusion test (Auditec of St. Louis). A comparison of the two spectrograms shows that the filtering process has removed much of the acoustic energy in the frequency range of F1 and F2, while some energy is still present around and above F3. Therefore, it is not surprising that the most common "incorrect" response from a group of thirty-eight normal young adults who took the binaural fusion test was "van" (Harris et al., 1992). In fact, "van" could be considered the correct response. The speech filters had removed the acoustic transitions and formant frequencies characteristic of the vowel /ai/, and many of the listeners perceived /ae/ due to the filtered spectrum (Peterson and Barney, 1952).

It is straightforward to anticipate that interactions between specific speech filters and the acoustic spectra of words can influence perception. However, there may also be similar influences associated with background noise or even dichotic listening. Figure 8.4 shows numbers of errors for stimulus words frequently missed on the SCAN Auditory Figure-Ground Subtest (Keith, 1986). Listeners were the same thirty-eight normal young adults mentioned above (Harris, Cannito, Descouzis, and Stiritz, 1992). The data in the figure indicate that the stimulus most frequently misidentified was the word "loud" (pre-

sented monaurally to the left ear against a background of speech babble). Listeners who failed to identify "loud" commonly responded with either "love" or "law." The high degree of consistency for these two responses may be based on an acoustic-phonetic context that increased the probability of perceiving the phonemes /ʌ/, /v/, and /a/, while reducing the probability of perceiving /au/ and /d/.

An additional influence leading to the narrow set of two common misidentifications may be due to the fact that "love" and "law" occur more often in spoken English than "loud" (Berger, 1977). Thus, listeners who were uncertain about what they heard may have guessed at a common word that was feasible according to their attempts to analyze the signal. The fact that this same pattern of narrow sets of misidentifications was observed for the other stimulus words shown in Figure 8.4, supports the notion that acoustic, phonetic, and semantic (word frequency) factors might interact to influence the probability that a particular response will occur. It is important to remember that probability is a continuum, but the scoring of test items as correct or incorrect is not. A child who happens to misidentify most or all of the words listed in Figure 8.4 could be on the way to an abnormal numerical score. Yet, one might wonder what the actual probability of an auditory processing disorder really is.

Figure 8.5 shows a spectrogram of the stimulus pair "are-cow" from the SCAN Competing Words Subtest (Keith, 1986). It can be seen that a relatively steady-state band of energy is present in the F1 and F2 frequency range commonly associated with the vowel /a/ (as in "car") whereas a formant transition more characteristic of /au/ (as in "cow") is not as apparent (Peterson and Barney, 1952). The word "car" was a very frequent response among the thirty-eight normal young adults for either or both stimulus words. Even though the Competing Words Subtest is a dichotic task, it seems that some of the listeners analyzed the different words presented to each ear and ended up with a singular unit made up of the pho-

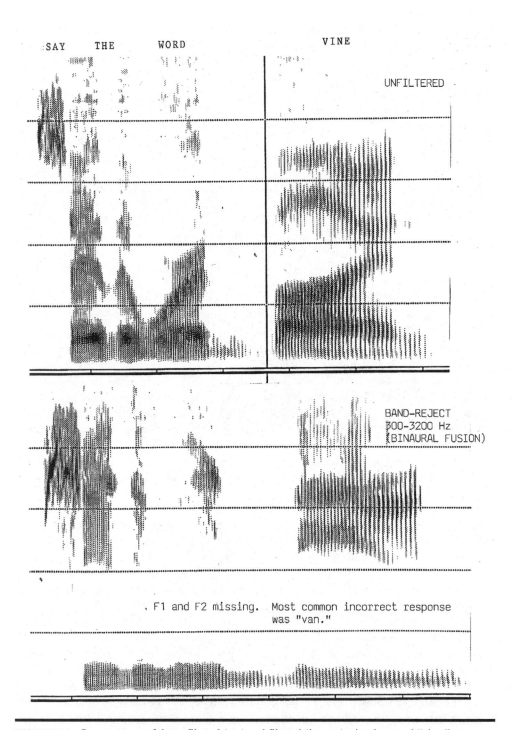

**FIGURE 8.3**   Spectrograms of the unfiltered (*top*) and filtered (*bottom*) stimulus word "vine."

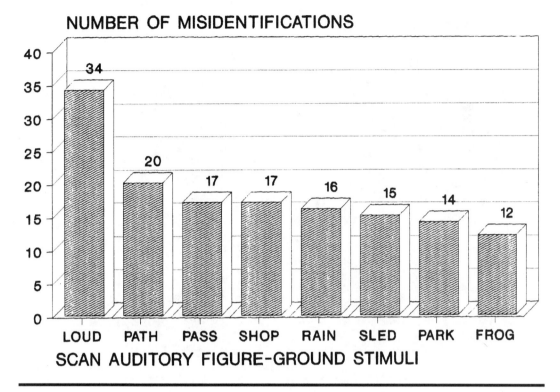

**FIGURE 8.4**   Numbers of errors for stimulus words frequently missed on the SCAN Auditory Figure-Ground Subtest.

nemes /k/, /a/, and /r/. The fact that "are" and "car" also occur more frequently than "cow" in spoken English, cannot be ignored as a possible influence (Berger, 1977). In contrast, the stimulus pair "fire-you" in the Competing Words Subtest was not misidentified by any of the thirty-eight listeners. It may be that the particular phonetic differences between these two words, as well as their relatively high frequencies of occurrence, ensured the intended identification.

The data in Figures 8.4 and 8.5 present only isolated illustrations of the generality that stimuli used to sample auditory processing may have complex interactions with the individual child's auditory and linguistic functioning. Several more examples involving widely used tests such as the Staggered Spondaic Word Test (Katz, 1962), Competing Sentences Test (Willeford, 1985), Se-

lective Auditory Attention Test (Cherry, 1980), and Compressed Speech (Willeford, 1985) could be presented. However, it already should be clear that the journey between a stimulus and a child's response may be treacherous, regardless of the type of test. Much more research is needed on the paths that must be followed and those that must be avoided to effectively assess auditory processing. Carrying out such research will be difficult, because the acoustic signals of speech, and the linguistic and cognitive systems that underlie perception, are inherently redundant and highly integrated (Lieberman, 1977). Therefore it is very hard to isolate individual features of normal or disordered auditory processing.

Anyone who doubts the difficulty of isolating elements of auditory processing should examine the data in Figure 8.6, which shows the pattern of

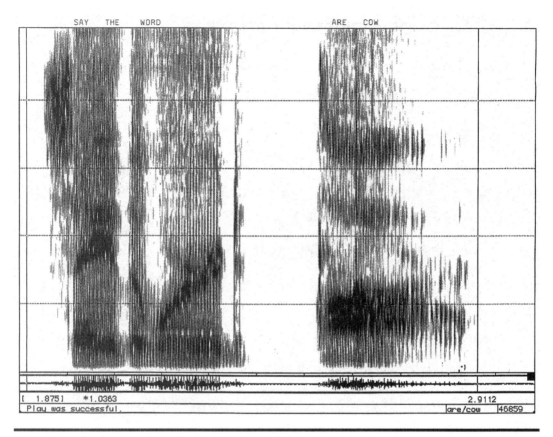

**FIGURE 8.5** Spectrogram of the stimulus pair "are-cow" from the SCAN Competing Words Subtest.

errors made on the Dichotic Digits Test (Musiek, 1983) by thirty-eight young adults with traumatic brain injuries (Harris et al., 1992). The test employs only the numbers listed along the abscissa of the graph as stimuli (1, 2, 3, 4, 5, 6, 8, 9, 10). Every test item consists of two pairs of numbers presented in succession, so that each ear simultaneously receives one member of each pair. The listener is instructed to repeat both pairs of numbers presented in each item. "Seven" is not used as a stimulus because it has two syllables.

The bars in Figure 8.6 show the percentage of misidentifications that occurred for the individual stimulus numbers, relative to the total amount of times each number was presented. For example, 10 percent of presentations of the stimulus "ten"

resulted in misidentifications. The data in the figure included only substitution responses (one number for another), so that omissions did not influence the percentages. The surprising result drawn from the data is that significant differences existed between the amount of substitution responses for some of the stimuli. "Five," "nine," and "ten" were misidentified much more often than "three," "four," "six," and "eight," even though responses were limited to a small closed set. To add to this mystery, there were no significant trends in substitutions. The thirty-eight young adults with brain injuries used all numbers in the set as substitutions about equally as often. This result emphasizes the general conclusion that it is very difficult to account for interactions be-

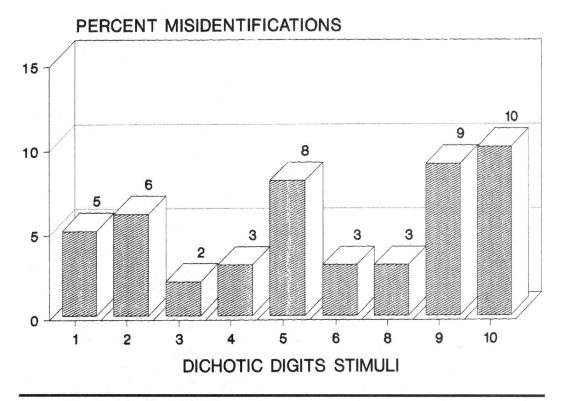

**FIGURE 8.6**   Pattern of errors made on the Dichotic Digits Test by thirty-eight young adults with traumatic brain injuries.

tween stimulus-specific conditions and the auditory functioning of the individual, and perhaps even more difficult to isolate individual features of normal or disordered auditory processing.

Although the ideal test conditions for assessing auditory processing in children have yet to be developed, some suggestions could be offered to address the foregoing concerns about current methods. The following ideas may be worth considering:

**1. Focusing test construction on developing items that sample specific auditory–linguistic responses.** For instance, if we are interested in a child's ability to identify speech sounds under a certain test condition, we could select the stimuli and design the condition to have as consistent an

effect as possible on acoustic and phonetic contexts. One example of such a design would involve matching filter or noise spectra to sets of words with specific phoneme features (manner, voicing, place, etc.). Thus, words composed of fricatives or plosive consonants might have a different filter or noise condition than words composed of nasalized or lateralized consonants (Lieberman, 1977).

The current clinical practice of maintaining one filter or noise condition throughout a particular test is exactly the opposite of what has just been described. Maintaining a uniform spectrum without regard to variations in the acoustic and phonetic properties of the stimulus words inevitably leads to major differences in stimulus identification probabilities. An extreme example of such current test construction is the use of a constant filter setting for phonetically balanced word lists like NU-6.

Test construction may also be focused on sampling auditory–linguistic behaviors above the level of speech sound identification. Possible semantic influences for word stimuli may be addressed by developing items that have more equivalent frequencies of occurrence in the language. For example, the Staggered Spondaic Word Test, List EC (Katz, 1962) has several items such as "washtub" and "whitewall" that are misidentified by young adults with brain injuries significantly more often than other stimuli from the same test (Harris et al., 1992). It may be no coincidence that "washtub" and "whitewall" are also disappearing from the lexicon of young Americans in general (Berger, 1977).

Possible syntactic influences could be dealt with similarly by attempting to equate grammatical structures in test items involving multi-word constructions. To illustrate the problem, the Competing Sentences Test (Willeford, 1985) has several stimulus sentences containing past tense verbs competing against sentences containing present tense verbs. Furthermore, there are large differences in the number and classes of nouns and modifiers between some sentence pairs. This situation makes it difficult to determine the extent to which grammatical structures may be challenging enough to cause the child to misidentify words and/or fail to extract the intended message. It also affords no direct information on the role of syntax, apart from other linguistic functions, as a factor in auditory processing.

**2. Using speech science laboratory approaches to develop test items.** Once an auditory–linguistic behavior has been defined for assessment, the technology and experimental methods commonly used in the speech science laboratory can be adapted to devise stimuli and estimate their potential for sampling the defined behavior. Some of these methods already have been discussed in this chapter. Many others will be familiar to the audiologist formally trained in speech science. By now it should be clear to all that objective measures of acoustic and phonetic stimulus contexts can be of great assistance to those interested in understanding the responses of children above the level of "right" and "wrong" answers on auditory processing tests.

**3. Conducting item analyses on prospective tests of auditory processing.** An important step in the development of any test that will be used repeatedly for groups of subjects is to analyze the pattern of scores for each item. For particular tests, items that are missed very frequently or very infrequently across all subjects contribute little to the process of discriminating among levels of performance. Such items may be replaced with those having more representative distributions of scores across performance levels, thereby improving the distribution of scores over the test as a whole. In other words, subjects who score higher on a test should produce the correct response for a given item relatively more often than subjects who score lower on the same test.

**4. Using weighted scoring methods to compensate for test item variations in discriminating among levels of performance.** To date, it appears that the process of item analysis has not been systematically applied in the development of many auditory processing tests widely used with children. Admittedly, it would be very difficult to ultimately create sets of speech stimuli composed of items that uniformly discriminate among levels of performance. However, the more the process is attempted, the greater the probability that defined auditory–linguistic behaviors can be sampled.

Until such efforts are completed, the use of weighted scoring methods may provide a way of compensating for the effects of individual item scores on test score distributions (Barcikowski, 1983). Hypothetically, scores for items in a particular assessment could be weighted according to their accuracy in discriminating performance. Similarly, mean scores of subtests could be weighted according to their relative contributions to discriminating performance on the test as a whole. Finally, total scores could be weighted across tests assembled into a given battery. This process would certainly consume much time and effort, and therefore it may be best accomplished by a team of professionals with individual skills in hearing and speech, test construction, and statistics.

**5. Using assessment methods that approximate as closely as possible listening conditions children encounter in the real world.** Earlier in this chapter it was pointed out that sound rooms, audiometers, earphones, and prerecorded sets of stimuli provide consistent listening conditions that are to some degree unlike conditions children typically experience in daily living situations. In fact, much of the equipment used today in clinical audiology is primarily designed to detect ear disease, auditory CNS pathology, and/or hearing loss, none of which is an inevitable cohort of disordered auditory processing. As a result, we have nothing to lose and everything to gain by experimenting with assessments that involve more naturalistic auditory environments. This is not to say that current test methods should be discarded, only that different approaches may also be helpful in describing and remediating pediatric CAPDs.

Sound-field listening tasks may be the approach most familiar to the audiologist for doing away with the unnatural conditions imposed by earphones. Several studies have investigated sound localization, speech in noise, and dichotic listening tasks performed in sound field, under the theory that such tasks can yield information on auditory processing not available by methods limited to earphones (Bergman, Hirsch, and Solzi, 1987; Jerger, Johnson, Jerger, Coker, Pirozzolo, and Gray, 1991; Jerger, Martin, and Jerger, 1987; Papso and Blood, 1989). The results of these studies generally support such a hypothesis.

Dispensing with technology altogether may also open the way to other useful methods for assessing auditory processing in children. A few behavioral scales focused on auditory processing recently have been developed (Smoski et al., 1992), and there is no written rule stating that audiologists are forbidden from observing children

in daily living and contributing to the completion of behavioral surveys. Doing so may be a good way to increase the audiologist's participation in the professional team effort required for optimal remediation of pediatric CAPDs. Furthermore, until the relationships between the results of auditory processing tests, behavioral surveys, language evaluations, and cognitive assessments are investigated, cohesive team approaches will be difficult to coordinate.

### *Reporting and Use of Assessment Results*

No matter how sophisticated assessment methods may become, test results will be of little value unless they lead to effective, practical strategies for managing childhood CAPDs. The following excerpts from the results of two auditory processing assessments (A and B) performed for the same child by different clinicians illustrate approaches to reporting test results that either limit or increase the amount of useful information available. The child is an 8-year-old normal-hearing male with a history of developmental delays in articulation, language, and motor skills. He has been in special education programs since the age of 3. Results for the same auditory processing tests are interpreted in A and B.

A. It may be difficult for Sam to hear and understand speech, even though he has no peripheral hearing loss. Under these circumstances, his failure to respond should not be construed as a behavior problem or lack of motivation, but as a true organic disorder.

B. Specific auditory discrimination deficits [are indicated] for plosive and fricative consonants, when noise or other distracting stimuli are present. In particular, the voiceless consonants f, p, th, t, and s are identified. This pattern is consistent with some of Sam's articulation problems noted by [speech-language pathologist] in her report.

The difference in specificity between A and B is due to the fact that A is based solely on interpretation of numerical scores, while B is based on phonetic transcriptions of Sam's test responses, along with numerical scoring. As a result, therapy recommendations from assessment B could be focused on strategies to improve Sam's ability to discriminate target sounds in controlled steps of increasing noise, along with using an FM system and arranging preferential classroom seating, whereas recommendations from assessment A were limited to the latter strategy.

The foregoing example highlights one of the most powerful tools currently available for assessing pediatric auditory processing and making the best use of test results. The value of transcribing and scrutinizing each "incorrect" response that a child produces cannot be overstated. In doing so we can sample what the child perceives and identify factors important in shaping specific responses. This approach also is conducive to individualizing remediation for the child and to including other professionals in treatment planning. Additionally, it focuses attention on auditory-linguistic functioning and reduces the temptation to make potentially confusing or alarming pronouncements on the organicity of any deficits.

## SUMMARY

Hopefully, this chapter has demonstrated that the relationships between auditory processing stimuli and test responses may be influenced by many factors that can vary according to the construction of the stimuli and the auditory–linguistic functioning of the child. Efforts to understand what the child actually perceives, and to interpret auditory processing test results from that perspective, will lead to challenging opportunities for innovations in assessment and remediation methods. Audiologists who wish to meet these challenges should have special preparation in neuroanatomy and neurophysiology, child psychology, speech and language development, speech science, and test construction. Also, teamwork with other professionals should be increased to maximize our efforts in serving children with auditory processing disorders.

## REFERENCES

Barcikowski, R. S. (1983). *Computer Packages and Research Design* (vol. 2, SAS). Lanham, MD: University Press of America.

Barkley, R. A. (1990). *Attention-Deficit Hyperactivity Disorder: A Handbook for Diagnosis and Treatment.* New York: Guilford Press.

Berger, K. W. (1977). *The Most Common 100,000 Words Used in Conversations.* Kent, OH: Herald Publishing House.

Bergman, M., Hirsch, S., and Solzi, P. (1987). Interhemispheric suppression: A test of central auditory function. *Ear and Hearing, 8*(2), 87–91.

Breedin, S. D., Martin, R. C., and Jerger, S. (1989). Distinguishing auditory and speech-specific perceptual deficits. *Ear and Hearing, 10*(5), 311–317.

Chalfant, J. C., and Scheffelin, M. A. (1969). Central processing dysfunctions in children. National Institute of Neurological Disease and Stroke Monograph 9. Bethesda, MD: U.S. Department of Health, Education, and Welfare.

Cherry, R. S. (1980). *Selective Auditory Attention Test.* St. Louis: Auditec of St. Louis.

Flavell, J. H. (1963). *The Developmental Psychology of Jean Piaget.* New York: D. Van Nostrand Company.

Hall, J. W. III, and Harris, D. P. (1994). Auditory evoked responses in acute brain injury and rehabilitation. In J. T. Jacobson (ed.), *Principles and Applications in Auditory Evoked Potentials* (pp. 477–516). Needham Heights: Allyn and Bacon.

Harris, D. P., Cannito, M., Descouzis, D., and Stiritz, L. (1990). Distinctive feature confusions in responses to filtered speech stimuli. Paper presented at the 17th Annual Meeting of the American Auditory Society, Seattle, WA.

Harris, D. P., Cannito, M., Descouzis, D., and Stiritz, L. (1992). Central auditory test results: Are we listening? An unpublished paper presented at the 19th Annual Meeting of the American Auditory Society, San Antonio, TX.

Harris, D. P., and Hall, J. W. III (1990). Feasibility of auditory event-related potential measurement in brain injury rehabilitation. *Ear and Hearing, 11,* 340–350.

Henri, B. P. (1994, January). Graduate student preparation: Tomorrow's challenge. *Asha, 36,* 43–46.

Jerger, J., Johnson, K., Jerger, S., Coker, N., Pirozzolo, F., and Gray, L. (1991). Central auditory processing disorder: A case study. *Journal of the American Academy of Audiology, 2*(1), 36–54.

Jerger, S., Martin, R. C., and Jerger, J. (1987). Specific auditory perceptual dysfunction in a learning disabled child. *Ear and Hearing, 8*(2), 78–86.

Jirsa, R. E. (1992). The clinical utility of the P3 AERP in children with auditory processing disorders. *Journal of Speech and Hearing Research, 35,* 903–912.

Jirsa, R. E. and Clontz, K. B. (1990). Long latency auditory event-related potentials from children with auditory processing disorders. *Ear and Hearing, 11*(3), 222–232.

Katz, J. (1962). The use of staggered spondaic words for assessing the integrity of the central auditory nervous system. *Journal of Auditory Research, 2,* 327–337.

Keith, R. W. (1986). *SCAN: A Screening Test for Auditory Processing Disorders.* San Antonio: The Psychological Corporation.

Knopman, D. S., Rubens, A. B., Klassen, A. C., and Meyer, M. W. (1982). Regional cerebral blood flow correlates of auditory processing. *Archives of Neurology, 39,* 487–493.

Kraus, N. and McGee, T. J. (1994). Mismatch negativity in the assessment of central auditory function. *American Journal of Audiology, 3*(2), 39–51.

Kuhl, P. K. (1980). Infant speech perception: Reviewing data on auditory category formation. In P. J. Levinson, and C. S. Sloane (eds.), *Auditory Processing and Language* (pp. 35–59). New York: Grune & Stratton.

Lieberman, P. (1977). *Speech Physiology and Acoustic Phonetics.* New York: Macmillan Publishing Company.

Mayer, R. E. (1977). *Thinking and Problem Solving: An Introduction to Human Cognition and Learning.* Glenview, IL: Scott, Foresman and Company.

Miller, G. A. and Nicely, P. E. (1955). An analysis of perceptual confusions among some English consonants. *Journal of the Acoustical Society of America, 27*(2), 338–352.

Musiek, F. E. (1983). Assessment of central auditory dysfunction: The dichotic digit test revisited. *Ear and Hearing, 4,* 79–83.

Musiek, F. E. (1985). Application of central auditory tests: An overview. In J. Katz (ed.), *Handbook of*

Clinical Audiology (3rd ed., pp. 321–336). Baltimore: Williams & Wilkins.

Musiek, F. E. and Baran, J. A. (1987). Central auditory assessment: Thirty years of challenge and change. *Ear and Hearing, 8*(Suppl. 4), 22S–35S.

Musiek, F. E. and Chermak, G. D. (1994). Three commonly asked questions about central auditory processing disorders: Assessment. *American Journal of Audiology, 8*(3), 23–27.

Netter, F. H. (1975). *The CIBA Collection of Medical Illustrations: Vol. I. Nervous system.* Rochester, NY: The Case-Hoytt Corporation.

Papso, C. F. and Blood, I. M. (1989). Word recognition skills of children and adults in background noise. *Ear and Hearing, 10*(4), 235–236.

Peterson, G. E. and Barney, H. L. (1952). Control methods used in a study of the vowels. *Journal of the Acoustical Society of America, 24*(2), 175–184.

Sloane, C. S. (1980). Auditory processing disorders in children: Diagnosis and treatment. In P. J. Levinson, and C. S. Sloane (eds.), *Auditory Processing and Language* (pp. 117–133). New York: Grune & Stratton.

Sloane, C. S. (1985). Auditory processing disorders: What are the implications regarding treatment? *Human Communication Canada, 9,* 117–126.

Sloane, C. S. (1986). *Treating Auditory Processing Difficulties: Theory and Practice* (pp. 5–19). San Diego: College-Hill Press.

Smith, E. C., Stapleton, J. M., and Halgren, E. (1986). Human medial temporal lobe potentials evoked in memory and language tasks. *Electroencephalography and Clinical Neurophysiology, 63,* 145–159.

Smoski, W. J., Brunt, M. A., and Tannahill, J. C. (1992). Listening characteristics of children with central auditory processing disorders. *Language, Speech, and Hearing Services in Schools, 23*(2), 145–152.

Willeford, J. A. (1985). Assessment of central auditory disorders in children. In M. L. Pinheiro, and F. E. Musiek (eds.), *Assessment of Central Auditory Dysfunction. Foundations and clinical correlates* (pp. 239–255). Baltimore: Williams & Wilkins.

Zimmerman, R. L. (1985). Neurologic considerations for audiologists. In J. Katz (ed.), *Handbook of Clinical Audiology* (3rd ed., pp. 39–53). Baltimore: Williams & Wilkins.

# PART THREE

# COUNSELING
# CONSIDERATIONS

# CHAPTER 9

# PARENT AND FAMILY COUNSELING

*FREDERICK N. MARTIN*

## INTRODUCTION

For most people the rearing of children is the single-most difficult venture of their lives. There is no challenge, large or small, for which most of us are more poorly prepared. The law makes no demands of would-be parents in terms of credentials, preparation, skill, knowledge, or even dedication. There are no manuals or required courses. It probably seems to most parents that common sense, personal experience, observation of other people's approaches to child rearing (both positive and negative), perhaps some reading, and a bit of good luck, will see them through the rigors of conceiving, bearing, rearing, and educating their children. Even under the most ideal circumstances, bringing up children is one of the most difficult and frustrating ongoing activities imaginable. When a child is physically or mentally challenged that task can be mind boggling.

In recent years the sensitivity to counseling issues has been raised, in large measure because of the work by Kübler-Ross, *On Death and Dying* (1969). She describes the difficulty physicians experience in dealing with the loss of their patients. Other clinicians also have difficulties in coping with the nontechnical management of patient disorders that involve *empathic* responses. This most assuredly includes working with children who have hearing loss. Our first task is to recognize the emotional needs of patients and their families. The second is to find ways to confront these needs.

## COUNSELING DEFINED

The word "care" is one of the primary dictionary definitions of counseling. The way counseling is usually defined by health-care providers is as a system of information transfer, in which the counselor (audiologist, physician, hearing aid dispenser) provides directions that the patient or family is expected to follow. This is no surprise since the word "client" comes from the Latin *cliens,* a follower, or one who bows, or leans on another (such as one's master) for protection. The alternative word "patient," which is the one I reluctantly prefer, is not much better, since its root is in the Latin *patiens,* to suffer, or to be a person passively receiving care. It is little wonder then that the clinician usually operates from a position of authority and the family from one of subservience.

Many clinicians have depended upon common sense and patient feedback to allow them to customize their emotional support to parents who must cope with rearing a child with a hearing disorder. Relying on skill at predicting or "reading" the emotional reactions of another can be unwise (Martin, Barr, and Bernstein, 1992). For example, we tend to believe that there is a linear relationship between the severity of a disorder and the intensity of the reaction families have when learning of that disorder. This is often untrue. I have seen parents accept the news of a severe hearing loss in their children in apparently calm and unemotional ways, while other parents go to pieces when they find their child needs a myringotomy.

Hodgson (1994) avers that counseling by audiologists should be concerned with two major areas. The first of these has to do with the disposition of information. This naturally includes interpretation of the tests that have been done, the medical and (re)habilitative aspects of the hearing loss, implications for education, amplification, social integration, and so forth. All of this is very logical to the clinician/counselor, and often it is falsely assumed that it is equally logical to the family. There is ample evidence, however, that at the time of the initial diagnosis of hearing loss, logic often takes a back seat to emotion, and families are incapable of assimilating and processing new and stressful facts. As important as it is that families are given the data they must have to base decisions regarding their child, it is useless to force-feed individuals who cannot digest those facts that carry an emotional message. The sensitive clinician recognizes this and may opt to stage the information given over a period of several sessions, at which time the accuracy of the original hearing tests can be verified. Even when emotions do not appear to dominate the counseling session, information is often misinterpreted or forgotten (Martin, Krueger, and Bernstein, 1990).

The second area Hodgson describes relates to the effects that emotion exerts on the counseling session. It has already been said that emotions can cloud logical thinking and perception. Audiologists must determine that families are prepared to accept and understand new ideas and information before they embark on the passage of this information. The important choices presented to families should not be made under pressure. With some exceptions, most families reach a time wherein they can be offered the diagnostic information needed to make the difficult decisions that must be made in the interest of the child with a hearing loss.

Parents react differently to bad or disappointing accounts about their children depending, to a large extent, on their personality styles. While audiologists do not deliver the same kinds of catastrophic health news that physicians often report, the news of their child's hearing loss may affect parents in much the same way as "the loss of the perfect child" (Rose, 1987, p. 82). Much has been written in recent years on the belief that people go through a series of stages in learning to cope with untoward situations. The dynamics of human behavior do not, for the most part, allow for such a simplistic approach to adjusting to situations that

can alter the future in dramatic ways. The concept of a series of stages of adjustment conjures up the notion of linear movement along a time line, beginning in the first stage, working through to the last stage, and, if all comes out well, winding up with a satisfactory adjustment. It seems to me that in reality, this progression is more like a flow chart, with "yes loops" and "no loops" along the way, and feedback to phases already passed through as likely as procession to the next phase.

An early phase encountered by most parents is the *shock* of learning that their child has a hearing loss that may be permanent and that this loss has totally unanticipated ramifications. It is often not possible to recognize when parents are in shock because their affects may become flat, and what they show outwardly is no emotional reaction at all. When in shock, people are incapable of processing new information. For the audiologist to explain the technical aspects of test results and then go on to discuss what must next be done for the child may be like forcing the parent to listen to a foreign language. The parents may appear to listen politely but may be uncomfortable and anxious to escape from what they perceive as a dire situation.

*Denial* is often manifested when parents say to the clinician, to each other, or to themselves: "This can't be true. It must be a mistake. A different audiologist will give us a different (better) answer to our questions." Many people remain in denial for long periods of time, which can be vexing to the audiologist who wants to get on with the business of habilitation for the child. Parents in denial may shop for rosier diagnostic findings, may seek out a variety of healers to make the child's symptoms go away, or may turn to religion as the sole answer to their problems. At a conference on counseling families Luterman (1987a) was asked by an audiologist what one is to do when religious parents use prayer and waiting rather than the advice they have been given for getting on with amplification and therapy. His answer was "God always wins," suggesting that it is not only unwise, but useless to try to argue with strong religious beliefs. Personal experience has led me to the same conclusion. Ultimately it is the right of the parents to determine the methods to be used in assisting their child and, indeed, whether any intervention takes place at all. Referral to a counselor with similar religious beliefs may result in less zealous views and may help the parents put issues into perspective.

It is common for parents to become angry when they learn of special difficulties that face them and their child. This *anger* need not be logical and can be directed at anyone and everyone. Parents may become angry at the obstetrician for not warning them of what was to come, at the pediatrician for suggesting they wait for a hearing evaluation when hearing loss was suspected earlier, at the audiologist who made the diagnosis and concretized what they were fearing in the abstract, at the grandparents for what they might feel is interference, at each other for just being there, and at the child, for it is the child who has to be addressed in unanticipated ways. What often accompanies or follows illogical anger is *guilt.*

It is natural for people to look upon a serious condition in their child as a form of punishment for past deeds or obligations not met. The comment, "Why did this happen to *me?*" is not uncommon. It does little good to advise parents that guilt will accomplish nothing, that they should put these emotions behind them and get on with things, and so forth. Parents may have some real reasons to feel guilty, such as the mother who ignored her physician's advice to quit smoking during her pregnancy, the use of drugs, or other violations of acceptable prenatal care. Often the guilt lessens as parents are encouraged to speak about their concerns for their children, and a caring audiologist can function as a good listener and help to ameliorate this. Talking with other parents who have been there may be extremely helpful. If guilt is persistent, neurotic, or damaging to progress, the audiologist should consider a referral for more in-depth psychological counseling.

The phase of *acknowledgment* allows parents to accept the problem and recognize that it does,

in fact, exist. However, acceptance does not imply that parents are ready to launch into those activities that are necessary for their child's aural habilitation. When parents can enter into *constructive action* they can see themselves intimately involved in the management of their child's hearing loss. I am impressed with the title of Luterman's (1987b) book, *Deafness in the Family,* for it implies that hearing loss is a condition that affects much more than the patient, but rather all those with whom the patient interacts.

It is a mistake to conclude that emotional turmoils are over once families have reached a point at which they can objectively deal with the difficulties associated with children who have hearing impairments. Often the early emotions reemerge, sometimes for no apparent reason and often when children move into new phases of their lives, such as beginning school, reaching adolescence, completion of education, entering into the workplace, and so forth. Even parents of adult, relatively unchallenged children will attest to the fact that parenting and concern over children never ends and, while emotional reactions may attenuate, they never really disappear.

## THE ROLE OF THE AUDIOLOGIST-COUNSELOR

The goal of audiologists is to help parents to achieve independence and learn to solve problems engendered by their child's hearing loss. It is tempting for audiologists to perform as case managers as they did during the all-important diagnostic phase. Luterman (1984) was one of the first to point out that audiologists should define their activity as *facilitators* when functioning in a guidance role.

The role of the audiologist as diagnostician of hearing loss in children is quite clear, and most clinicians and graduate students-in-training are comfortable in this personification. Counseling is, of course, a natural follow-up to diagnosis. Before diagnostic information can be imparted in ways that will be meaningful, it must first be determined whether parents may suffer adverse reactions to what they are told. Hearing parents naturally want to have children with normal hearing, just as many parents with profound hearing loss themselves might be disappointed to learn that their child's hearing is normal. Parents are often confused even before their children are brought for the diagnosis, and the technical jargon that follows may confuse them further.

Parents naturally become worried about their family's futures based on the discovery of hearing loss which, more often than not, is unanticipated. The fear sets in that family lifestyle changes are inevitable and that the future is uncertain. While allaying anxiety and fear in parents is an important part of the audiologist's responsibility, false expectations and promises, no matter how well intended, may eventually change the attitude of the parents from joyful support to angry disappointment.

Clark (1994) defines both the responsibilities and limitations of audiologists who function as counselors. To present information in matter-of-fact ways may result in less-than-satisfactory receipt and use of that information. Since audiologists may be said to be generally more at ease as diagnosticians than as counselors, there may be a conscious or unconscious desire to abrogate counseling duties. Many have a "that's not my job" attitude on this subject, or believe that "telling the facts" is all that is needed. The reality is that audiologists are the ideal persons to help families work with a child's course of action after diagnosis, since they are at the epicenter of the nonmedical management of hearing impairment. The question of academic and emotional preparedness naturally arises.

With very few exceptions audiologists are not well trained as counselors. They are not alone in this regard, other professionals whose responsibilities include counseling are equally unprepared. These "nonprofessional counselors," as Clark (1994) calls them, also include physicians, dentists, teachers, attorneys, the clergy, and friends. They may be contrasted sharply with "professional counselors" like psychologists and psychiatrists, although many of the latter group function

primarily as neurochemists. Whoever works with the families of children seen in audiology clinics must be prepared for ongoing interpersonal dialogues, both with children, if they are old enough, and with significant others.

## Counseling Theories

All counseling theories are based on a "therapeutic alliance" (Van Hecke, 1994) between the audiologist and patient or family. Most of the parents we see are psychologically normal but are trying to cope with a major disruption in their lives. Before audiologists embark on efforts to counsel families they should determine that the families are not facing deep emotional problems which, no matter how unintentional, might be exacerbated without referral to a professional counselor.

### Person-Centered Therapy

Also called *nondirective psychotherapy,* this is the approach originally advanced by Carl Rogers (1959). Its basic tenet is that, at some level of consciousness, patients know what is best for them. By careful listening and paraphrasing what families say, the audiologist helps them to tap their own inner resources. The audiologist avoids posing as an expert and tries to sidestep clear recommendations as solutions to problems. Above all, the audiologist/counselor never assumes an authoritarian role and allows the person being counseled to reach independent decisions.

Person-centered therapy also avoids the use of labels. The authors of the various chapters of this book have attempted to adopt the *people first* approach when discussing patients. "Person with a hearing impairment" is preferred to "hearing-impaired person" because it helps to keep individuals from fixating on their disability, thereby making it the reality of their self-image. Individuals do not want to be defined by their disabilities, and the growth we hope to see in the family is greater when they elevate their children's assets above their disabilities.

Many individuals with disabilities object to the use of the word "handicapped," although that word is seen and heard in many places. I have been told by a usually reliable source that the word comes from the time when beggars soliciting alms held out their caps in their hands. This is not an image desired by clinicians or the families they serve. Even if this etymology of the word "handicapped" is not correct, if the perception remains, the word should be avoided. Although I see problems with the word "disabled" it appears to be preferred as of this writing.

Since one of the objectives of patient-centered counseling is to increase the family's sense of self-worth, a nonjudgmental attitude on the part of the clinician is essential. Families should be helped to perceive that the audiologist's office is a place to which they can come and say anything they feel without fear of being judged. However, before families can be comfortable with audiologists, audiologists themselves must be comfortable in their roles.

The practice of person-centered therapy is virtually useless unless the clinician has a feeling of self-congruence. When this exists there is no need to hide behind an air of inflated professionalism. The audiologist can come out from behind the barrier of the office desk and sit close to and facing the family. This makes the exchange more intimate and need not lead to a lessening of respect. The words used by the clinician must be chosen carefully and tailored to individual circumstances. The use of jargon, which nonprofessional people cannot be expected to know, is often a clue that the clinician is insecure or insensitive. However, families can only be helped to find tangible solutions for their difficulties; no one else can resolve them.

Person-centered therapy requires, above all, good listening skills. Finding a good listener in any situation is difficult, for most people merely maintain their silence politely until they can make their own comments. Often little effort is spent at truly attending to what the other person says, and if the family senses this, a valuable link may be broken. Our ability to appreciate how people perceive their problems allows us to absorb the problem and then reflect it back in a supportive way.

## Behavioral Counseling

It was through the work of B. F. Skinner (1953), that we learned the principles of operant conditioning. A behavior is learned when it is followed by circumstances that are rewarding. This is called *positive reinforcement.* When a family does not allow a child to wear hearing aids to church or family gatherings because of their self-consciousness, this behavior may be reinforced by a decrease in anxiety or embarrassment. To extinguish this kind of behavior it must be demonstrated to the family that these rewards are illusions and that anxiety is raised when these behaviors are carried out.

Unlike the Rogerian approach, behavioral counseling is a direct method. The family is advised that they can derive rewards by making environmental changes that produce positive behavioral changes. The behavioral approach involves telling people what one thinks, as opposed to paraphrasing what the family has said, as used in the Rogerian method.

## Combining Counseling Methods

With some practice the two methods described above can be combined. Audiologists have a moral and legal obligation not to get in over their heads when counseling families. They should know the availability of professional counselors in their areas and visit with them to learn of their approaches before making referrals. It is extremely valuable to find a counselor who understands some of the problems associated with hearing impairment. On rare occasions counselors are available who have at least a rudimentary knowledge of sign language, which is very much appreciated by people who communicate manually. No mention is made in this chapter of more sophisticated psychotherapeutic approaches because I believe that without proper training they can be misused and dangerous. For in-depth reading the suggested list of books at the end of this chapter may be consulted. Readers who are interested in other psychotherapeutic methods are urged to research those areas.

Although it is often difficult for audiologists to make referrals for professional counseling, in some cases such referrals are imperative. It is most important for audiologists to make referrals before they get into situations that they do not fully understand and from which they might find it difficult to extricate themselves. Red flags should wave when families come to depend on audiologists for decisions, not only about their children, but about other, sometimes intimate aspects of their lives.

Audiologists must learn to recognize depression in parents and to determine whether that depression has reached clinical significance. Parents have been told: "Of course you are depressed, who would not be at learning all you have learned about the problems of your child?" Depression has been defined as "anger turned inward," and so long as parents struggle with this they may be incapable of working with and for their children. Other signals that referral is needed include persistence in denial, anger, or guilt; withdrawal from everyday activities; sleep or appetite disturbances; difficulty concentrating; excessive procrastination (as in putting off the purchase of hearing aids); or unrealistically high expectations (Clark, 1994).

Relatively little is known about the reactions of siblings of children who have hearing loss. While Trevino (1979) recommends involvement of the entire family of a challenged child in the counseling process, Murphy (1979) specifically advocates support groups for siblings. Such meetings allow for the ventilation of pent-up emotions about the disabled sibling, along with opportunities to obtain new information. A recent study using the Sibling Inventory of Differential Experience (SIDE) failed to show significant differences between siblings of children with hearing loss and a control group of siblings of children with normal hearing with regard to such logical emotions as jealousy, affection, and antagonism. (Martin, Grace, and Vangelisti, unpublished ms). The fact that these differences did not reach significance does not mean that they do not exist or that sibling emotions should be ignored, only that more needs to be learned on this issue. Parental suggestions

for the siblings of children with hearing loss may be found in Appendix 8.

In making a referral for a parent, sibling, or patient for professional counseling it is wise to anticipate the possibility of adverse reactions. The audiologist must be prepared for such responses as: "Why are you sending me to a psychologist? Do you think I'm crazy?" When referring to other professionals I prefer the term "counselor" to other kinds of labels because it does not connote mental illness in any way. If the family objects to the referral or reacts negatively to it, all clinicians can do is share their concerns for the best treatment of the child and answer questions as kindly and honestly as they can.

Both in and out of their professional roles, audiologists, like everyone else, have developed their own social styles. Many of us emulate the styles of professors or supervisors we admired during our education and training. As we accrue our own experiences we develop systems that work best for us and with which we are most comfortable. When we step away from communication systems with which we are comfortable we run the risk of appearing insincere and losing the rapport with families that is so important.

Some clinicians are comfortable with the use of humor in counseling. I consider humor to be hazardous for no matter how well intentioned it can be perceived as trivialization of the families' concerns. Audiologists must not only understand their own social styles, but must be able to recognize those of the families so that the two can be blended.

## Preparing for Dialogue

Psychotherapy is generally held to mean the application of any form of mental treatment in the interest of achieving or maintaining psychological well-being. Such treatments can range from hypnosis to psychopharmacology, from suggestion to psychoanalysis, or from directive measures to supportive listening and reflection. It is obvious that audiologists without specific training have no business meddling in what may be the explosively troubled lives of others. However, psychological support counseling can be carried out by persons with little formal training as long as they function as sensitive listeners.

Stream and Stream (1978) advise the audiologist, before embarking on counseling, to stop, look, and listen. They believe that the audiologist must *stop* long enough to review audiometric data and to make a plan on what information is to be conveyed and the best ways to interpret it to the family. They should *look* for feedback from the family for verbal and nonverbal cues about how the process is proceeding and make adjustments as they go along. Finally, they must *listen* for specific questions that may be broken down into three types: content questions (requests for specific information), confirmation questions (searching for support of positions that the parents may have already established), and affect questions (those that may be a guise for emotions). Except for specific questions of content, like "How much hearing loss does my child have?", there are no absolutes, no correct or incorrect responses, only those that are appropriate to the situation (Luterman, 1976).

### Support Counseling

Support counseling is a part of the ongoing interaction between the audiologist and the family, for it addresses the concerns of those most closely involved with the child. The apprehensions of parents must be recognized even if they are unstated. It is natural for audiologists to be uncertain in many cases just how far to go in counseling.

Like all counselors, audiologists must recognize their own shortcomings. Counseling coursework is usually limited or absent, and practice is varied based on experience and work setting. In the process of designing a study on the perceptions of professionals dealing with patients with hearing loss, we (Martin, et al., 1992) interviewed a number of audiologists and otolaryngologists while we were designing our questionnaires. What surprised us was the number of people we initially interviewed who thought that the results

of our study would not be particularly revealing since they did not perceive patients as having emotional difficulties when dealing with the news of an irreversible hearing loss. One very excellent otologist stated: "I just tell them what is wrong and what they need to do about it. I never see anything like shock, disappointment or depression." This takes us back to the earlier statement about how difficult it often is to learn from facial expressions and body language just how troubled families may be about disappointing news, even if that news was anticipated. Results of our studies both in the United States and Australia supported the hypothesis that many individuals are troubled at the time they receive the diagnosis of hearing loss. They either condemn clinicians whom they perceive to be insensitive or appreciate those who appear to care about their feelings (Martin, George, O'Neal, and Daly, 1987; Martin, Abadie, and Descouzis, 1989).

Another reason audiologists are often uncomfortable as counselors is that we, too, are human and prefer to avoid unpleasant encounters. It is doubtful that too many people like to go to the dentist and maybe, for some patients, seeing us is just as dreaded. What we often tell parents truly hurts. We may reduce our own anxieties by consciously or unconsciously ignoring parents' difficulties in coping. Audiologists may further avoid dealing with adjustment problems in hopes that other professionals will be seeing the family down the line and do what we were uncomfortable in doing. The "others" may have similar anxieties and so the family falls between the cracks, with no one to see to their needs for support.

For audiologists to function successfully as counselors, certain realities must be faced. Clinicians should not hold out impossibly high standards for themselves or the families with whom they work. Often family expectations must be scaled down to avoid later disappointment, even if those expectations are required to maintain the enthusiasm needed to carry out (re)habilitation. Audiologists must realize that none of their efforts can make up to parents for the loss of communication and disappointment about hearing loss in a child. To function adequately audiologists must be comfortable in their roles as counselors. However, they should not consider themselves to be long-term therapists, particularly if emotional aspects of confronting a child's hearing loss appear to be intense, or if initial adverse reactions do not subside.

### Content Counseling

When most clinicians think about working with patients and families, it is probably content counseling that comes to mind. Here audiologists are comfortable, for it appears to involve conveying the results of their tests along with their interpretations. It also includes laying out plans for the future treatment of the child with an auditory problem. However, studies (e.g., Martin et al., 1987) show that families often tend to feel that they have not been given all the information they require at the time of diagnosis or shortly thereafter. Clinicians, on the other hand, may either present too much technical information for families to comprehend, or may hold back in fear that the parents will understand very little.

A sensible place to begin content counseling is simply to ask families what they know about the child's hearing problem and what they wish to know. Clinicians may be surprised by some families who say that they do not wish to be told any more than what they must know to understand the rudiments of the hearing problem and what must be done about it. In such cases a clear diagnosis isall that should be told to them at the evaluation, and further explanations should be made at a later date when the family is ready. There are sometimes conflicts between parents when one is anxious to leave and the other wishes more information.

Sooner or later, however, careful explanation of test results must be imparted to the family. The more families understand about hearing loss in general, and the particulars of their children's problems, the better they are able to cope with their future lifestyle. Education of the family is es-

sential if they are to accept their roles as authorities in the management of their children and come to understand the facilitator role assumed by the audiologist.

If an audiogram has been obtained, it should be explained clearly, starting with the graph itself and what the coordinates mean. What is often said is something like: "This is pitch and this is loudness. This is your child's threshold in decibels at each frequency." If neophytes are not confused and bewildered by this jargon, they are unusual. No proposed monologue is suggested here, for thinking audiologists will need to find their own words. Audiologists should recall that it probably took several weeks into the first course in audiology before many of these concepts became clear to them and that it is expecting far too much of families to understand and retain such new and technical information.

A variety of pamphlets and videotapes can be loaned or given to families, which will allow them to review what is said in the clinic in the privacy of their own homes. This has the additional advantage of allowing other interested parties to participate in the learning process. At the time of the next visit the materials can be reviewed and questions answered. Results of electrophysiologic tests, including otoacoustic emissions, auditory evoked potentials, and acoustic immittance, along with their implications, should also be reviewed.

It is difficult for parents facing the problems of rearing and educating a child with a disability not to feel terribly alone. Though such feelings defy logic they may be present in the most intelligent parents. Under ideal circumstances, group meetings can be set up with other parents, preferably in the evening, so that if there are two parents, both can attend (Atkins, 1994). Lectures can be delivered on such topics as anatomy and physiology of the auditory system, interpretations of test results, habilitative options, amplification systems, and so forth. The knowledge available in such situations, coupled with the group psychotherapeutic value, can be immeasurable.

## AUDIOLOGIC COUNSELING

### When Counseling Begins

Many people believe that the counseling process begins before the child arrives at the clinic (e.g., Luterman, 1987c; Martin, 1994). There is often a time delay between when parents request an appointment for their child's hearing evaluation and their actual appointment date. This is unfortunate in many ways because it may have taken the family a while to become convinced that they should address their concerns for their children. Nevertheless, the time interval can be used constructively.

Many audiology clinics send information through the mail to families of children to be seen for hearing evaluations. Often included are maps or directions to the audiology clinic, information about fees for services, instructions regarding what will take place, and a history form (see Appendix 3). Parents can complete the history on their child in an unhurried fashion in their homes, checking on dates of important matters such as illnesses and developmental milestones. One of the first tasks that can be done when the parents arrive at the clinic is to review the history and obtain clarification of certain facts that are incomplete or obscure. Consideration of the history in advance of the child's arrival can help the audiologist plan the appropriate diagnostic path in terms of the hierarchy of procedures to be used. It should not be prejudicial in the ultimate diagnosis, for histories can be quite misleading.

When the family arrives at the clinic and faces the audiologist, the first real opportunity for developing rapport presents itself. It is frequently best to begin with a statement of the problem as perceived by the family. A good way to commence is "Why did you bring your child to the clinic today?" or "What questions do you want answered about your child today?" These are obviously preferable to leading questions like "Tell me about your child's hearing loss." What the parents say and the manner in which they say

it can provide insights not only in terms of diagnosis, but also in approaches to counseling that will follow.

Although some parents are uncomfortable in watching their children's hearing evaluations, it is very often desirable to have them observe. If both parents are present, which is highly preferable but often impossible, one can remain in the patient room with the child and audiology assistant (if the child is very young), while the other can sit with the audiologist at the audiometer. Often a useful dialogue can be set up so that questions are asked and answered while the test is in progress.

### The Conference

The time for conferencing usually comes after hearing tests have been completed. Often young children are tired and fretful at this point and it is best if someone can tend to them in a separate room to avoid distraction. A good way to begin is to ask the parents what they thought of the evaluation and the ways in which the child behaved. Often they will state that the child appeared to have difficulty in hearing, which allows the clinician to agree with parental statements, dignifying their opinions. It may be necessary to probe the parents for statements, for often they say that they do not know what to conclude. The audiologist may decide at this juncture to offer either direct or indirect counseling, based on the perception of the parents' ability to comprehend the diagnosis and its ramifications.

It goes without saying that the family and the child must be treated with the utmost respect at all times. If children are old enough and have sufficient language to allow for verbal communication it should be aimed directly at them in the presence of the parents. In other instances the parents are addressed directly and their opinions sought at strategic points during the conversation.

It is unwise for audiologists to adopt airs of detachment, which is sometimes done to avoid personal involvement and to convey professionalism. Parents also do not enjoy the "small talk" that some clinicians use to "break ground" for the serious business to follow. The goal, of course, is to establish rapport with the family and this is best accomplished by showing interest and concern. Encouraging questions from the family is an excellent way of communicating what is essential, using topics of their choosing.

All answers to family questions should be made honestly. Content questions deserve content answers. It often happens that on the first examination of a young child only an approximation of the extent of an auditory disorder is known (see Chapter 6). That should be admitted honestly and plans made to pursue the testing. Some information asked for by parents is either not known or unwise to convey. For example, many parents wish to know the percentage of their child's hearing loss. This is generally a very misleading concept; for example, using the American Academy of Ophthalmology and Otolaryngology (1979) percentage of hearing impairment formula, an average hearing loss of 92 dB computes to a 100 percent hearing impairment. This would suggest to parents that no usable hearing remains, bringing into question why the audiologist may be suggesting amplification and aural habilitation. Most audiologists would agree that a 92-dB hearing loss can constitute a lot of residual hearing. Conversely, the same formula shows that an average hearing loss of 25 dB HL computes to zero percent hearing impairment, indicating normal hearing. Audiologists frequently provide amplification and rehabilitative strategies for children with a 25-dB hearing loss because it is needed. Percentage of hearing impairment is not a useful concept in counseling parents despite its apparent simplicity.

At times, despite everyone's good intentions, hostility develops between the audiologist and the family. The audiologist may feel threatened by comments made by the family, and the family may feel defensive about comments made by the audiologist about their child. Good clinicians should never have a reason to feel threatened by patients or families, but it is natural for families to feel threatened at the thought of their lives changing following delivery of upsetting news by an audiologist.

One reason for parental hostility is their sense that insufficient progress is being made with their child. They may feel that it is taking too long to make a precise diagnosis, or that once remediation has begun the child is not making the kind of advancement they anticipated. Their concerns must be heard with empathy and acceptance. Rogerian counseling can be very useful here, with such expressions as, "You don't feel that your daughter is getting enough help from her hearing aids." This shows the family that you understand their concern, that you care about them, and that you wish to hear more. If the family is referred as soon as possible to an appropriate program, support counseling should be available on a regular basis so they can talk through their feelings.

It is tempting to give parents "pep talks," both at the counseling following initial diagnosis and during remediation. It is unwise to make promises of an excellent outcome but, short of this, optimism should be expressed. Parents dislike being told that a clinician "understands" how they feel, so this should never be stated. No one can truly understand the deep emotions of another. Careful reflection of the parents' words can convey empathy, however.

One of the major complaints that parents make is that they feel rushed, both during and after evaluations of their child's hearing. This resentment is probably justified in many cases, even if the audiologist never intended to slight the family in any way. Whether true or not, the perception that the family is rushed through a difficult time can damage a relationship that is important to the child. Often there is no easy way to solve this problem, but knowing that it might exist can help the audiologist to find practical ways to deal with it. If it is not possible to complete a conference because of imminent time constraints, another appointment should be set up at the earliest possible time.

There are times during meetings with parents when seemingly interminable periods of silence occur. When this happens it appears neither party has anything to say to the other. This can be disquieting, especially when audiologists sense that they are losing control and may feel that they must plunge in to fill the gaps with information and advice. At times families just need time to gather their thoughts, and patient waiting is very much appreciated. If it appears that nothing more can be accomplished at this meeting, the next one should be scheduled.

Counseling families is an ongoing process that continues throughout the professional association the family develops with the audiologist. Clinicians may never fully realize the impact they may have on the lives of the patients they assist and their families. This can be rewarding and fulfilling or terribly frustrating. Many families find in the audiologist the first person who truly paid attention to their concerns for their children and remain eternally grateful for what they have done. Although the demeanor of the audiologist should not change, the precise information that is conveyed to families about a child's hearing loss will naturally vary, depending on a number of factors, including the age at onset and type and degree of the impairment.

### Severe Prelinguistic Sensorineural Hearing Loss

Counseling is most challenging when parents are told that their child has a severe hearing loss that is probably irreversible. Even if the diagnosis has been anticipated it can be devastating. Although details may be staged over several interviews, parents must be told of the options that are open to them on the ways in which their child may be educated (Johnson, 1994). As soon as they can handle the information they should learn how to interpret their child's audiogram. At the earliest feasible time parents should be advised to speak with parents of other children with hearing losses similar to their child's, so that the sense of being alone can be lessened (Atkins, 1994). Although this process cannot be rushed, audiologists should not fail to seize every opportunity to move families along

in the interests of their child. If an oral/aural approach is to be taken, amplification systems should be discussed (see Chapters 11 and 14). At the appropriate times, parents may need to be educated on some of the less traditional approaches to amplification such as cochlear implants or vibrotactile instruments (see Chapter 13). If the parents so desire, referral may be made so that they can speak with members of the deaf community on manual communication approaches for their child.

### Adventitious Sensorineural Hearing Loss

When a child acquires a postlinguistic sensorineural hearing loss it is usually due to illness or trauma, of which the parents are aware, although audiologists must always be on the lookout for heritodegenerative hearing losses. When the hearing loss is postlinguistic and the child has developed language concepts and skills, the parents should be encouraged, again as soon as they are capable of managing the important information, to embark on speech and language conservation procedures. The use of amplification should be introduced as soon as possible. If the child attends school the efficacy of FM transmission systems should be discussed and, if and when the parents are ready, the audiologist should be prepared to introduce the system to the teacher and perform demonstrations in the classroom (see Chapter 14). Such systems have proved to be highly successful for a variety of hearing losses, including cases of unilateral hearing loss.

### Congenital Conductive Hearing Loss

In those cases of hereditary or early acquired conductive hearing loss, such as those due to external auditory canal atresias, the best approach may be to prescribe a bone-conduction hearing aid. Parents must understand enough about aural anatomy to realize why such recommendations are being made. If an implantable bone-conduction device seems in order it should be discussed, but the parents must be made aware early in these discussions that the final decision on such matters is always left to the ear surgeon. If they are interested, parents should be helped in making an appointment with an otolaryngologist who has experience with such surgery.

### Conductive Hearing Loss Secondary to Infection

There are many times when audiological and immittance measures reveal the presence of conditions that require immediate medical attention. Otitis media with effusion is an illustration of a situation where time may be of the essence. Protracted nondirective counseling may result, in some cases, in tympanic membrane perforation. The child's health and safety may need to take precedence over the family's difficulty in accepting the fact that an abnormality exists. When the audiologist is fearful that waiting may result in unfortunate medical sequelae, a direct approach should be taken and, short of frightening the parents, they should be urged to follow up immediately.

There are some awkward times when audiologists see children with chronic ear conditions that they feel are either mismanaged or handled too conservatively. This presents a counseling dilemma, for the audiologist must balance the concept of ethics (which can be defined strictly in this case as not crossing the barrier into the practice of medicine), with a moral point of view (which dictates that the audiologist cannot stand by and watch the child being deprived of proper medical care). In such cases, the counseling skills of the audiologist are sorely tested. Whenever a child is referred for medical treatment of a conductive hearing loss, arrangements should be made for audiological and tympanometric follow-up. Ears can look perfectly normal following medical treatment, even if a conductive hearing loss persists.

### Genetic Counseling

It has been said that approximately half of all profound hearing loss in children is genetically based. For many reasons, less is known about the statistics involving mild to severe losses. Genetic counseling related to hearing loss is designed to assist potential parents in their decisions regarding family planning.

It is difficult for many audiologists to address the results of genetic analysis objectively because we may bring our own philosophies to the topic. As mentioned earlier, it is common for most parents with normal hearing to want children with normal hearing, and for many parents with severe hearing losses to want children with severe hearing losses. This has to do with what has come to be a sometimes unfortunate alienation between the "hearing community" and the "deaf community." Individuals who identify with the latter may feel that the efforts of audiologists to force children with severe hearing loss into the former are misplaced. At the extreme are those who believe that there is an almost genocidal attempt to do away with the "deaf community," which has its own systems of communication and philosophy.

The genetics associated with hearing loss in children are discussed in Chapter 2. Endeavors such as the American Genome Project hold forth a mixture of positive and negative concerns. If, as predicted, all 100,000 human genes will have been mapped by the year 2005, parents will be able to determine, even before conception, whether an hereditary hearing loss will be present in their child. This raises a myriad of ethical considerations that may boggle the minds of modern philosophers. Should a pregnancy be terminated because the child may have a hearing loss? Can health insurance companies refuse to cover a fetus whose life will be complicated by expensive and complicated procedures? Will parents *want* to know the potential hearing status of their children?

In many cases, the audiologist is the tie between the family and the genetic counselor. This means that the audiologist must know who to call upon or refer to when genetic counseling is needed. The purpose is not just to supply information necessary to help parents make important decisions, but to support the family in dealing with the information that may be forthcoming.

Genetic counseling is best accomplished through the team approach. Such a team ideally includes the geneticist, the counselor, usually a person with a master's or RN degree with special interests in genetics, and other specialists who have expertise in specific disorders such as cleft palate or hearing loss (Smith, 1994). It is important that audiologists bring up the possibility of genetic counseling whenever that might be helpful. This is important for professional, moral and legal reasons.

If referral for genetic counseling is not made, important information may not become a part of the decision-making process. To deprive parents of information they may not even know they have available to them is unfair. Finally, failure to make appropriate referral might lead, as it has before, to legal action against the audiologist for failing to point out potential hearing loss.

## SUMMARY

All of the diagnostic expertise of the audiologist may be for naught if families are not helped to understand their children's hearing disorders and what must be done to ameliorate them. Despite outward appearances to the contrary, many parents are emotionally fragile when it comes to dealing with their child's hearing loss. The audiologist must display warmth and concern for the family and apply humanity along with science. What is most important, and what all caring clinicians can bring to counseling, is patience and understanding, and a recollection of what it is like for all of us to feel alone, confused, and frightened.

## REFERENCES

Atkins, D. V. (1994). Counseling children with hearing loss and their families. In J. G. Clark and F. N. Martin (eds.), *Effective Counseling in Audiology: Perspectives and Practice* (pp. 116–146). Englewood Cliffs, NJ: Prentice-Hall.

American Academy of Ophthalmology and Otolaryngology Committee on Hearing and Equilibrium and the American Council of Otolaryngology Committee on the Medical Aspects of Noise. (1979). Guide for the evaluation of hearing handicap. *Journal of the American Medical Association, 241,* 2055–2059.

Clark, J. G. (1994). Audiologists' counseling purview. In J. G. Clark and F. N. Martin (eds.), *Effective Counseling in Audiology: Perspectives and Practice* (pp. 1–17). Englewood Cliffs, NJ: Prentice-Hall.

Hodgson, W. R. (1994). Audiologic counseling. In J. Katz (ed.), *Handbook of Clinical Audiology* (pp. 616–623). Baltimore: Williams & Wilkins.

Kübler-Ross, E. (1969). *On Death and Dying.* New York: Macmillan.

Johnson, C. D. (1994). Educational consultation: Talking with parents and school personnel. In J. G. Clark and F. N. Martin (eds.), *Effective Counseling in Audiology: Perspectives and Practice* (pp. 184–209). Englewood Cliffs, NJ: Prentice-Hall.

Luterman, D. (1976). The counseling experience. *Journal of the Academy of Rehabilitative Audiology, 9,* 62–66.

Luterman, D. (1984). *Counseling Parents of Hearing-Impaired Children and Their Families.* Boston: Little, Brown & Company.

Luterman, D. (1987a). Counseling parents of hearing-impaired children. In F. N. Martin (ed.), *Hearing Disorders in Children* (pp. 303–320). Englewood Cliffs, NJ: Prentice-Hall.

Luterman, D. (1987b). *Deafness in the Family.* Boston: Little, Brown & Company.

Luterman, D. (1987c). Counseling the Communicatively Disordered and Their Families. Symposium of the National Student Speech-Language-Hearing Association, The University of Texas at Austin.

Martin, F. N. (1994). Conveying diagnostic information. In J. G. Clark and F. N. Martin (eds.), *Effective Counseling in Audiology: Perspectives and Practice* (pp. 38–69). Englewood Cliffs, NJ: Prentice-Hall.

Martin, F. N., Abadie, K. T., and Descouzis, D. (1989). Counseling families of hearing-impaired children: Comparisons of the attitudes of Australian and U.S. parents and audiologists. *Australian Journal of Audiology, 11,* 41–54.

Martin, F. N., Barr, M., and Bernstein, M. (1992). Professional attitudes regarding counseling of hearing-impaired adults. *The American Journal of Otology, 13,* 279–287.

Martin, F. N., George, K., O'Neal, J., and Daly, J. (1987). Audiologists' and parents' attitudes regarding counseling of hearing-impaired children, *Asha, 29,* 27–33.

Martin, F. N., Grace, M. B., and Vangelisti, A. (1994). Perceptions of siblings of children with hearing impairment: Siblings, parents and peer relations. Unpublished manuscript.

Martin, F. N., Krueger, J. S., and Bernstein, M. (1990). Diagnostic information transfer to hearing-impaired adults. *Tejas, 16,* 29–32.

Murphy, A. (1979). *The Families of Hearing Impaired Children.* Washington, DC: A. G. Bell.

Rogers, C. R. (1959). A theory of therapy personality and interpersonal relationships. In Koch, S. (ed.), *Psychology: A Study of Science* (vol. 3, pp. 184–256). New York: McGraw-Hill.

Rose, D. (1987). The psychological world of the hearing-impaired child and the family. In F. N. Martin (ed.), *Hearing Disorders in Children* (pp. 81–111). Englewood Cliffs, NJ: Prentice-Hall.

Skinner, B. F. (1953). *Science and Human Behavior.* New York: Free Press.

Smith, S. (1994). Genetic counseling. In J. G. Clark and F. N. Martin (eds.), *Effective Counseling in Audiology: Perspectives and Practice* (pp. 70–91). Englewood Cliffs, NJ: Prentice-Hall.

Stream, R. W. and Stream, K. S. (1978). Counseling the parents of the hearing-impaired child. In F. N. Martin (ed.), *Pediatric Audiology* (pp. 311–355). Englewood Cliffs, NJ: Prentice-Hall.

Trevino, F. (1979). Siblings of handicapped children: Identifying those at risk. *Social Casework: The Journal of Contemporary Social Work, 60,* 488–493.

Van Hecke, M. L. (1994). Emotional responses to hearing loss. In J. G. Clark and F. N. Martin (eds.), *Effective Counseling in Audiology: Perspectives and Practice* (pp. 92–115). Englewood Cliffs, NJ: Prentice-Hall.

## SUGGESTED READING

Arbuckle, D. S. (1970). *Counseling: Philosophy, Theory and Practice* (2nd ed.). Boston: Allyn and Bacon.

Clark, J. G., and Martin, F. N. (eds) (1994). *Effective Counseling in Audiology: Perspectives and Practice.* Englewood Cliffs, NJ: Prentice-Hall.

Hoffman, L. (1981). *Foundations of Family Therapy.* New York: Basic Books.

Kennedy, E. (1977). *On Becoming a Counselor: A Basic Guide for Nonprofessional Counselors.* New York: Continuum.

Kopp, S. (1972). *If You Meet the Buddha on the Road Kill Him!* Palo Alto: Science and Behavioral Books.

Kübler-Ross, E. (1969). *On Death and Dying.* New York: Macmillan.

Lieberman, M., Yalom, I., and Miles, M. (1973). *Encounter Groups: First Facts.* New York: Basic Books.

Mearns, D. and Thorne, B. (1988). *Person Centered Counseling in Action.* London: Page Publications.

Minuchin, S. (1974). *Families and Family Therapy.* Cambridge: Harvard University Press.

Murphy, A. (1981). *Special Children, Special Parents.* Englewood Cliffs, NJ: Prentice-Hall.

Peck, S. (1978). *The Road Less Traveled.* New York: Simon and Schuster.

Schein, J. (1982). *Group Psychotherapy and Counseling with Special Populations.* Baltimore: University Park Press.

Schneider, J. (1983). *The Nature of Loss, the Nature of Grief. A Comprehensive Model for Facilitation and Understanding.* Baltimore: University Park Press.

Schneider, J. (1984). *Stress, Loss, & Grief.* Baltimore: University Park Press.

Siegel, B. S. (1986). *Love, Medicine, & Miracles.* New York: Harper & Row.

Skinner, B. F. (1953). *Science and Human Behavior.* New York: Free Press.

Stewart, M., and Roter, D. (eds.) 1989). *Communicating with Medical Patients.* Newbury Park, CA: Sage.

Thrower, P., Casey, A., and Dryden, W. (1988). *Cognitive-Behavioral Counseling in Action.* London: Page Publications.

Webster, E. (1977). *Counseling with Parents of Handicapped Children.* New York: Grune and Stratton.

Yalom, I. (1989) *Love's Executioner.* New York: Basic Books.

# CHAPTER 10

# MEETING THE NEEDS OF ADOLESCENTS WITH IMPAIRED HEARING

*ELLYN ALTMAN*

## INTRODUCTION

The year was 1973. The child in the rear of the car was 9 years old. Her audiologist of eight years had finally found hearing aids he thought sufficiently powerful for her profoundly impaired hearing. He had given her the opportunity to remove her body aids and replace them with hearing aids that fit behind her ears and under her hair. Finally she felt she could be just like all her other hearing impaired friends and almost like the other kids at school who could hear. Gone were the unnatural protrusions through her shirt, embarrassing her with the premature announcement of breasts that would take years to develop. Gone was the weight of the "boxes" against her flat chest. No longer did unattractive wires compete with her lovely long dark curls. She had been ecstatic.

But something was wrong. She had struggled for days with the reality that these behind-the-ear aids—the most powerful yet manufactured according to her audiologist—were insufficient to help her use her residual hearing to complement what her speech reading missed. They could not help her maintain the good quality of her speech and voice that her body aids did. Though impaired, she valued her hearing and needed it so that she could function in the world in which she had become a full-fledged member. She could not and would not deny the reality. These hearing aids were not right. From the rear of the car she called sadly to her parents: "We need to stop the car and get my aids out of the trunk. These don't work for me."

This child was Stephanie, my daughter, who is now an oral deaf adult. Her statement at 9 years of age demonstrated her commitment to, reliance on, and appreciation of her residual hearing and her hearing aids.

There have been other young people with hearing impairments who have entered my life since Stephanie: her friends, my patients, and their families, and the participants in research I have conducted (Altman, 1988). Their stories describe varying experiences with hearing impairments. This chapter is about their adolescence. Indirectly they will be your teachers as I share what they, my training, and my clinical experiences have taught me.

This chapter has been designed to discuss the tasks of adolescence and the resources adolescents have developed through childhood and bring to this period to negotiate their way through the challenges they encounter. The role of the audiologist as a service provider is discussed with regard to developing a collaborative relationship with the adolescent.

## ADOLESCENCE—A PURPOSEFUL TRANSITIONAL PERIOD CONNECTING CHILDHOOD TO YOUNG ADULTHOOD

Adolescence begins at preadolescence (10–12 years) and may continue through an extended adolescence into the twenties. It includes young people who are dependent and in college and those still clarifying their occupational goals. This bridge between childhood and adulthood is the time during which the competencies needed to maintain a self-sufficient existence are developed. It is the period of change wherein complementary developmental phenomena including physiologic changes, emotional and social maturation, intellectual development, sexual development, and cultural forces intertwine.

The physiologic changes and cognitive developments that lead to a sense of personal identity and social growth during adolescence take place in the cloistered environment of adolescent society, located in schools and community-centered sites. By the conclusion of adolescence, young people are expected to have passed through and overcome the emotional instabilities of adolescence and to enter young adulthood with a meaningful perspective on the world, an appreciation for their culture, and a sense of purpose.

As we proceed we will consider the contributions that pediatric audiologists and workers from related professions can make to ensure, whenever possible, that the adolescent with impaired hearing is prepared to enter adulthood with the greatest possibilities for success and satisfaction.

## THE CHILD WITH HEARING LOSS AND THE EFFECTS OF EARLY EXPERIENCE ON PREPARATION FOR ADOLESCENCE

### Important Variables Impacting on Development

Because so may variables operate to distinguish one child from another, broad brush strokes to describe the development of "the" hearing-impaired child will not suffice. We will consider many variables that influence development to obtain as much understanding as possible to empathize with the developmental challenges facing young children who have impaired hearing.

Among the many important influences that will have a differential effect on the course of development is the time of onset of the hearing im-

pairment. There is a difference between children who have a congenital impairment and those who are postlinguistically deafened at an early age. There is also a difference between those who progressively lose their hearing in childhood and those who lose their hearing after a serious illness. The personal sense of loss is qualitatively different as is the nature of the depression that may underlie emotional development. It is also a decidedly different experience when the perspective is taken that deafness is not a disability or a handicap but rather a characteristic that qualifies a person for membership in deaf culture where hearing is not needed in order to function (Bienvenu, 1989).

The degree of hearing impairment determines the amount of residual hearing available for language and speech development. Children who are hard-of-hearing or moderately hearing impaired will have an easier time developing verbal communication skills than children who are severely and profoundly deaf.

For those who are self-conscious about their hearing impairments it is easier to relinquish the use of a hearing aid and residual hearing, if the hearing aid is only minimally helpful. For adolescents struggling with identity and body image, in-the-ear hearing aids may seem as obtrusive as the protrusions made by the body aids described in the first vignette.

The impact of the diagnosis on the emotions of the parents and family as well as the family's behavioral responses initially and over time have a potentially differential affect on the course of the child's development. While hearing parents may undergo a profound sense of distress, many deaf parents are often relieved and even pleased when their child is deaf. They want to pass their knowledge and culture onto their children to preserve their cultural heritage (Bienvenu, 1989).

The family's financial and educational resources as reflected in socioeconomic status can influence the stresses and strains of managing the care needed by the hearing-impaired child and the other siblings. Families with modest incomes may have fewer options available to solve their problems and less money to spend on child care services, assistive devices, or equally important, recreation for refueling, rest, and relaxation.

These are some of the major variables that affect the development of children with hearing loss (Cohen, 1978; Meadow, 1980). Many of these children will enter our offices in need of services.

## Early Childhood—Emerging Language and Social and Emotional Development

Some parents are alerted to potential hearing problems because of acquaintance with people who are deaf or hard-of-hearing. Other parents who have experienced early childhood development through their older children are aware of the normal course of speech and language development. They are usually able to identify developmental delays. As discussed further in Chapter 5, for those parents who are uninformed, there are programs mandated by some states to assess high-risk potential for hearing impairments among newborns and to assist identified children and their families with referrals and resources.

During their first year, most babies who have hearing loss, but no coexisting handicaps, progress normally in motor development and some social behaviors, achieving their first year developmental milestones. They learn to suckle, communicate through crying and cooing, roll over, sit, crawl, and eat solid food. Some will have begun to walk and talk. Toward the end of the first year they come to know their caregivers well enough to feel anxiety with strangers. With each new achievement their innate sense of competence is increasingly reinforced and a healthy core self develops (Stern, 1985).

Like children with normal hearing, those with hearing loss exhibit personality characteristics that reflect their individual temperaments. The "goodness of fit" or interpersonal harmony between parent and baby is desirable. When the "fit" is poor, parents may need help to adjust to their role.

The achievement of speech and language milestones will vary among children with hearing

impairments. Often this depends on the age of identification of hearing loss, severity of the impairment, family support, and the extent and quality of the auditory stimulation and language enrichment that the child receives.

During the first year of life, most babies receive extensive stimulation because their parents hold them, play with them, and talk to them. They receive tactile, visual, kinesthetic, proprioceptive, and olfactory stimulation. They begin to make gurgling and cooing sounds that become increasingly complex babbling. However, those that lack auditory stimulation and the reinforcement provided by their own hearing will need assistance to hear through the use of hearing aids and other enrichment interventions if their babbling is to progress to verbal language.

Most toddlers, even those with hearing loss, experience a time of rapprochement during which a sense of confidence permits movement away or separation from the caregiver to explore the world, followed by a return to make sure that there is a caregiver present in case of need. This process of individuation and separation, characteristic of healthy toddlers (Mahler, Pine, and Bergman, 1975), is also characteristic of healthy adolescents.

In contrast to children with moderate to severe hearing impairments born to hearing parents, the deaf child of deaf parents may make an early entrance into the world of the Deaf Culture. Even though isolated from the neighborhood children, the deaf child may be very involved in Deaf Social Club activities. The deaf child often may not be included in group play or invited on play dates by the neighborhood hearing children due to communication problems. Instead of feeling excluded, the deaf child and his or her family may reject association with members of the hearing world.

## Middle Childhood

By the time children enter elementary school they are social creatures wanting to be with other children. At this stage, parents may be concerned if there are no other hearing-impaired children in school with whom their hearing-impaired child can associate. They may recognize also that their child is not as mature as hearing children despite their similar chronological ages. Children who have hearing loss at this early age may be very much aware of being different from the other children as they recognize their own need for special services. We will consider below the value of a support group for mainstreamed students from other schools to provide an avenue for meeting other children like themselves.

## Later Childhood to Preadolescence

By preadolescence (the period from approximately 10 through 12 years) children may be at varying levels emotionally. However, chronologically they are at the threshold of adolescence. It is very important that we appreciate that there are additional stresses on preadolescents with hearing loss that create inner tension and turmoil, requiring more effort to adapt than is required of the typical hearing preadolescent. If we forget this, we will be insufficiently appreciative of the extra effort we need to expend for meaningful and satisfactory interactions.

If "good enough" parenting has been provided these children through the course of their development (Winnicott, 1975), they will develop the important human capacity to affiliate with and trust people to assist them when they are in need. No matter how trying the adolescent challenges, if they have known security from their caregivers through the years up to their preadolescence, they are likely to have a basic sense of inner security and inner trust, accompanied by a willingness to engage with others (Erickson, 1968). If they have felt rejection, unkindness, criticism, and indifference they will be inclined to expect a repetition of this treatment. This expectation can lead to defensive rejecting behaviors toward professionals and other adults.

If an adequate means of communication has not been developed, frustration is likely to interfere with the development of interpersonal relationships over and above the normal frustrating

trials and tribulations that are expected during adolescence. If a school environment is provided that adequately meets the social, language, and academic needs of children, a useful system of communication is likely to develop.

Between the ages of 6 and 10 or 11 children normally develop friendships that provide feedback about their appealing and offensive personal qualities. Upon entrance into adolescence proper, this self-awareness will become increasingly integrated and facilitate entrance into a peer group that will further affect the development of personality.

When children with hearing loss are in a special school program for those with impaired hearing, there will be many others like themselves. However, when these adolescents are mainstreamed and there are few if any others like themselves in their schools, the sense of being different can be disturbing. The capacity to adapt to the mainstream is a notable achievement, because many difficult challenges accompany the process. Some mainstreamed students get used to feeling comfortable with being unique. In fact, the ability to succeed contributes to the development of self-esteem and self-confidence. Others who are mainstreamed may find integrating socially to their satisfaction extremely difficult.

The family's internal harmony often influences the hearing-impaired preadolescent's sense of security. Parents' attitudes towards their children, especially to their hearing impairment, often influences their preadolescents' fundamental attitude toward themselves and their disability.

## ATTITUDES ON THE USE OF RESIDUAL HEARING FOR COMMUNICATION

There are many alternative positions that encourage the employment of residual hearing in conjunction with other resources adolescents with hearing loss can bring forth to enhance their functioning. Some alternatives include auditory–oral, auditory–verbal, cued speech, and total communication. Duffy (1990) developed an integrated system that he calls multisensory verbal communication. This approach makes use of the auditory, visual, and oral modalities in combination with a form of modified cued speech. Proponents of these approaches seek to optimize each person's potential for a life of increased options and self-determination. These multisensory orientations support the acquisition of as many skills, resources, and competencies as possible.

These approaches may involve risks for the child with hearing loss, because there are no guarantees for success or for acceptance by others. For teens with hearing loss it takes a strong sense of self to risk the inconsideration, impatience, and/or indifference of one's peers or adults.

Some members of Deaf Culture criticize parents of hearing-impaired children who decide in favor of cochlear implants to foster the use of residual hearing and the use of oral language for communication. They object to the importance placed upon hearing and speech reading for communication. They argue that deaf people have a language that does not require audition and that communicating to a hearing-impaired person the importance of the use of hearing is inherently incorrect, unnecessary, and demeaning. As discussed in Chapter 13, these attitudes seek to generate pride in the Deaf Culture. Many members of Deaf Culture are angry over society's responses to them and their own difficulties interacting within a society in which hearing and oral language are basic to the common language and daily functioning (Bienvenu, 1989, 1991; Rosen 1991).

When deaf adolescents and their families from Deaf Culture seek the assistance of audiologists for the purpose of employing their residual hearing, it may be viewed as a departure from the current orthodoxy of Deaf Culture. Interest in technical aids to make use of residual hearing represents a more flexible attitude that professionals are well-advised to nurture.

I am working with Donna, a 16-year-old mainstreamed adolescent with a severe hearing loss. Her speech fluctuates from fair to good, influenced not only by her severely impaired hearing but also by her level of anxiety. She is timid and self-effacing, eager to be accepted but reticent to push herself into peer groups in which she would be the only hearing-impaired person. Like many, she worries about being accepted and included. She struggles with feelings of discomfort.

Donna is an example of many adolescents who are dealing with the social challenges of living in a world with others from whom she feels very different. As we look into the adolescent challenges described below, we can begin to understand the pressures on adolescents that might influence their attitudes toward themselves and others.

## ADOLESCENT HURDLES

As we consider the hurdles through which adolescents pass, we need to remember that the adolescent patients we see are not only adolescents with typical adolescent challenges but they are also hearing impaired with the additional formidable challenges that accrue from having auditory disability. Unless we too are hearing deprived, we cannot know how much higher they need to rise to overcome the ordinary hurdles that life presents.

### Autonomy

Adolescence is the time during which teens experiment with strivings for independence and struggle with more familiar childlike needs for protection from adults, including parents, teachers, coaches, principals, neighbors, and so forth. To be or not to be a child represents a serious conflict, sometimes conscious, about taking personal responsibility. When parents' ambivalence about their adolescent's impending independence is added to the conflict, family life can become quite volatile.

By 14 years teens are questioning parents' authority, expectations, and their interpretation of arbitrary rules (Baumrind, 1991). The experience of being able to simultaneously emulate and reject parental standards is important to the development of self-respect for one's ability to think and then to assert the products of one's thinking.

If parents and other authority figures are able to engage in open-minded discussions, adolescents can remain connected and potentially collaborative. Otherwise, in the face of perceived disrespect and rejection by parents and other adults, adolescents can become enraged and retaliate with reciprocal rejection. This state of affairs can place adolescents in an uncritical dependence on their peer group as they seek refuge from the narcissistic injuries experienced from authoritarian adults.

Interdependence rather than complete dependence or complete independence is an alternative means for establishing autonomy. Interdependence provides an opportunity for participation in decision making and rule making and, as a consequence, greater self-determination. Adolescents can function more comfortably and more effectively with increasing self-reliance as opposed to rebelliousness toward authority and inappropriate reliance on peers (Steinberg and Silverberg, 1986).

At the entrance into young adulthood adolescents who are individuated usually exhibit a balance between their individuality and connection to others, are capable of self-assertion and clear presentation of their viewpoints, and can distinguish their own point of view from the views of others. Their capacity for connection enables responsiveness and respect for the views of others including peers and adults (Baumrind, 1991). This leads to a more equal balance in the power structure and reduces the dependency bonds of childhood. Adolescents who achieve autonomy can renegotiate their roles and responsibilities more rationally. And of great importance, with these competencies they can maintain their self-esteem, which permits self-assertion with peers as well as with adults.

It is clear that to achieve this degree of autonomy a capacity for communication is required. Adolescents with hearing loss will have great difficulty achieving a healthy degree of autonomy if they do not feel others will take them seriously. They may also feel inhibited if they believe others will have difficulty understanding their expressed ideas because they have speech or language problems. If others do not know the language they use (e.g., American Sign Language or Signed English) communication will be even more difficult and/or labored.

Their belief in their capacity to function independently can be seriously and sometimes realistically affected by the difficulties in negotiating the everyday tasks of the world in which they live. Feelings of inadequacy generated over years of frustration can interfere with the energy needed to declare independence. Years of dependence on parents to intervene and advocate for them in the mainstream may have precluded the development of needed competencies.

The resulting anxiety about having the requisite communication skills is likely to be shared by the adolescent and the parents. When adults have advocated for their hearing-impaired child, they perform a much needed service. If the parents are successful they reinforce their competencies. However, if the child has not been a participant in the process, then that child who has become an adolescent will not have had the opportunity to witness the advocacy process and share in the development of these competencies. This is unfortunate because these experiences form the foundation of a sense of belief and faith in one's own capacity to manage challenges.

## Identity of the Self

Another of the core adolescent tasks is identity formation. With a firm sense of self, individuals can move from the safe, predictable, and protected reality of childhood into the unpredictable, challenging reality of adulthood where there are no guarantees of security.

Although the subject of autonomy and identity of the self are treated separately, they are intertwined. Within the concept of self there is an important need for self-esteem. It contributes to a sense of psychological well being and involves self-acceptance, self-liking, and self-respect with attendant feelings of competence and efficacy. We are concerned with the identity of adolescents with hearing loss who begin life with an impairment that can impair self-esteem.

Initially our sense of our "self" is strongly influenced by the perceptions of others and how they see us. During later childhood the capacity to take on another's point of view expands our self-concept and self-knowledge. This is often facilitated by having a friend who can give feedback about our pleasant or offensive behaviors (Sullivan, 1953.)

Since there are many factors that affect the growing sense of identity of adolescents who are hearing impaired, a reconsideration of these factors may be helpful. From birth through preadolescence the attitudes of parents have a vital impact on the emerging sense of self. What parents plant may be viewed as seeds, and how they nurture the seeds affects the development of their child. Very often parental attitudes toward themselves have been input and nurtured by experiences with their own parents. These experiences will influence the developing identity of their own hearing-impaired child. If the parents have a relatively good sense of themselves imparted by their own parents, they are likely to convey positive attitudes toward their children and contribute to a relatively healthy sense of identity.

Frequently, parents have much recovering to do after discovering their child has a hearing impairment. The diagnosis can seriously damage the anticipated bliss of parenthood for an undetermined period of time. Parents' adjustment to the hearing problem is likely to influence the developing sense of identity of their children and have some affect on the emotional equipment with which these children enter adolescence and solidify their identity.

Parents are not the only ones to input attitudes. There are other family members, extended family, important family friends and neighbors, and other adults in authority including teachers, principals, clergy, therapists, and audiologists. By their attitudes they influence, either positively or negatively, the esteem, interest, and affection felt toward the adolescent with hearing loss.

The preteen years are a difficult time for girls and boys. Girls tend to want to talk more during this period and be less physically active than they may have been before. Boys are also playing with more rules and discussion attendant to their games. Those preteens with hearing impairments may have difficulty engaging in these preadolescent challenges. They may therefore have less opportunity for social interactions.

Especially promising about the adolescent period is the time available for further development, fulfillment, and evolution no matter what the emotional status of the adolescent at the onset of this period. The adolescent's sense of self is defined and then redefined through identification with and imitation of the characteristics of a reference group as well as peer group interactions.

## Affiliation with a Peer Group

The peer group gives adolescents opportunity to connect to others who are similar in order to share their inner world of dreams, hopes, and fears that exist privately and apart from their families (Atkins, 1994). Responses from peers provide information from which are derived self-attributions.

Peer groups provide opportunity to experiment with social roles and decisions about the present and future, as peers play the roles of models, mirrors, and helpers. In the process of being together, being seen with one another, and talking and walking together, adolescents derive a sense of self-value. The interpersonal sphere in which this takes place contains intense levels of intimacy in which adolescents take joy from finishing each other's sentences, reading each others minds, and sharing a sense of simpatico (Kinney, 1993). The peer group enables the adolescent to become a person who feels secure in functioning as an individual with respectable thoughts and feelings.

The importance of peer relations becomes of even greater significance in the development of romantic relationships. In these important relationships, often as steeped in "ecstasy" as they are visited by "agony," are the lessons of being intimate, loving, and sexual. These are important precursors to a sense of interpersonal fulfillment in adult life and the capacity, if desired, to create a family of one's own.

Teens who have no sense of actual peer group membership often affiliate with a reference group and identify with its characteristics: for example, heavy metal music, environmental conservation, amnesty advocation, or old-fashioned "hippies." Although the adolescents may not have actual membership within the chosen reference group, its values and standards can be adopted and used to guide behavior. Others who are not peer group–affiliated rescue themselves by becoming more conspicuous through participation in school activities.

Establishing relationships with older students tends to validate those who may not be affiliated with their age-related peers. The affirmation by the older student helps to reduce the feelings of being alone and of self-consciousness and increases feelings of adequacy and self-confidence.

It is important to appreciate the possibilities for students with hearing loss to re-define their social and psychological reality by participation in school activities and/or establishing relationships with older students. This is often more easily accomplished in high school where there are more groups and activities to choose from and more flexibility among the boundaries of the age groups than in junior high school. It is also easier to re-define one's social existence during the first year of college when students are away at school or at a school out of their immediate community. As students mature they become more open to people who are different. When hearing-impaired adolescents enter college, the eagerness among freshman to make friends with one another can open up a social world never before experienced.

Within the mainstream high school, students with hearing loss can often feel lonely, rejected, and socially isolated because they may be the only person in their school with a hearing impairment. There is much to be done by professionals to help teens integrate into the mainstream environment: for example, fostering acquaintances between students with hearing loss and older students could have a reciprocal benefit.

Multiple efforts are needed to help adolescents with hearing loss to build friendships. Helping mainstreamed students develop the skills to further integrate into the mainstream would probably contribute even further to their existing competencies, personal satisfaction, achievements, and contributions. Unfortunately, this service is not viewed often enough by professionals as a worthy investment of their time.

Proponents of residential schools for the deaf, day schools for the deaf, and day programs for the deaf often point out that the social limitations for mainstreamed hearing-impaired students could outweigh whatever advantages the mainstream school might provide. They talk of the social advantages of their programs in which many peers are clustered and in which social and emotional satisfaction may be more available (Leigh and Stinson, 1991). Within the deaf community organized teen groups provide peer group socials. The links among the adolescents that connect them are their deafness and their age (Cohen and Long, 1991).

## Physiologic Changes

The pubescent changes of adolescence often result in increases in self-consciousness, accompanied by mood changes and a sense of uncertainty about self with great concern about appearance (Rosenberg, 1986; Hauser, Borman, Powers, Jacobson, and Noam, 1990). Most adolescents feel best when they are sharing the timing of puberty with their peers. The rate of biologic maturation—precocity or delay—affects self-esteem and interpersonal comfort (Cohen, 1978; Meadow, 1980). The hormonal changes in themselves affect emotions by stirring feelings, impulses, and sensations on a physiologic level that are unfamiliar.

Accompanying the onset of physiologic changes is the growing interest in romantic attachments. To continue healthy emotional development adolescents need to disengage from the beloved significant people of their earlier life and replace them with an age-appropriate person to love (Blos, 1967).

Adolescence has become a time for teens to experiment sexually. Integrating physiologic maturation, social and cognitive development, and emotional needs for intimacy is a major adolescent task. With the hazards of promiscuous or unprotected sexuality during this time of AIDS and venereal disease, adolescents have many formidable hurdles.

Finding an attractive person with whom to explore developing romantic and sexual feelings is often a difficult challenge for hearing adolescents. We have considered the challenge of acceptance of the hearing-impaired mainstreamed student by hearing peers. When we add to this the goal of finding a peer who is attractive, we entertain another significant challenge. Making this even more difficult for the mainstreamed student is the limited number of students with hearing loss in the neighborhood school with whom to develop a relationship.

Sexual sensations can be very confusing and extremely difficult to discuss with a peer, a family member, or a professional. It is desirable nevertheless that an opportunity be provided the adolescent with hearing loss to talk about these matters. I remember the relief of one adolescent when he finally found a place to discuss his turmoil. He seemed even more frustrated by the absence of someone to discuss his yearning for a girlfriend than his not having a girlfriend. He understood that he had few social skills and that he needed to cultivate them by having a place to discuss his sense of inadequacy and how to overcome it.

Feelings of emerging sexuality are an important part of the lives of the adolescents with whom we come in contact. They may not be able to articulate what is going on internally but these are factors that impinge on them as we attempt to be involved in our respective roles with them.

For some adolescents with hearing loss whose physiologic time clock is ticking, bodily changes can further challenge the blossoming sense of self. Becoming comfortable with secondary sexual characteristics that are intrinsic to sex role identification is an important accomplishment. Hearing aids, if valued, are a conspicuous extension of the body. Many adolescents who are hard of hearing but function better with their hearing aids prefer at this time to forget them, remove them, misplace them, et cetera. Being different is a difficult condition for adolescents in general and especially so for many hearing-impaired adolescents. Audiologists need to be sensitive to this issue when they are asking, insisting, or cajoling the adolescent to use hearing aids or other assistive devices in the mainstream class. As discussed in Chapter 11, less conspicuous amplification, although electroacoustically inferior, may be an interim solution during this period.

## Occupational Preparation

Adolescence is also the period for developing capacities, talents, and interests in preparation for an occupation. Part of the identity crisis for many adolescents is the uncertainty about their future, their opportunities, and their occupational goals. In an economy in which there is significant unemployment, the pressures to make decisions about the future can be overwhelming for insecure teens.

For some adolescents college attendance provides a chance to spend time constructively and prepare for employment opportunities. There is a proportionately higher number of hearing adolescents who go on to college than hearing-impaired adolescents. Adolescents with hearing loss who opt for higher education, rather than technical school or employment upon graduation from high school, have probably come through their education with a sense of self-confidence consolidated from their adolescent and earlier life's experiences. Having had a camp or other experience away from home during earlier adolescence can serve as a head start for the adjustment to college or technical school.

## THE AUDIOLOGIST'S RELATIONSHIP WITH THE HEARING-IMPAIRED ADOLESCENT

Adolescents bring with them a history and well-established patterns of behaving, thinking, and feeling about their lives, including their hearing impairments. We are well advised to respect the already existing personality framework with which they greet us. Our interactions with them are determined not only by who we are but also by the character they are developing and presenting to us along with their perspectives on the world. Despite our good intentions, our mission to be of help may be thwarted. There are no guarantees when we work with adolescents that they will want what we want to give. It is an interpersonal challenge requiring professional skill and sensitivity.

### Establishing a Relationship

Foremost among the guiding principles of dealing with adolescents is the acceptance of who they are. We may feel attracted, neutral, or repelled by them, but we would do well to accept them as they present themselves to us. If adolescents feel this acceptance, we have a chance of being accepted by them. This mutual acceptance is the key to the secret of continued interaction that is the foundation upon which sharing of thoughts and feelings is built. The best yardstick to determine that rapport is being established is a personal sense that the adolescent is connecting and interacting with the clinician as demonstrated by communication in some manner. It is a great advantage to have cultivated sign language skills for those patients who communicate manually. The ability to sign when necessary will probably make a significant impact on the relationship that develops and the ability to be of assistance to deaf adolescents.

Rapport can often be established with adolescent patients by talking about anything of mutual interest: exempli gratia, an article of clothing they are wearing, a book they are carrying, the state of football or basketball championships, et cetera. The willingness of adolescents who are hearing impaired to converse can be viewed as a gift. They have worked hard to cultivate their language. If they give it to professionals, it is because they feel comfortable enough to talk with them, or because they have not been given any reason to be rejecting. It is important, however, to recognize that an unwillingness to communicate may be a reflection of their own insecurity or the way they have learned to treat people in positions of authority.

### The Adolescent as Consultant to the Service Provider

To be effective it is to the audiologist's advantage to learn as much as possible about the adolescent's attitudes. If the adolescent does not want to wear hearing aids and is present because of the parents' insistence, a recommendation of hearing aids may be an exercise in futility. A healthy respect for this resistance and some relationship building can influence the eventual participation in assessment and acceptance of recommendations.

Learning about the adolescent's attitude toward hearing, hearing aids, and other assistive devices is a worthwhile investment of professional time. It is possible to determine early on if the adolescent is a cooperative or resistant patient. Exploring attitudes toward the use of hearing aids will uncover some of the problems that have interfered with a more positive attitude toward the use of hearing aids and other assistive devices.

For example, if an audiologist encounters an adolescent who has recently lost hearing after 15 years of being a hearing person, there are innumerable emotions that may be experienced from anger through depression to victimization to self-pity. Learning beforehand the adolescent's state of mind and how the provision of services is viewed can contribute to knowing if a collaborative field to work within can be established.

When working with adolescents in the throes of an identity crisis who have discovered that they aspire to be members of Deaf Culture and have established it as their reference group, hearing aids may not be a top priority. In fact, if parents are insisting on new and more effective hearing aids, those adolescents may be exceedingly resistant and see the professional as the enemy. For those adolescents it may be important to explore the propensity for identity with Deaf Culture and provide help to them and their families to examine the adolescents' needs more openly.

I recall a 13-year-old boy brought to me because of great difficulty adjusting to his class in which oral language was the means of communication among the hearing-impaired children. His speech was difficult to understand, and he had great difficulty understanding oral language. His hearing impairment was severe but with hearing aids, moderate. His parents were insistent that his hearing aids be changed to improve his hearing and that the teachers work harder with him. The faculty believed he needed a program that employed total communication. The parents resisted the teachers' recommendations. The boy was miserable. No one had consulted with him about his problems. This was a difficult problem that took a long time to resolve, because the parents, rather than the adolescent, were so resistant to making a change he very much needed.

In each case an observant and sensitive audiologist can conceivably provide verbal reflection that a problem exists and that the adolescent could benefit from some discussion of the problem. The audiologist can serve as a catalyst in bringing problems into the open of which the family is aware but has not actively addressed. While a family may resent intrusion, it is possible for the audiologist to request permission to make an observation about an apparent problem. In that way family and audiologist are agreeing to discuss the issue before it is introduced.

These suggestions are not designed to encourage audiologists to intervene and provide services for which they are not trained. Audiologists would benefit from training in the fundamentals of counseling and assessment. With these competencies they can provide a service to help adolescents and their families find the help they may need to address some of the problems characteristic of the adolescent period.

## Modeling Problem-Solving and Decision-Making Skills

Professionals who contribute to the development of their patients problem-solving and decision-making skills are performing an important service. When professionals permit patients to experience the problem-solving process in which they engage as they conduct an assessment, they serve as a model for patients to observe, learn from, and possibly incorporate. This can be even more beneficial to patients when professionals engage them directly in the problem-solving process by defining the problem and examining alternative approaches to solving it with them, including the consequences or potential advantages and disadvantages of one option as compared to another option.

This active involvement facilitates the selection of a decision and its execution by the patients directly. If the relationship with the patient endures over time, it is possible to follow up to examine the results of the decision made or solution selected. This is all part of problem-solving and a fine bonus to give patients in addition to audiometric services.

Professionals who set unrealistic goals for themselves (and their patients) are apt to be defeated when working with adolescents who are exercising autonomy, struggling with a sense of identity, and highly resistant. Professionals cannot control another person's behavior. However, when professionals behave responsibly they serve as models of responsible behavior with which patients can identify.

A teenage boy who was driving his parents and teacners to distraction through his refusal to use an FM system was referred to me by his audiologist. As a result of our discussions, he was able to communicate to his parents and teachers that he had other developmental challenges with which he was coping. His serious consideration of the need for and use of the FM system would have to wait.

This case illustrates the occasional need to accept one adaptive behavior and let another go. Finding this adolescent the best possible hearing aid and encouraging him to use the hearing aid because it would help him were worthy investments of professional effort. Informing him of and providing the FM system was another important service. Those were three professional successes. His choosing not to use the FM system was a decision he made and was deserving respect. The professional's job was done. This adolescent had received knowledge and demonstrated how he chose to be in control.

## Assessment and Referral

During the interaction with adolescents, audiologists may observe a need for services that they are unable to provide. For example, if an adolescent is awkward or seems to have some motor difficulty, some form of physical therapy or occupational therapy might be helpful. Adolescents can have a wide spectrum of social problems including painful isolation. They may also have frustrated social needs because of deficits in social skills or severe interpersonal problems because of emotional pathology. Adolescents may have physical problems manifested by symptoms of severe acne, offensive body odor, bad breath, or early balding. Sensitive inquiry about making a referral could be in order.

Another important area in which the perceptive audiologist can perform an important role is in assisting parents to identify problem areas in which they can improve their relationship with their child. Many parents have unfinished business with their acceptance of their adolescent's hearing impairment. Oftentimes parents have been so busy trying to help their child that they have not allowed themselves to take stock of their feelings. They are sometimes ashamed of their child and of themselves. Sometimes their guilt is so persistent it offers no respite in spite of the many years they have lived with the diagnosis. Their hurt feelings may still operate, causing insidious negative effects on the adolescent, on the marital relationship, and on the other members of the family. The tensions between adolescents and their parents are often observable to a perceptive audiologist, who can gently encourage parents to express themselves. In the development of trust the audiologist could help them determine if professional help for themselves and/or the family might be in order.

Making a proper referral to a mental health professional is an important service that an audiologist can provide. Because the audiologist is by definition a helper to the adolescent and the family, it is less likely that the audiologist's interest would be perceived as offensive. Asking for permission to express an observation that is unsolicited is a good way to start. Sometimes simply bringing a problem into the open for discussion may be enough for the family to mobilize.

It is especially important for audiologists to remain connected to their patients. It is very comforting for people to know there is someone out there who is in their corner and cares about their welfare. The belief in the audiologist's interest facilitates rescheduling for follow-up assessment. It is also very gratifying for audiologists to have the conviction that they are behaving in professionally appropriate ways and that their patients appreciate their efforts.

## Identifying and Becoming Instrumental in Providing Needed Programs

Adolescents who attend schools for the deaf usually have opportunities for social activities. Those who are too shy or withdrawn to attend these events might need the assistance of a counselor to whom an audiologist can make a referral. If the audiologist works within the school setting, the school counselor can be easily engaged to help encourage and support more involvement by the adolescent.

There are times when audiologists provide services to a number of adolescents who are unacquainted and come from different locations to a speech and hearing center. Often these adolescents are educated in the mainstream and are the only students with hearing loss in their respective schools. With the adolescents' and parents' permission, it is possible to share names of these adolescents with one another so that they could meet and become acquainted. Providing the site and hosting an initial meeting can be a very important and very much appreciated service by the facility in which the audiologist is employed.

An alternative way of handling this intervention could be to arrange for a psychologist, social worker, or counselor to organize a group to enable these adolescents to come together to work on their interpersonal issues. It is very possible that their isolation has social scars beneath it. These isolated teens could benefit from sharing ideas in the presence of a competent mental health professional. Bringing together adolescents with similar needs is a very special service.

For those mainstreamed adolescents, it is crucial that professionals do everything they can to help them to develop relationships within the mainstream. Five means to this end include:

1. Establish school programs that provide information about hearing impairments including hearing aids and other assistance devices. Such programs can demystify some of the anxieties of hearing teens, anxieties that may alienate them from mainstreamed students with hearing loss.
2. Establish a buddy system between hearing older students and mainstreamed younger students with hearing loss that can serve as a means for involvement and integration.
3. Establish support groups comprised of students with disabilities and students without apparent physical problems.
4. Establish support groups comprised of students with disabilities of different types.
5. Provide opportunities for students with hearing loss and hearing students to meet older hearing-impaired people including college students and adults engaged in a variety of careers. Such meetings serve to enlighten and inform students about future prospects and the lives of successful hearing-impaired people (Atkins, 1994).

## SUMMARY

The process of collaboration between audiologist and adolescent will contribute to a sense of interpersonal comfort and a good working relationship with the possibility of a longer term investment by audiologists in the welfare of their patients. Behaving professionally requires that we adjust our approach whenever possible to be better able to deliver our services. We further credit our respective professions when we stretch ourselves into creative pursuits in behalf of our patients.

For those of us involved with adolescents, we may choose to engage with them in their growth process by making helpful contributions that allow us the opportunity to grow professionally and personally alongside them. As consumers they empower us to the degree that we are able to help them consider, process, and accept our knowledge and services.

## REFERENCES

Altman, E. (1988). *Talk with Me!: Giving the Gift of Language and Emotional Health to the Hearing-Impaired Child.* Washington, DC: A. G. Bell.

Atkins, D. (1994). Counseling children with hearing loss and their families. In J. G. Clark and F. N. Martin (eds), *Effective Counseling in Audiology: Perspectives and Practice* (pp. 116–146). Englewood Cliffs, NJ: Prentice Hall.

Baumrind, D. (1991). Effective parenting during the early adolescent transition. In P. A. Cowan and E. M. Hetherington (eds), *Advances in Family Re-*

*search* (vol. 2, pp. 111–163). Hillsdale, NJ: Erlbaum.

Bienvenu, M. J.(1991). Can deaf people survive "deafness"? A Deaf American Monograph, 21–25.

Bienvenu, M. J. (1989). Disabled: Who? *The Bicultural Center News*-Riverdale, MD, *13,* 1.

Blos, P. (1967). The second individuation process of adolescence. In R. Eissler et. al. (eds.) *Psychoanalytic Study of the Child* (vol. 15, pp. 162–186). New York: International Universities Press.

Cohen, O. (1978). The deaf adolescent: Who am I? In A. Neyhus and G. Austin (eds.), *Deafness and Adolescence.* Washington, DC: Alexander Graham Bell Association for the Deaf.

Cohen O. and Long, G. (1991). Introduction. In O. Cohen and G. Long (eds.), *Selected Issues in Adolescence and Deafness.* Washington, DC: Alexander Graham Bell Association for the Deaf.

Duffy, J. K. (1990). *The Multisensory Verbal Communication Method.* Port Washington, NY: Duffy Publications.

Erikson, E. (1968). *Identity: Youth and Crisis.* New York: Norton.

Hauser, S. T., Borman, E. H., Powers, S. I., Jacobson, A. M., and Noam, G. G. (1990). Paths of adolescent ego development: Links with family life and individual adjustment. *Adolescence: Psychopathology, Normality, and Creativity, 13,* 489–510.

Kinney, D. (1993). From nerds to normals: The recovery of identity among adolescents from middle school to high school. *Sociology of Education, 66,* 21–40.

Leigh, I. W. and Stinson, M. S. (1991). Social environment, self-perceptions, and identity of hearing-impaired adolescents. *The Volta Review, 93,* 7–22.

Mahler, M., Pine, F., and Bergman, A. (1975). *The Psychological Birth of the Human Infant.* New York: Basic Books.

Meadow, K. P. (1980). *Deafness and Child Development.* Berkeley: University of California Press.

Rosen, R. (1991). *Some Thoughts on Deafness.* A Deaf American Monograph, 127–129.

Rosenberg, M.(1986). Self concept from middle childhood through adolescence. In J. Suls and A. Greenwald (eds.), *Psychological Perspectives on the Self* (vol. 3, pp. 107–138). Hillsdale, NJ: Erlbaum.

Steinberg, L. and Silverberg, S. (1986). The vicissitudes of autonomy in early adolescence. *Child Development,* 57, 841–851.

Stern, D. (1985). *The Interpersonal World of the Infant: A View from Psychoanalysis and Developmental Psychology.* New York: Basic Books.

Sullivan, H. S. (1953) *The Interpersonal Theory of Psychiatry.* New York: Norton.

Winnicott, D. W. (1975). *Through Paediatrics to Psychoanalysis.* New York: Basic Books.

# PART FOUR

# AMPLIFICATION AND AUDITORY STIMULATION

# CHAPTER 11

# PEDIATRIC AMPLIFICATION: SELECTION AND VERIFICATION

*JOHN GREER CLARK*

## INTRODUCTION

Perhaps the greatest challenge to audiologists comes when attempting to apply the principles of selection and fitting corrective amplification to the pediatric population. Yet, admittedly, no other professional challenge we face is likely to have more far-reaching consequences, since the future of these children will be directly influenced by the decisions we make. By providing a detailed overview of those factors that influence the selection and verification of personal amplification for children, this chapter is presented as part of a continuing and critical examination of options presently available.

## PRESELECTION OF PEDIATRIC HEARING AID CANDIDATES

In the best interests of the child and consistent with regulations of the Food and Drug Administration (1977), the fitting of hearing instruments for children should always be preceded by a comprehensive otologic consultation. Such consultation can only add further to the etiologic picture, since it will assess the child's general otologic health, determine the possibility of any correctable disorders, and rule out any potential medical contraindications to the use of amplification.

Early appropriate amplification is fundamental to the success of any auditory-based (re)habilitation program with children. Yet in spite of all that can be done to assess the nature of a child's hearing loss, an accurate diagnostic picture can rarely be obtained before children are 2 or 3 years of age. As we proceed toward the selection of am-

plification for young children, certain intrinsic variables cannot be immediately determined, such as innate intelligence, central auditory intactness, language facility, et cetera. Nor can all of the extrinsic variables, including family support and dynamics, family financial responsibilities and burdens, and the consistency of the child's exposure to language, be fully uncovered in the early stages of our work with children (Clark, 1983). Regardless of these factors, however, the early fitting of amplification is paramount if we are to minimize the effects of sensory deprivation and maximize use of audition during the child's early developmental years.

Occasionally, hearing levels are judged to be so poor that one might question whether amplification is a viable option. This judgment, however, must not be made prematurely. Although in full agreement with the position held by the deaf community that a non-oral deaf child is of equal worth to any other human being, we must nevertheless recognize that the ability to function in the world today is largely dependent on spoken communication. For this reason, until we can demonstrate that a child cannot benefit from amplification, it is essential that we treat that child as one with some useful residual hearing.

Conversely, we must question whether a child's hearing is ever so minimally impaired that amplification is not necessary. There exists a large cadre of research documenting adverse developmental consequences for both conductive and sensorineural hearing losses of minimal degree. For some children with minimal hearing loss, it may certainly be justifiable to recommend the part-time use of personal amplification in the classroom

(Bess, 1985; Mueller and Grimes, 1987). Mueller and Grimes point out that the sole recommendation of preferential seating, even for children with unilateral hearing impairment, may not fulfill our professional responsibility to these children. Sound-field amplification within the classroom as discussed in Chapter 14 is certainly another viable option to consider.

## PARTNERSHIPS IN HEARING AID SELECTION

The appropriate age for the fitting of amplification will largely be dictated by how early the hearing loss is identified. Even once identified, though, it is impossible to proceed with the selection of amplification without the parents' support. If the audiologic (re)habilitation program is to meet with success, audiologists will find their counseling skills are integral to building the requisite understanding, acceptance, and commitment of parents or other appropriate caregivers (Clark and Martin, 1994).

Familiarizing parents with the tests being utilized and the expectations from the child creates active partners in the selection of amplification; partners whose later observations of maturing auditory behavior become increasingly valuable. Parent involvement in subsequent hearing aid fittings should continue through adolescence as this involvement can provide a valuable carryover during adjustment (Thibodeau, 1994).

As children mature, they, too, should be included in the hearing aid selection process. Children have a much greater sense of contribution, and subsequently of responsibility, if their opinions are not only considered, but actively encouraged. Brightly colored hearing aid casings are available for behind-the-ear instruments, and young children are often eager to help with this selection (Johnson, 1994). Older children may have definite preferences for how their hearing instruments interface with FM systems. Eliciting preferences like these increase feelings of "ownership" toward the hearing instruments and, at the same time, make children feel more in control of their own situation.

Thibodeau (1994) points out the value of discussing with parents the possible differing opinions among audiologists as they pertain to a particular child's amplification requirements. Such discussions not only raise the credibility of the audiologist, which might otherwise be undermined if alternate recommendations are later revealed through another source, but also serve to increase parental involvement and thus facilitate their development as an advocate for their child's needs.

## UNILATERAL VERSUS BILATERAL FITTINGS

Since a primary goal of any hearing aid fitting should be to restore hearing to as near normal a state as possible, it only stands to reason that every attempt to restore binaural hearing should be made. Given that binaural hearing is a goal that is not always attainable with two hearing aids, the term bilateral is used here as more descriptive of the actual fitting (Byrne, Nobel, and LePage 1992). With young children, it may be a number of years before audiologists know if the goal of binaural hearing has been even approximated by a bilateral fitting.

When true binaural hearing is attained, or approximated, through bilateral hearing aid fittings, the listener experiences a number of listening benefits. Through the auditory phenomenon of binaural summation the binaural threshold is approximately 3 dB lower than is the threshold of the better ear alone (Hirsh, 1948). This summation effect has been shown to be even greater at suprathreshold levels with sensorineural hearing loss (Hawkins, Prosek, Walden, and Montgomery, 1987). The immediate benefit of binaural summation is an equivalent loudness at a lower volume setting resulting in less feedback. The improved aided threshold attained through binaural summation will also result in an increase in the dynamic range because the loudness discomfort level is not significantly different for a binaural signal than for a monaural signal.

In addition to the loss of sound localization abilities with a unilateral hearing aid fitting, unilateral fittings can result in a loss of high-frequency gain of 10 to 18 dB on the unaided side (Feston and Plomp, 1986). By eliminating this head shadow effect, bilateral fittings result in improved speech recognition. When binaural hearing is attained with a bilateral fitting, speech recognition is further improved because of the auditory system's ability to *squelch* the adverse effects of noise and reverberation.

Continued evidence suggests that a unilateral hearing aid fitting may result in auditory deprivation effects to the unaided ear (Gelfand and Silman, 1993). Although recent investigation suggests the reduction in speech recognition through auditory deprivation may be reversible (Boothroyd, 1993; Silman, Silverman, Emmer, and Gelfand, 1992), the potential for long-term consequences lends further credence to bilateral hearing aid recommendations.

Only if later testing reveals one ear to be nonfunctioning should the audiologist consider a unilateral hearing aid fitting. Until this is fully determined, audiologists should proceed on the premise that all children should receive bilateral fittings because of the proven superiority of this fitting arrangement.

## HEARING AID STYLE CONSIDERATIONS

### Body Style Gives Way to Behind-the-Ear Instruments

Not too many years ago the most common hearing aid for children was the body style hearing aid fit either bilaterally or with a "Y" cord to ensure bilateral stimulation. Today, the advantages of ear level hearing instruments (Figure 11.1) has led to a sharp decline in the fitting of body instruments. Ear level hearing instruments eliminate the body baffle effects and improve perception of acoustic temporal and spatial cues. These instruments are

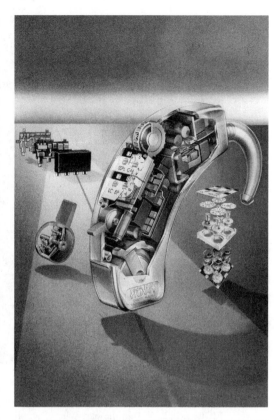

**FIGURE 11.1**   Advances in BTE technology, permitting greater gain and more accessibility to the coupling requirements of assistive listening devices, has greatly reduced the use of body style amplification. (Photo courtesy of Phonak.)

further enhanced by continuing improvements of behind-the-ear (BTE) hearing aid design that permit higher gain and greater electroacoustic flexibility. Body level amplification may still be viewed as appropriate, however, for the severely multihandicapped child whose inadequate neuromuscular control precludes adequate head support, resulting in acoustic feedback with ear level amplification.

### In-the-Ear Hearing Aids for Children

In-the-ear (ITE) instruments (Figure 11.2) are not recommended for children nearly as frequently as

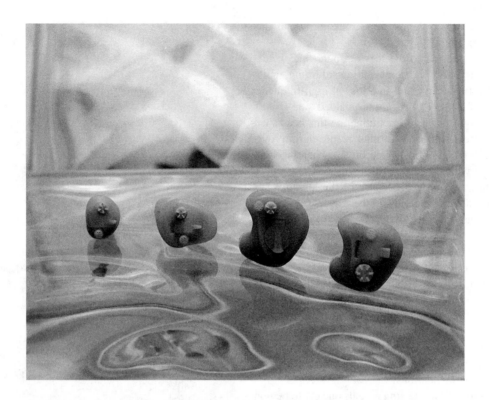

**FIGURE 11.2**   Within-the-ear styles of amplification from left to right: full shell (ITE), low profile, half-shell, and canal. While ITE and low-profile hearing aids can be modified for tele-coil and direct audio input circuitry, half-shell and canal hearing instruments have serious constraints in pediatric fittings. (Photo courtesy of Rexton.)

are BTE instruments. However, even these small instruments have overtaken body style hearing aid fittings in the pediatric population. The small size of these instruments becomes increasingly attractive to children as they get older. When audiometric profiles permit, even children in kindergarten and early elementary grades may be fit with ITE instruments.

Caution is necessary, however, because of the unpredictable, but inevitable, growth of children's ears. To maintain a satisfactory fit to the ear, ITE instruments may need to be recased as often as every 6 months for some young children. If the manufacturer does not include recasing costs within

an extended warranty program, this expense can become significant for parents.

In-the-canal (ITC) and half-shell hearing instruments are even smaller than ITE instruments (Figure 11.2). Typically, these are not considered appropriate for children, because of even greater constraints to the coupling with assistive listening devices and the potential for increased acoustic feedback with the greater proximity of the microphone and receiver. Unfortunately, during adolescence, some children reject the use of amplification for cosmetic reasons and their perceptions of peer acceptance/rejection. If ITC instruments or completely-in-the-canal (CIC) instruments will be worn, and if they will provide some benefit, the audiologist should consider that hearing instrumentation that is electroacoustically underfit, but worn daily, is superior to a more ideal fitting that is rejected.

An alternative to ITC or CIC fittings that provides similar cosmetic appeal to ITC instruments is low-profile ITE hearing aids with camouflaged faceplates. This design can address some of the cosmetic complaints of older children while allowing for telecoil interfacing with assistive devices (Clark and Clark, 1994).

## Bone-Conduction Hearing Aids

Bone-conduction hearing aids are selected for children with significant conductive hearing loss and otologic conditions that preclude the use of air conduction amplification (Figure 11.3). Such

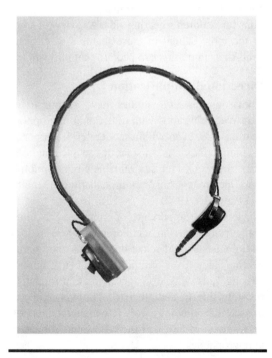

**FIGURE 11.3** The vibrating receiver of bone-conduction hearing aids sends sound waves to the cochlea through the bone-conduction auditory pathways of the scull. (Courtesy Starkey Laboratories.)

conductive hearing loss may include those accompanied by persistent or recurrent ear drainage, or hearing loss resulting from congenital ear canal or middle ear anomalies. The transducer is a vibrating receiver pressed firmly against the skin of the mastoid process. This transducer may be incorporated within an eyeglass-style hearing aid, a post-auricular instrument worn with a headband, or coupled to a body style hearing instrument.

For some patients, due to pressure irritation from conventional bone-conduction hearing aids or inconsistent signal strength resulting from shifting of the transducer, implanted, or bone-anchored hearing aids (BAHA), may be an option (Mylanus, Snik, Jorritsma, and Cremers, 1994). Yellin, Meyerhoff, and Roland (1988) state that candidates for such devices should have bone-conduction pure-tone averages no poorer than 30 dB HL with no single frequency poorer than 40 dB HL. The success of BAHA fittings with young children has not been fully demonstrated. However, potential problems with magnetic retention may limit its usefulness for this age group (Roush and Gravel, 1994).

## CROS/BiCROS Configurations

When there is a unilateral absence of functional hearing, a microphone may be placed on the non-functioning ear to pick up sounds that may then be transmitted via direct attachment or FM transmission to a hearing instrument on the normal ear. This contralateral routing of signals (CROS) was first successfully reported by Harford and Barry (1965) and has proven beneficial in many unilateral hearing loss fittings. The most frequent modification of the CROS principle, the BiCROS fitting (Harford and Dodds, 1966), allows for the addition of amplification directly to the better ear when this ear does not have normal hearing (Figure 11.4).

In true CROS hearing aid fittings with children, audiologists should keep in mind that improved hearing within the educational environment is of greatest importance. For the enhancement of classroom signal-to-noise (S/N) ratios, the

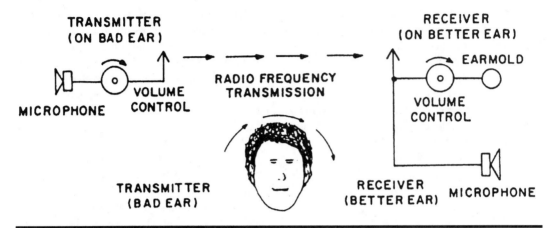

**FIGURE 11.4**    CROS hearing aids permit the routing of sound from the side of a nonfunctioning ear over to the better hearing ear. The BiCROS instrument adds additional amplification into the better ear when this ear is not normal. Signal routing is accomplished through either a direct wire connection or FM transmission. (Courtesy of Telex Communications.)

use of FM systems or sound-field amplification as discussed in Chapter 14 will be a more beneficial recommendation than a CROS hearing aid.

### Frequency Transposition Hearing Aids

The transposition of high-frequency speech information to the lower frequencies allows detection and, with training, recognition of high-frequency consonant sounds for those with residual hearing limited to lower frequencies. Although this has been attempted with varying degrees of success for more than 30 years, Penn-Davis and Ross (1993) described a transposition hearing aid that lends greater (re)habilitative promise to this concept than have past transposition units.

Certainly not all individuals with an absence of usable high-frequency hearing will benefit from frequency transposition hearing aids. However, if candidates are properly selected and are provided with appropriate audiologic follow-up, the results can provide significant improvement.

## CIRCUIT CONSIDERATIONS

When working with children, it is especially important to take advantage of available circuitry options to provide the most optimal signal possible.

Table 11.1 provides a summary of desirable options for children's hearing aids. A review of some of the more salient of these features quickly reveals their importance to pediatric amplification.

### Directional Amplification

Numerous research studies have demonstrated improved S/N ratios with directional microphone hearing aids, even within moderately reverberant listening conditions. In spite of this fact, audiologists rarely consider this valuable circuit option in their electroacoustic recommendations (Mueller and Hawkins, 1990).

Given the importance of enhanced S/N ratios in the (re)habilitation of children with hearing loss, audiologists should select directional microphone hearing aids over omnidirectional microphone hearing aids whenever possible. Unfortunately, possibly due to audiologists' failure to embrace this useful technology, very few manufacturers offer a variety of hearing instruments with directional microphones.

### Telecoil Circuitry

As discussed further in Chapter 14, the telecoil circuit within a hearing aid allows the instrument to pick up signals through electromagnetic induc-

**TABLE 11.1**   Recommended Options for Pediatric Amplification

---

1. Direct input capability for FM-only and FM/environmental microphone.
2. Neck loop induction coupling for FM-only and FM/environmental microphone (with strong telecoil).
3. FM reception circuitry built directly into BTE instrument (Numbers 1 and 2 above unnecessary if child has such fitting. FM-only and FM/environmental microphone signal options remain critical).
4. Direct audio input for coupling to auditory learning aids.
5. Directional microphone for enhanced S/N ratios.
6. Compression circuitry to avoid peak clipping distortion.
7. Extended warranty with loss and damage coverage.
8. Tamper-resistant battery compartment and volume control.

---

tion, thereby permitting an enhanced interface with the telephone or greatly improved S/N ratio through induction coupling to assistive listening devices. While a "T" switch can be put onto most styles of hearing aids, its strength and positioning within the instrument may limit its usefulness with ITE hearing aids.

A preamplifier to strengthen the telecoil signal and the provision of clear communication with the manufacturer for positioning of the electromagnetic inductive coil will help overcome some of the telecoil limitations associated with ITE hearing aids. Horizontal positioning of the telecoil permits the best magnetic pickup for telephone use, while a vertical orientation will enhance signal reception for room loops and neck loops. An angling of the induction coil between horizontal and vertical permits good signal reception for all three conditions (Preves, 1994). From an educational standpoint, the hearing aid should be able to function in the microphone only, telecoil only, and combined microphone telecoil modes. Not all manufacturers can provide ITE hearing aids wired to this specification.

Given the value of telecoil circuitry, its importance in hearing aid design and selection can-

not be overstressed (Beck, 1991; Gilmore, Beck, Compton, Hanna, Lederman, Marshal, Asprino O'Brian, Preves, Stone, Teder, and Wilber, 1993). However, telecoil coupling with assistive devices can alter the output signal considerably, necessitating probe–microphone measures to verify the adequacy of the received signal.

## Direct Audio Input

It has been more than 20 years since the Education for All Handicapped Children Act of 1975 (Public Law 94-142) brought an influx of children with impaired hearing into regular classrooms. Yet generally, these classrooms have still not provided the acoustic treatments necessary to enhance S/N ratios and reduce reverberation.

However, even when classroom acoustic treatments have been completed, one of the most effective means to improve the S/N ratio and to decrease the effects of sound reverberation remains the use of FM amplification systems. It is therefore imperative that all pediatric hearing aids either have circuitry for FM reception built into the hearing instruments themselves or have the requisite circuitry to allow FM systems to be coupled to the hearing instruments. Such coupling circuitry is readily available on BTE instruments and on many ITE instruments when needed modifications are requested.

## Compression Circuitry

As research findings and clinical observations bear out, patient loudness discomfort levels are not increased by the amount of an individual's hearing loss. Therefore, it is clear that loudness recruitment will be present to some degree with all patients who have sensorineural hearing loss. Although loudness discomfort measures are not always attainable on children, some degree of compression to avoid distortion through peak clipping is advisable in pediatric fittings.

## Digital Programmability

Although truly digital hearing aids have yet to become marketable, the use of digital programming to help shape the electroacoustic characteristics of analog hearing instruments is increasing rapidly. The multiband signal processing and compression circuitry of these hybrid hearing instruments (digitally programmed analog circuits) has been shown to provide improved sound quality and hearing performance within a number of listening situations compared to conventional hearing instruments (Stypulkowski, Hodgson, and Raskind, 1992).

Certainly the greatest advantage of programmable hearing instruments is their high flexibility allowing for future modifications as more audiometric information becomes available for the child. However, when considering programmable instrumentation for children, audiologists must remain cognizant of the important features that are desirable to pediatric hearing aid fittings and ensure that these benefits are not sacrificed (Table 11.1).

## ACOUSTIC COUPLING

Variations in the acoustic coupling of a hearing instrument to the ear can either adversely or advantageously affect the final electroacoustic product delivered to the ear. Therefore, particular attention should be given to the selection of earmold style for BTE instruments and to shell modifications for ITE instruments.

### Acoustic Venting

A vent may be created by drilling a hole from the lateral face of the earmold or ITE hearing aid either parallel to, or intersecting with, the sound channel (Figure 11.5). When canal diameter permits, a parallel vent is preferred because it maintains more amplification in the higher frequencies than does an intersecting vent. The primary purpose of the vent is to modify the low-frequency response of the hearing aid to varying degrees depending on the vent's length and diameter. Unfortunately, the small size child's ear canal may preclude the use of any venting larger than a vent for pressure relief. This should not present a problem, however, as electronic circuit modifications

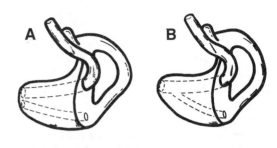

**FIGURE 11.5**   Earmold or hearing aid shell vents of varying lengths and diameters can attenuate amplification of the lower frequencies. (*A*) Parallel venting. (*B*) Intersecting venting. (Courtesy of Westone Laboratories.)

through programmable changes or potentiometer adjustments are superior to acoustic venting.

### Acoustic Damping

Acoustic dampers or filters placed at the end of the earhook of postauricular hearing instruments can smooth the mid-frequency response peaks of hearing aids that normally result from the interactive effects of the hearing aid and the earmold tubing (Figure 11.6). If peaks in the electroacoustic response of hearing aids are not reduced, their presence can limit the volume setting and add to the potential for acoustic feedback. Placement of acoustic dampers within the sound bore of ITE instruments may also be desirable, but the effects are somewhat less predictable. Acoustically tuned continuous flow adapter earmolds eliminate the need for acoustic dampers in BTE hearing aids, thereby avoiding the problems of periodically replacing moisture-blocked dampers.

### Sound Bore Diameter

Doubling the internal diameter of the last 10 mm of the medial segment of the earmold tubing (from the typical 1.93 to 4 mm) can increase the response above 3000 Hz by approximately 10 dB. Decreasing the standard diameter by one-half will have the opposite effect and can be put to effective use with patients who have a reverse (rising) slope to the audiometric curve.

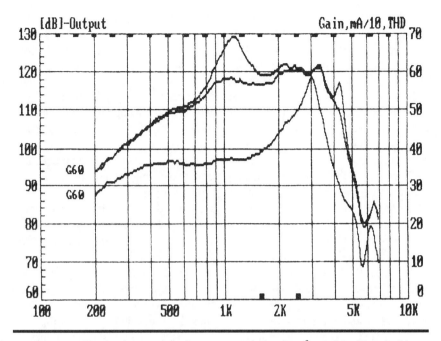

**FIGURE 11.6** Hearing instrument gain as measured via a 2-cm³ coupler with and without acoustic damping. Dampers and filters help to smooth undesirable mid-frequency response peaks. Bottom curve results from a blocked filter.

Given the importance of high-frequency hearing to speech and language processing, a step-bore fitting should be standard for ITE or BTE fittings whenever ear canal size permits. Continuous flow adaptor earmolds provide similar high-frequency advantage without the accompanying constraints due to ear size.

## Acoustic Feedback

The presence of acoustic feedback not only decreases the usable gain of hearing instruments but increases the likelihood of instrument rejection. The natural lifetime growth of the pinna is most rapid during the first decade of life. To prevent acoustic feedback, children's earmolds should be replaced every 3 to 6 months in the early years and annually after about age 5 years.

Although not intended as a supplement for appropriately fitted earmolds, digital feedback-suppression (DFS) circuitry reportedly can allow an increase in gain of 10 dB or more before the hearing instrument will feed back (Smriga, 1993). The benefit could be substantial for children with severe to profound hearing loss whose hearing aids' gain is often set to a point just below feedback rather than at a more optimal setting.

## SELECTION AND VERIFICATION OF ELECTROACOUSTIC DIMENSIONS

The selection of the electroacoustic dimensions of amplification systems for a child, by necessity, is an ongoing process encompassing the full range of the child's listening environments. For this reason, parents and teachers must realize that periodic changes may need to be made to the amplification system as a more definitive audiologic picture evolves. Toward this end, the audiologist must select instrumentation with a high degree of flexibility in electroacoustic parameters.

After selecting the appropriate hearing aid style and circuit options, and before assessing the performance of any hearing instruments on a child, it is paramount that audiologists carefully preselect the electroacoustic response. This selection is based on what is already known of the $2\text{-cm}^3$ coupler electroacoustic characteristics of the instruments and what is known of the child's hearing. The goal of this selection process is to obtain electroacoustic parameters that will optimize auditory learning for the child. The verification process is the time in which the audiologist assesses the in situ (as worn) performance of the selected amplification and then fine-tunes the instruments through potentiometer adjustments, programmable modifications, and/or changes in the acoustic response of the earmold coupling. Verification of performance is paramount to the success of any fitting as $2\text{-cm}^3$ coupler measures are truly useful only for monitoring the functional status of hearing aids or for comparison with manufacturers' technical specifications. Little valid data are available from these measures to accurately predict hearing aid performance in the ear. If direct verification of hearing aid performance cannot be completed due to a lack of child cooperation, performance predictions can be made through knowledge of the real ear coupler difference (RECD) as discussed later.

## Frequency Response/Gain Selection and Verification

A variety of prescriptive measures for frequency response/gain selection are reviewed by Hawkins (1992a). The very existence of a wide number of prescriptive formulae attests to the fact that the ideal procedure to determine the appropriate hearing aid response is yet to come. Certainly one drawback to the threshold-based procedures is that they do not account for the implications of loudness recruitment. Yet frequency response/gain selection based upon suprathreshold measures (Cox, 1983) may not be of use as these measures cannot be attained reliably with very young children. The fact that prescriptive formulae were designed for frequency response/gain selection

for linear hearing aids presents a further limitation when fitting nonlinear hearing instruments. In spite of the limitations of prescriptive selection procedures, they can provide a good working format when selecting electroacoustic parameters. Prescriptive measures are especially useful when working with a population that cannot always provide meaningful feedback efficacious to the selection process.

The various target gain procedures use a variety of defining values for the speech spectrum. Any set of these values can only approximately represent the variations in speech spectrum resulting from differences in such factors as talker age, gender, distance, and vocal effect (Seewald and Ross, 1988).

In addition when using target gain formulae to assess the frequency response/gain requirements for a child's hearing loss, the audiologist must keep in mind that these formulae make use of the external ear resonance properties of the median adult ear. Kruger (1987) has demonstrated that the primary external ear resonance frequency decreases from approximately 6000 Hz for newborn children to the average adult value of 2700 Hz by about 2 years of age (Figure 11.7). To avoid overamplification in the 2000 to 3000 Hz range, and underamplification in the higher frequencies, it becomes imperative that a given child's probe–microphone real ear unaided response (REUR) be accounted for in the frequency selection process (Tecca, 1990). As the child's REUR matures, the selected amplification must be flexible enough to compensate for the loss of gain between 2000 and 3000 Hz when the natural resonance peak is lost through placement of the earmold in the ear (insertion loss).

Seewald and his colleagues (Seewald, Zelisko, Ramji, and Jamieson, 1991) have developed a computer-based hearing aid selection/verification protocol for use with infants and young children. Their Desired Sensation Level (DSL) approach permits a fitting that considers the audiometric data, the electroacoustic characteristics of the selected device, and the parameters of verification. This procedure makes possible a prescriptive

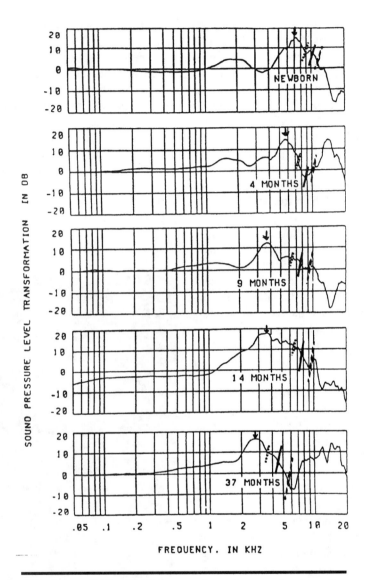

**FIGURE 11.7**    Diffuse field to ear canal sound pressure level transformation for a newborn, and 4-, 9-, 14-, and 37-month-old children. (From Kruger, 1987, used with permission.)

approach that can provide an initial fitting based on the limited audiometric data that audiologists are often restricted to with infants and young children. In addition, it accounts for the real ear properties of the child's ear through probe–microphone measures and considers the need for amplification to provide audibility of others' speech as well as the child's own speech for self-monitoring purposes.

In addition to the DSL, which is designed specifically for children, many defensible approaches exist for the prescriptive selection of amplification. Indeed, the approach chosen will vary with circumstance. However, regardless of the approach used to select the frequency response/gain requirements for a child's hearing loss, audiologists must rely on their own knowledge of the acoustics of speech and environmental sounds to ensure an optimum fitting.

Audiologists must take full advantage of the extended high frequencies available in today's newer amplifiers. For children who rely on the full complement of acoustic energy, not just for speech recognition, but also for the development of speech production and eventual deciphering of the linguistic code, such high-frequency information becomes critical.

At the same time, audiologists must remain cognizant of both the positive and negative implications of low-frequency amplification. Sufficient low-frequency amplification can have a significant bearing on the perceived quality of the human voice, and thus on the voice-monitoring abilities of the child. However, excessive amplification of the lower frequency first formants of the speech signal may adversely affect perception of the higher frequency formants and their transitions that add to consonant perception (Danaher, Osberger, and Pickett, 1973). Chapter 1 presents further discussion of the importance of speech acoustics on the speech perception of those with hearing loss.

## Obtaining Probe–Microphone Verification of Gain

The most efficient and reliable means of verifying the performance of a child's amplification system while it is being worn is through comparison of a target gain to real ear probe–microphone measures using a speech spectrum input. The advantages of probe–microphone measures in the verification of hearing aid fittings has been delineated in some detail (Mueller, Hawkins, and Northern, 1992; Tecca, 1990). With children, these would include the need for only passive cooperation from the child; the provision of an objective measure with very good test-retest reliability; a rapid means of obtaining accurate results across the *entire* frequency range; a rapid assessment of the effects of electroacoustic and

earmold "plumbing" adjustments not readily attainable through sound-field behavioral measures; and a means of assessing the adequacy of meeting target gain levels and avoiding overamplification.

Counteracting the advantages of probe–microphone measures with children is the not insignificant difficulty audiologists may face when attempting to insert the probe tube into the ear canal of a less than cooperative child or obtaining measures from a vocalizing child. Success with these measures is heightened when attempted with a drowsy or sleeping child or a child who is kept quiet and passive with a visual distractor (Figure 11.8).

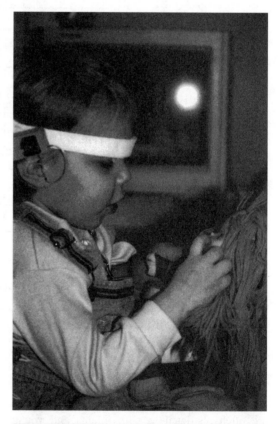

**FIGURE 11.8** Probe–microphone measures are completed by inserting a soft silicone tube in the ear canal. A visual distraction is helpful when testing young children. (Photo courtesy of Hear Care, Inc.)

If a single aided probe–microphone response can be measured with the child, the decibel difference between discreet frequencies in the probe–microphone response and the 2-cm$^3$ response can be determined. Knowing this real ear coupler difference (RECD) allows for all subsequent hearing aid modifications to be measured in the 2-cm$^3$ coupler. Adding the RECD to the 2-cm$^3$ coupler response will then yield a valid prediction of hearing aid performance in the child's ear. This procedure can substantially reduce the time and cooperation needed from the child. Moodie, Seewald, and Sinclair (1994) present a means of obtaining the RECD with an insert earphone coupled to the child's earmold thereby further eliminating some of the variability associated with sound-field probe microphone measurements in children. Substituting an insert earphone for the probe–microphone system's sound-field speaker necessitates a correction for head diffraction and microphone location effects.

## Reporting Probe–Microphone Verification of Gain

Maintaining a hard copy of the obtained probe–microphone measures, or storing these measures within the computer's memory, allows for future hearing aid performance comparison. However, explaining the resultant graphs to parents, and the often unresolved limitations of amplification systems in fully matching a target response, can be difficult for the audiologist and confusing for the parents.

Presenting all hearing test data and hearing instrument assessment data on a single graph in SPL can provide a more accurate description of the factors considered in fitting amplification. This approach can be very useful with parents who have not been previously indoctrinated to dB HL audiometric notations. However, an SPL test presentation can be confusing for parents or (re)habilitation professionals who have been brought up on the more conventionally plotted aided and unaided threshold audiogram.

While output verification is of extreme importance in hearing aid fittings as discussed later,

it is the verification of frequency response/gain that is of greatest consequence to the (re)habilitation team. Therefore, it is important that audiologists report data related to both hearing loss and hearing aid benefit in a fashion that is both comprehensible and useful. The use of the Articulation (audibility) Index can provide a readily visual and comprehensible portrayal for parents, teachers, physicians, speech-language pathologists, and others who may not be well versed in the interactive dynamics of speech acoustics and amplification.

In keeping with the reasoning of Killion, Mueller, Pavlovic, and Humes (1993), I favor the term *audibility index* over Articulation Index. The audibility index was devised to represent the amount of average intensity of conversational speech energy that can be heard with a given hearing impairment at a distance of 3 to 6 feet. Clark (1992) and Killion and colleagues (1993) have recommended eliminating the computational steps proposed in the original articulation index formulae for ease of comprehension of the resultant value. Following these recommendations, the audibility index is computed by simply counting the number of dots below the hearing levels plotted on the audiogram. This number may then be interpreted as the percentage of speech energy available to the listener when speech is spoken at normal conversational levels.

The software of some probe–microphone computer systems automatically overlay measurement curves on a portrayal of the audibility index. When this feature is not available (or when responses have been predicted with the RECD as discussed previously) the insertion gain response values (or predicted values) can be plotted on the "count-the-dot" audiogram at octave and interoctave values to readily depict the effectiveness of selected amplification in reaching the goals of making the acoustics of speech audible (Figure 11.9).

When substituting for sound-field measures by plotting real ear insertion gain values in this way, audiologists should be cognizant of possible estimation errors for individuals with unusual real

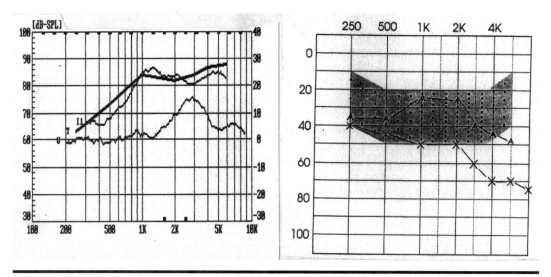

**FIGURE 11.9**    Aided hearing levels extrapolated from probe–microphone measures and displayed on an audibility index (count-the-dot) audiogram portray the effectiveness of amplification in making audible the energy of conversational speech at a 1-meter distance.

ear unaided responses (Mueller, 1992). In addition, an overestimation of gain is likely when insertion gain values are plotted for frequencies where no measurable hearing exists. Further, it is important to remember that these are gain measures for a set input signal and that actual realized gain will vary somewhat as mentioned earlier on the basis of individual speaker differences as well as listener/talker proximity. For example, children seated on a caregiver's lap will receive typical speech inputs at the hearing aid microphone 20 dB higher than the level assumed from prescriptive measures based on a 1-meter distance (Stelmachowicz, Mace, Kopun, and Carney, 1993).

In spite of these limitations, plotting probe-tube insertion gain on an audibility index audiogram is a superior means of visual depiction of aided performance than is sound-field audiometry in response to frequency specific stimuli. Even so, as discussed in Chapter 16, audiologists should always provide some detail of information in their reports on the amplification system's ability to make audible specific speech sounds.

While many parents will ask for a percentage hearing loss, audiologists would be wise to advise them of the weaknesses of such numbers, which are only confounded by the multiple formulations for computing percent hearing loss (Clark, 1981, 1982). It should be made clear that the audibility index is not a percentage of hearing loss, but rather the percentage of conversational speech energy received. One cannot judge the suitability of amplification on the basis of how close the aided threshold approximates normal threshold levels. It may prove impossible to attain normal threshold levels, or even full audibility of the speech spectrum with some severe or profound hearing losses, because of the constraints of acoustic feedback and tolerance levels associated with the individual hearing loss. Table 11.2 provides aided threshold goals for various degrees of sensorineural hearing loss. Ears with conductive or mixed pathologies will tolerate more gain than pure sensorineural pathology. A cursory inspection of Table 11.2 quickly reveals that restoration of normal hearing levels is not an attainable goal for the child with hearing loss.

**TABLE 11.2**   Aided Threshold Goals

| AVERAGE HEARING THRESHOLD[a] dB HL | | + | AVERAGE AIDED REAL-EAR GAIN | = | AIDED THRESHOLD GOAL[c] dB HL |
|---|---|---|---|---|---|
| *Hearing loss descriptor[b]* | | | | | |
| –10–15 | Normal hearing | | NA | | NA |
| 16–25 | Slight hearing loss | | 4–10 | | 12–15 |
| 26–40 | Mild hearing loss | | 10–20 | | 16–20 |
| 41–55 | Moderate hearing loss | | 20–30 | | 21–25 |
| 56–70 | Moderately severe loss | | 30–40 | | 26–30 |
| 71–90 | Severe hearing loss | | 40–45 | | 31–45 |
| 91+ | Profound hearing loss | | 46+ | | 45–55 |

[a]Average 0.5, 1, and 2 kHz re: ANSI-1989

[b]From Goodman (1965) modified by Clark (1981), Goodman recommended normal hearing from –10 to 25 dB

[c]Goal based on sensorineural hearing impairment. Conductive and mixed pathology will tolerate more gain resulting in a lower threshold goal.

NA = not available.

## Sound-Field Gain Verification

The traditional alternative to probe–microphone measures as a verification of hearing aid benefit is the measurement of functional gain in the sound field. The clinical availability of probe–microphone analysis has increased rapidly in recent years, all but making sound-field gain measures passé except when a child will not tolerate probe–microphone measures. In the absence of probe–microphone measures, sound-field gain can be plotted on the count-the-dot audiogram and presented to parents and rehabilitation team members in the same manner as already discussed. However, several serious limitations exist with this practice.

Sound-field gain measures provide a comparison of a child's sound-field responses with and without amplification. The first limitation appears when functional gain measures are completed with nonlinear hearing instruments. The higher level input signals or everyday communication will often activate compression circuitry that will not be activated during sound-field threshold measures that may have been obtained at a lower SPL. The resultant overprediction of hearing levels and hearing abilities can be misleading for both parents and educators.

Another significant limitation of functional gain measures with small children is the sometimes high test-retest variability, a problem that can only increase during the lengthy sessions required for the assessment of different hearing aid modifications. Further, the fact that functional gain is typically measured in 5-dB steps may preclude observation of small electroacoustic changes following hearing aid adjustment.

However, probe–microphone measures should not preclude behavioral sound-field speech recognition measures in instances when the child's age, verbal abilities, and cooperation permit. Such speech audiometric verification procedures become more meaningful when one considers that probe–microphone measures do not assess the cognitive processing abilities of sound. Parental and educational/(re)habilitation observations of aided listening performance can also provide useful information on the performance of hearing aids (Appendix 11).

## Alternate Objective Gain Verification

Using the Audibility Index to display probe–microphone insertion response (REIR) requires more unaided frequency-specific knowledge of a young child's hearing status than may be available during the early stages of hearing aid fitting. Two alternative methods of verifying benefit from amplification are available that do not require full knowledge of hearing status. These are accomplished through the use of acoustic reflex testing and auditory evoked potentials (Hall and Ruth, 1985).

Comparison of aided and unaided acoustic reflex thresholds provides the advantage of an easily attained, accurate assessment of amplification as worn by the child, accounting for both earmold acoustics and external ear canal volume. However, its use does have prerequisites. If reflexes are to be observed, the child's hearing loss must be purely sensorineural and no greater than moderately severe. Further, unless the child can sit without vocalizing, some mild sedation becomes a necessity.

While a variety of auditory evoked potentials have been used to verify the benefits of amplification, the auditory brain stem response (ABR) has been utilized most extensively. Although responses generated further up the auditory pathways may be more frequency-specific, they are also more susceptible to the effects of sedation. Generally, the more normal the ABR response with amplification appears, the more appropriate the hearing aid system is judged.

## Output Selection and Verification

As with frequency/gain response selection, the audiologist must also give close consideration to the selection of hearing aid saturation sound pressure levels. The final output selection must not only ensure that the upper end of the amplified speech spectrum remains audible, but it must also ensure that residual hearing is protected and that amplified sounds do not exceed levels of comfort. Comparing the gain given to the average speech signal to the desired real ear saturation response (RESR) clearly shows how well the selected amplification

has fit within the child's dynamic range of residual hearing.

Research indicating the possibility of the development of further hearing loss from high levels of amplification (Rintelmann and Bess, 1977) has resulted in federal legislation that requires a warning to accompany all hearing aids with a maximum power output (MPO) exceeding 132 dB SPL (Food and Drug Administration, 1977). It is important for audiologists to remember that this level of 132 dB SPL should not be set based on 2-$cm^3$ coupler readings and manufacturer specification data sheets, but rather on the actual recorded (or estimated) SPL in the child's ear canal. Selection of hearing instruments with a gain control separate from the MPO or saturation sound pressure level (SSPL) control can help the audiologist to fit adequate gain without overamplification. While using the 132 dB SPL as a guideline, audiologists must also remember that in cases of profound hearing loss this may need to be exceeded to ensure that the amplified signal reaches audibility. *To remain below 132 dB SPL in the ear canal and deprive audibility defeats our purpose.*

When selecting maximum output levels for adults, the audiologist will select levels below measured loudness discomfort levels (LDL). Provided the concept of "too much" is appropriately conveyed, LDL can be obtained for children with a mental age as low as 5 to 7 years (Kawell, Kopun, and Stelmachowicz, 1988; MacPherson, Elfenbein, Schum, and Bentler, 1991) (see Figure 11.10.) Below this age, however, accurate measures of LDL cannot be attained. In the absence of LDL measures, target levels for sound pressure in a child's ear canal can be estimated from threshold data (Seewald et al., 1991).

To prevent overamplification, a direct measurement of hearing aid maximum output may be made with a probe–microphone system (Hawkins, 1992b; 1993). A prediction of RESR (Sullivan, 1987) may be obtained with the same RECD value used in the frequency response verification discussed earlier. This prediction may be obtained by adding the RECD to the hearing aid's measured 2-$cm^3$ coupler SSPL 90 response.

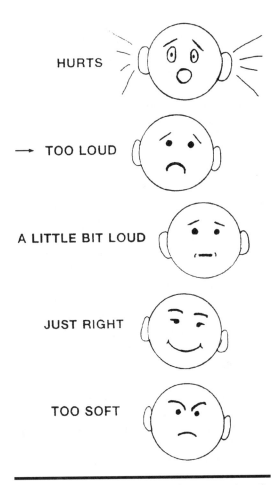

HURTS

TOO LOUD

A LITTLE BIT LOUD

JUST RIGHT

TOO SOFT

**FIGURE 11.10** Verbal and pictorial representation of the loudness categories used for the subject group ages 7 to 14 years. (From Kawell, M. E., Kopun, J. G., and Stelmachowicz, P. G. (1988). Loudness discomfort levels in children. *Ear and Hearing, 9,* 133–136.)

If probe–microphone measures cannot be obtained for direct or indirect setting of SSPL 90, the child's ear canal volume must be accounted for when setting the maximum output of amplification. A known increase in sound pressure levels accompanies a decrease in the physical space into which a sound is introduced. The volume between the medial tip of a child's earmold and the tympanic membrane is considerably smaller in young children than the 2-cm$^3$ coupler in which mea-

sures are made for the manufacturer's specification data sheets. For this reason, a higher sound pressure level occurs in the child's ear than the reported SSPL. This discrepancy between hearing aid SPL as measured in a 2-cm$^3$ coupler and the actual SPL in the ear canal has been known for more than half a century (Lebel, 1944), but is still unaccounted for in many pediatric hearing aid fittings today.

An approximation of the child's ear canal volume with an earmold in place may be obtained from immittance measures. Six dB may then be added to the manufacturer's stated SSPL 90 value (or conversely subtracted from desired RESR levels), as the volume is halved from the original 2-cm$^3$ cavity size. (For example, 6 dB may be added to the manufacturer's stated SSPL when ear canal volume is 1 cm$^3$; 12 dB may be added if ear canal volume is .5 cm$^3$, and so on.) *When working with manufacturers 2-cm$^3$ data, modifications must always be made to ensure that SPL in the ear canal is not higher than desired.*

As the knowledge of a child's true LDL is often uncertain, the child should be monitored closely for signs of loudness discomfort or overamplification. In addition, high levels of amplification that may place residual hearing at risk are not always judged uncomfortably loud (Hawkins, 1982). It is because of these factors that a child's hearing and hearing aids' performance should be monitored every 3 months during the child's first year with amplification (Hawkins and Northern, 1992).

It is clearly desirable to minimize even a temporary threshold shift from excessive SSPL in hearing aid fittings, since the child's auditory functioning will be commensurate with this greater hearing level when such shifts are present. Macrae (1993, 1994) calls fallacious the belief that decreasing the maximum power output is always appropriate if hearing aids are causing a temporary threshold shift. Unless the hearing aids are operating in saturation a large part of the time, reduction of the gain for a portion, or all, of the frequency response is the appropriate action. Reducing the output of a hearing instrument that has a high level of gain will quickly drive the hearing aid into saturation with a concomitant increase in harmonic distortion.

## HEARING AID MAINTENANCE

Regardless of the verification employed, long-term adequacy of the amplified response delivered to the child's ear is paramount to success with the auditory channel. Thus, proper hearing aid maintenance is as important as any aspect of the selection and verification process. A review of studies in hearing aid performance quickly reveals that audiologists continue to fall short in the effort to ensure that children are wearing appropriately functioning instruments (Clark, 1989b).

Although classroom teachers should ideally check the function of their students' hearing aids on a daily basis, surveys clearly indicate that this is not being done. Thus it is essential that audiologists ensure that the children under their care are working with a speech-language pathologist who is versed in the routine performance check of hearing instruments. Providing therapy to a child whose hearing aids are not functioning is at best an exercise in futility (Clark, 1989a, 1989b).

However, the final responsibility for maintaining the function of children's hearing aids must fall on the shoulders of the child's parents. Again, it would appear audiologists have been lax in stressing the importance of checking hearing aids and providing the training and support necessary to ensure that parents are confident in hearing aid operation and troubleshooting. It is unreasonable to depend on children below 6 years of age to monitor their own hearing aids. The young child who has never heard the normal, rich quality of sound as perceived by listeners with normal hearing cannot be expected to identify the acoustic deficiencies of a defective hearing aid (Riedner, 1978). This fact must be stressed repeatedly with parents. With an eye toward the goal of keeping children's hearing aids functioning, no pediatric hearing aid fitting should be considered complete without providing parents with a hearing aid stethoscope and battery tester and instruction in their use.

Certainly visual and listening inspections of hearing instruments as detailed by Ross in Chapter 12 cannot be considered a replacement for regular electroacoustic monitoring of hearing aids by an audiologist. Ideally, such monitoring of children's hearing aids should be completed every 3 to 6 months.

## SUMMARY

For a successful aural program for children with hearing loss, speech and language perception and production must be achieved through audition. Toward this end, the audiologist must select an electroacoustically flexible amplification system that will make audible as great a portion of the acoustic speech spectrum as is possible while keeping output at safe and comfortable levels.

The selection and verification of personal amplification is only a first step, albeit a crucial step, to the ultimate auditory success of the child with impaired hearing. The subsequent acceptance and proper use and maintenance of hearing instruments by the caregivers, and ultimately by the child, are critical. As Ross points out in the next chapter, the selection and verification of appropriate amplification is only the beginning of our responsibility to the child with a hearing loss.

## REFERENCES

Beck, L. B. (1991). Issues in the assessment and use of hearing aid technology. *Ear and Hearing, 12*(6), 935–965.

Bess, F. (1985). The minimally hearing-impaired child. *Ear and Hearing, 6,* 43–47.

Boothroyd, A. (1993). Recovery of speech perception performance after prolonged auditory deprivation: Case study. *Journal of the American Academy of Audiology, 4,* 331–336.

Byrne, D., Nobel, W., and LePage, B. (1992). Effects of long-term bilateral and unilateral fitting of different hearing aid types on the ability to locate sounds. *Journal of the American Academy of Audiology, 3*(6), 369–382.

Clark, J. G. (1981). Uses and abuses of hearing loss classification. *Asha, 23,* 493–500.

Clark, J. G. (1982). Percent hearing handicap: Clinical utility or sophistry? *Hearing Instruments, 33*(3), 37.

Clark, J. G. (1983). Beyond diagnosis: the professional's role in educational consultation. *The Hearing Journal, 46*(8), 20–25.

Clark, J. G. (1989a). The hearing-impaired child and speech-language therapy, or The challenge of Sisyphus. *Southwest Ohio Speech and Hearing Association Newsletter.*

Clark, J. G. (1989b). The speech-language pathologist and pediatric hearing aids. *Hearsay,* Spring, 45–46.

Clark, J. G. (1992). *The ABC's to Better Hearing.* Cincinnati: HearCare.

Clark, J. G., and Clark, S. M. (1994). Addressing adolescent cosmetic concerns through camouflaged instrumentation. *Hearing Review, 1*(8), 36, 38.

Clark, J. G., and Martin, F. N. (eds.). (1994). *Effective Counseling in Audiology: Perspectives and Practice.* Englewood Cliffs, NJ: Prentice Hall.

Cox, R. M. (1983). Using ULCL measures to find frequency/gain and SSPL 90. *Hearing Instruments* 34:17–21, 39.

Danaher, E. M., Osberger, M. J., and Pickett, J. M. (1973). Discrimination of formant frequency transitions in synthetic vowels. *Journal of Speech and Hearing Research, 16,* 439–451.

Feston, J., and Plomp, R. (1986). Speech reception threshold in noise with one and two hearing aids. *Journal of the Acoustical Society of America, 79,* 465–471.

Food and Drug Administration (1977). Hearing aid devices—Professional and patient labeling and conditions for sale. *Federal Register, 42,* 9286–9296.

Gelfand, S. A., and Silman, S. (1993). Apparent auditory deprivation in children: Implications of monaural versus binaural amplification. *Journal of the American Academy of Audiology, 4,* 313–318.

Gilmore, R., Beck, L., Compton, C., Hanna, W., Lederman, N., Marshal, B., Asprino O'Brian, J., Preves, D., Stone, R., Teder, H., and Wilber, L. (1993). Telecoils: Past present and future. *Hearing Instruments, 44*(2), 22–23, 26–27, 40.

Goodman, A. (1965). Reference zero levels for pure-tone audiometer. *ASHA, 7:* 262–263.

Hall, J. and Ruth, R. (1985). Acoustic reflexes and auditory evoked responses in hearing aid evaluations. *Seminars in Hearing. 6,* 251–277.

Harford, E. and Barry, J. (1965). A rehabilitative approach to the problem of unilateral hearing impairment: The contralateral routing of signals (CROS). *Journal of Speech and Hearing Disorders, 30,* 121–138.

Harford, E. and Dodds, E. (1966). The clinical application of CROS. *Archives of Otolaryngology, 83,* 455–464.

Hawkins, D. B. (1982). Overamplification: A well-documented case report. *Journal of Speech and Hearing Disorders, 47,* 382–384.

Hawkins, D. B. (1992a). Prescriptive approaches to selection of gain and frequency response. In H. Mueller, D. Hawkins, and J. Northern (eds.), *Probe Microphone Measurements: Hearing Aid Selection and Assessment* (pp. 91–112). San Diego: Singular Publishing Group.

Hawkins, D. B. (1992b). Selecting SSPL 90 using probe microphone measurements. In H. Mueller, D. Hawkins, and J. Northern (eds.), *Probe Microphone Measurements: Hearing Aid Selection and Assessment* (pp. 146–158). San Diego: Singular Publishing Group.

Hawkins, D. B. (1993). Assessment of hearing aid maximum output. *American Journal of Audiology, 2,* 13–14.

Hawkins, D. B. and Northern, J. L. (1992). Probe microphone measurements with children. In H. Mueller, D. Hawkins, and J. Northern (eds.), *Probe Microphone Measurements: Hearing Aid Selection and Assessment* (pp. 183–181). San Diego: Singular Publishing Group.

Hawkins, D. B., Prosek, R., Walden, B., and Montgomery, A. (1987). Binaural loudness summation in the hearing impaired. *Journal of Speech and Hearing Research, 30,* 37–43.

Hirsh, I. (1948). The influence of interaural phase on interaural summation and inhibition. *Journal of the Acoustical Society of America, 20,* 544–557.

Johnson, C. D. (1994). Educational consultation: Talking with parents and school personnel. In J. G. Clark and F. N. Martin (eds.), *Effective Counseling in Audiology: Perspectives and Practice* (pp. 184–209). Englewood Cliffs, NJ: Prentice-Hall.

Kawell, M. E., Kopun, J. G., and Stelmachowicz, P. G. (1988). Loudness discomfort levels in children. *Ear and Hearing, 9,* 133–136.

Killion, M. C., Mueller, H. G., Pavlovic, C. V., and Humes, L. E. (1993). A is for audibility. *The Hearing Journal, 46*(4), 29.

Kruger, B. (1987). An update on the external ear resonance in infants and young children. *Ear and Hearing, 8,* 333–336.

Lebel, C. (1944). Pressure and field response of the ear in hearing aid performance determination. *Journal of the Acoustical Society of America, 16,* 63–67.

MacPherson, B. J., Elfenbein, J. L., Schum, R. L., and Bentler, R. A. (1991). Thresholds of discomfort in young children. *Ear and Hearing, 12,* 184–190.

Macrae, J. H. (1993). Temporary threshold shift caused by hearing aid use. *Journal of Speech and Hearing Research, 36,* 365–372.

Macrae, J. H. (1994). An investigation of temporary threshold shift caused by hearing aid use. *Journal of Speech and Hearing Research, 37,* 227–237.

Moodie, K. S., Seewald, R. C., and Sinclair, S. T. (1994). Procedure for predicting real-ear hearing aid performance in young children. *American Journal of Audiology, 3,* 23–30.

Mueller, H. G. (1992). Insertion gain measurements. In H. Mueller, D. Hawkins, and J. Northern (eds.), *Probe Microphone Measurements: Hearing Aid Selection and Assessment* (pp. 113–143). San Diego: Singular Publishing Group.

Mueller, H. G., and Grimes, A. (1987). Amplification systems for the hearing impaired. In J. G. Alpiner and P. A. McCarthy (eds.), *Rehabilitative Audiology: Children and Adults* (pp. 115–160.) Baltimore: Williams & Wilkins.

Mueller, H. G., and Hawkins, D. B. (1990). Three important considerations in hearing aid selection. In R. E. Sandlin (ed.), *Handbook of Hearing Aid Amplification: Vol. II. Clinical Considerations and Fitting Practices* (pp. 31–60). Boston: College Hill Press.

Mueller, H. G., Hawkins, D. B., and Northern, J. L. (eds.). (1992). *Probe Microphone Measurements: Hearing Aid Selection and Assessment.* San Diego: Singular Publishing Group.

Mylanus, E., Snik, A., Jorritsma, F., and Cremers, C. (1994). Audiologic results for the bone-anchored hearing aid HC220. *Ear and Hearing, 15,* 87–92.

Penn-Davis, W., and Ross, M. (1993). Pediatric experiences with frequency transposing. *Hearing Instruments, 44*(4), 26–31.

Preves, D. (1994). A look at the telecoil: Its development and potential. *SHHH Journal, 15*(5), 7–10.

Riedner, E. D. (1978). Monitoring of hearing aids and earmolds in an educational setting. *Journal of the American Auditory Society, 4,* 39–43.

Rintelmann, W. and Bess, F. (1977). High-level amplification and potential hearing loss in children. In F. Bess (ed.), *Childhood deafness: Causation, Assessment and Management* (pp. 267–293). New York: Grune & Stratton.

Roush, J., and Gravel, J. (1994). Acoustic amplification and acoustic aids for infants and toddlers. In J. Roush and N. Matkin (eds.), *Infants and Toddlers with Hearing Loss: Family Centered Assessment and Intervention* (pp. 65–79.) Baltimore: York Press.

Seestedt-Stanford, L., and Bonta, R. (1993). Infrared programmables improve pediatric fittings. *Hearing Instruments, 44*(2), 20.)

Seewald, R., and Ross, M. (1988). Amplification for young hearing-impaired children. In M. Pollack (ed.), *Amplification for the Hearing Impaired* (pp. 213–271). Orlando: Grune & Stratton.

Seewald, R., Zelisko, D., Ramji, K., and Jamieson, D. (1991). *DSL 3.0 User's Manual.* London, Ontario, Canada: University of Western Ontario.

Silman, S., Silverman, C. A., Emmer, M. B., and Gelfand, S. A. (1992). Adult-onset auditory deprivation. *Journal of the American Academy of Audiology, 3*(6), 390–396.

Smriga, D. J. (1993). Digital signal processing to suppress feedback: Technology and test results. *The Hearing Journal, 46*(5), 28–33.

Stelmachowicz, P. G., Mace, A. L., Kopun, J. G., and Carney, E. (1993). Long-term and short-term characteristics of speech: Implications for hearing aid selection for young children. *Journal of Speech and Hearing Research, 36,* 609–620.

Stypulkowski, P. H., Hodgson, W. A., and Raskind, L. A. (1992). Clinical evaluation of a new programmable multiple memory ITE. *Hearing Instruments, 43*(6), 25–29.

Sullivan, R. (1987). Aided SSPL 90 response in the real ear: A safe estimate. *Hearing Instruments, 38,* 36.

Tecca, J. E. (1990). Clinical application of real-ear probe tube measurement. In R. E. Sandlin (ed.), *Handbook of Hearing Aid Amplification: Vol. II. Clinical Considerations and Fitting Practices* (pp. 225–255). Boston: College Hill Press.

Thibodeau, L. (1994). Counseling for pediatric amplification. In J. G. Clark and F. N. Martin (eds.), *Effective Counseling in Audiology: Perspectives and Practice* (pp. 147–183). Englewood Cliffs, NJ: Prentice-Hall.

Yellin, W., Meyerhoff, W. L., and Roland, P. S. (1988). A new development for conductive hearing loss. *Tejas, 14,* 44–45.

# CHAPTER 12

# PEDIATRIC AMPLIFICATION: USE AND ADJUSTMENT

*MARK ROSS*

## INTRODUCTION

There is a fundamental difference between the significance of hearing aids for adventitiously hearing-impaired adults and for congenitally hearing-impaired children. Hearing aids selected and used by adults are coupled to existing, auditory-based speech and language skills. The task for adults is simply to *recognize* a linguistic code learned and mastered in their early years. However distorted the acoustic signal may be, the intended linguistic message is within their developed competencies. Not so for children with congenital hearing losses.

For these children, the normal process of auditory-based speech and language development has been disrupted to a greater or lesser extent by the hearing loss (Ross, Brackett, and Maxon, 1991). For congenitally hearing-impaired children, *particularly those with significant degrees of residual hearing,* acoustic amplification is, or should be, the primary mechanism for the natural *development* of speech and language skills. This is a much more demanding task than that faced by adults; these children are attempting to *develop* auditory-based language skills through an impaired auditory system. Having developed a suitable auditory–verbal foundation—basically by providing them with an enriched and relevant pattern of linguistic inputs at optimal speech to noise ratios—they are then required to *recognize* oral messages in essentially minimal redundancy situations. That is, their hearing losses deprive them of some acoustic speech information, inappropriate hearing aids may eliminate additional poten-

tially available speech cues, while unfavorable acoustical conditions further impair the speech perception process (Ross, 1992a). That so many of these children function so well is not only a tribute to their determination and to the dedicated efforts of their parents and teachers, but evidence of the biologic potency of the auditory channel in the normal process of speech and language development (Fry, 1978).

The underlying assumption of this chapter is that amplified sound is the most effective therapeutic tool for minimizing or averting the usual linguistic and educational ramifications of a hearing loss, *for most, but not all,* hearing-impaired children. The consequences of inadequate or poorly functioning hearing aids for adults range from minimal to the serious; for children, these consequences may be catastrophic and seldom less than "very serious."

While the benefits of an amplified speech signal will, roughly, vary inversely with degree of hearing loss, some auditory contributions can almost always be realized. However, these contributions must not only be readily discernible to the parents and the professionals, but they must be apparent to the child as well. If hearing aids are viewed as a burden to be borne, and if amplified sound is, at best, irrelevant, and at worst, intrusive, then a successful adjustment to hearing aids will not be possible. The potential benefits of amplified sound will not be realized. Audiologists should know that when they are selecting and fitting hearing aids to young children they are engaged in a practice with repercussions extending over a child's lifetime.

## A TERMINOLOGICAL AND PHILOSOPHICAL DIGRESSION

To preclude any terminological confusions or misunderstanding, I should define what I mean by the term "hearing impaired" (Ross and Calvert, 1967; Wilson, Ross, and Calvert, 1974). I use the term in a generic sense, to refer to children with any type and degree of hearing loss. Qualifiers, such as "moderate" and "profound" add a degree of preciseness, while other terms, such as "deaf" and "hard-of-hearing" have more specific connotations (and may be preferable in many situations). I am making this point because many advocates of a unique deaf culture object to the use of the term hearing-impaired, arguing that neither they nor their hearing is "impaired," but that they are members of a unique visually oriented group. I would never argue that deaf people, *as people,* are "impaired"—indeed, that attitude is extremely repugnant to me—but I also think it unrealistic to hold that the absence of hearing is simply one of the normal variations found in the human species, akin to ethnicity. If you don't have any, or if it varies from normal to some significant extent, then one's hearing is "impaired" and no "politically correct" formulation will change that reality.

Children who have no residual hearing at all cannot benefit from acoustic amplification (see Chapter 13). Most hearing-impaired children, however, have some residual hearing. One of the primary responsibilities of audiologists, one that no other group is trained to do as effectively, is to exploit this residual hearing as much as is technically feasible. We do not practice our craft, however, in a vacuum. Except for a few exceptions, such as when a child's life is in danger, it is the parents who bear the responsibility, and have the authority, to make the crucial decisions that impact upon a child's life (Ross, 1992b). If parents, deaf or hearing, refuse to permit amplified sound to be employed with their children, then audiologists are obligated to adhere to and respect their

decision. But, on the other hand, our responsibility as professionals is to provide them with our best, and most objective, professional advice during the decision-making process.

## THE DETECTION FACTOR

It is instructive to place the audiologist's role within the context of a commonly cited auditory development hierarchy (Ling, 1978). There are four levels to this hierarchy: detection, discrimination, identification, and comprehension. For the most part, the audiologist is going to be concerned with detection, the most basic of all the levels. Within this framework, the detection level can be viewed as providing the acoustic raw material that "carries" the desired linguistic message. Another way of looking at the detection level is as amplified speech sensation levels. To an average speech spectrum input, this could be defined as the difference between unaided thresholds and the real-ear amplified output across frequency (the "audibility index").

To a great extent, performance levels achieved in the higher levels of the auditory hierarchy are going to be limited by our success in maximizing detection (within reasonable limits, of course [see Moodie, Seewald, and Sinclair, 1994]). For example, if children are unable to *detect* the acoustic energy that distinguishes such words as /room/ and /broom/, /bus/ and /but/, or /red/ and /head/—either because of an inadequate amplification pattern or because of insufficient residual hearing—then they will be unable to auditorily *discriminate* between them. Both words in the pair will be perceived similarly and the prerequisite condition for *identifying* an acoustic event—recognizing an acoustic difference between two stimuli—will not be realized. In selecting, and later modifying when necessary, the amplification pattern for a particular child, the audiologist is actually working on the detection level; the more successfully this can be accomplished, the greater the potential progress in the higher hierarchical levels.

Maximizing detection, however, is only the beginning of a process and not its conclusion. The most appropriately selected hearing aids will do a child little good in a world of silence. While trying to maximize detection, audiologists cannot ignore the higher levels of the auditory hierarchy. We do not only fit hearing aids and adjust their electroacoustic properties. Our professional responsibilities transcend this relatively superficial level of operation. We must also be concerned with the speech signals the child is hearing through our "prescribed" electroacoustic response. In other words, the linguistic nature of the input signals demands our attention as much as their acoustic spectrum does.

Although this chapter concentrates on the auditory channel, in real life, of course, the visual channel will be making its own complementary contribution. We know that bimodal (vision plus audition) speech *recognition* is usually better than either modality alone. It is also possible, for at least some children, that language *development* may be fostered by bimodal reception, given the fact that each channel does convey unique perceptual information (see discussion in Ross, Brackett, and Maxon, 1991, pp. 31–35). Nevertheless, the fact that vision plays a significant role in speech and language perception does not relieve us of the responsibility for optimizing the auditory channel. Audition is still the normal and most effective biologic route for language development.

## THE FIRST HEARING AID

Let us assume that appropriate hearing aid choices have been made, including a binaural fitting unless there are explicit contraindications. Furthermore, considering the state of present technology, I am going to further assume that the electroacoustic "targets" have been confirmed or developed through the use of real-ear measures whenever possible (Moodie et al., 1994),

## Setting Appropriate Amplification Targets

Getting a valid real-ear measure from a squirming, crying, fearful, and generally noncooperative child may be a difficult, and sometimes impossible, endeavor. But, as in any clinical practice, we do what we can and keep our priorities in order. We do *not* want to delay the onset of amplification until valid real-ear measures have been made (or even until we have precisely measured hearing thresholds across frequency in both ears). It is possible to utilize the norms developed by such hearing aid selection procedures as the Desired Sensation Level (DSL) (Seewald, Ramji, Sinclair, Moodie, and Jamieson, 1993) to arrive at acceptable estimates of the real-ear amplified frequency response and maximum output to a speech spectrum input.

A truism in hearing aid fitting, for adults as well as for children, is that the SSPL 90 should not exceed the person's tolerance level. Adults can, and will, complain if the signal is too loud. A congenitally hearing-impaired child is not going to be able to say, "hey, that hurts!" What such children will do is either fuss, cry, or pull at the hearing aid. A few unpleasant auditory experiences like this and we have set up an obstacle to a successful hearing aid fitting that is going to be very difficult to overcome. Since we cannot directly elicit loudness discomfort judgments from a child, we have to proceed cautiously, but not so cautiously that we *underamplify* a child, resulting in average speech inputs that produce inadequate amplified sensation levels.

The audiology profession, in my judgment, has been so traumatized by the fear of overamplification—concerned about the possibility of causing a permanent threshold shift by overamplification—that we often *unnecessarily* compromise the audibility of normal loudness input speech signals. There's little point of a child wearing a hearing aid if the average output falls *below* the child's hearing thresholds. It is my impression that loudness complaints seldom occur when a child has been fitted with hearing aids at a very young age (below age 1). I would speculate that this is related to the fact that the auditory system has not yet experienced the anatomic and physiologic effects of auditory sensory deprivation.

## Attending to the Fit of Earmolds

Once we have ensured that the SSPL 90 of the hearing aid is set at an appropriate level, not too high or too low, then the fit of the earmolds must be examined. It can be difficult to take acceptable ear impressions on some children. There may be a temptation to compromise if the impressions do not come out right the first time. This is not a good idea. Do not ask the earmold lab to build up or modify poor impressions in some way. It is advisable to take the time and trouble to make other impressions it you are not perfectly satisfied with the first pair (or second). The goal is a set of earmolds that do not call attention to themselves (by discomfort, pain, itching, etc), and that can be worn all day without the realization that they are even there.

Children will object—by all means, fair and foul—to wearing hearing aids when the earmolds hurt or are uncomfortable, and they will be right. Look for abrasions or pressure points (localized discolorizations) in the ear canal. One indication of an earmold problem is when the child objects to a hearing aid when the earmold has been inserted in the ear, but *before* the aid has been turned on. Don't underestimate the pain and discomfort an ill-fitting earmold can produce. A tiny welt can produce a big pain in the ear and essentially undercut all of our amplification goals with a child.

## Age as a Factor in Fitting

At the present time, the children with the most severe losses are detected earlier than those with less severe losses, and are candidates for amplification at a younger age. This situation may change if otoacoustic emissions (OAEs) become accepted as a universal mass hearing screening tool for neonates (Norton and Stover, 1994), particularly when coupled with ABR tests. This combination of tests has the potential of detecting not only deaf, but hard of hearing children at an early age, as indicated by the results of a statewide program in Rhode Island (White and Behrens, 1993).

This chapter, however, is written from the perspectives of current clinical practices, wherein only the severely and profoundly hearing-impaired children would be detected and managed at an early age (preferably less than 1 year of age, hopefully less than 2). Most of these children will not respond to hearing aids as an exceptional event in their young lives. They should not even be aware of them—*unless the parents and professionals make too big a deal of their presence.*

Of course many children receive their first hearing aids when they are older. These are primarily children with mild to moderate hearing losses, who have developed some auditory-based linguistic skills, albeit with varying degrees of abnormalities. Unlike the younger children, these older ones are well aware that their peers do not wear hearing aids, and the process of getting these older children to accept and to wear their first hearing aids is more involved. Fortunately, the advantages of amplification can easily be demonstrated with this population (e.g., hearing across the room, more accurate imitation of speech sounds, etc.). These advantages can be great "convincers" of the value of hearing aids to parents, teachers, and to the children themselves. Still, one should be prepared to be firm, while remaining sensitive to children's feelings, to ensure that they not only wear their hearing aids, but are happy with them (Schwartz, 1990). The essential point we must all accept is that *we have no choice.* Hard-of-hearing children *must* wear hearing aids if we are to minimize the speech, language, educational, and psychosocial problems the hearing loss *will* produce.

## Putting the First Hearing Aids On

Most pediatric audiologists agree that it is advisable for hearing-impaired children, particularly those with more severe hearing losses, to wear the hearing aids all day every day. There is some disagreement, however, on the rapidity and method of reaching this goal. Some audiologists prefer to increase use time over a period of some weeks (Downs, 1967), while others believe in total immersion (Ross and Tomassetti, 1980). There is no research evidence to support either approach. Some clinicians recommend gradually increasing the gain control over a period of time (Pollack and Downs, 1964), while still others recommend moving to the desired sensation level immediately (Seewald and Ross, 1988). For the most part, I favor the total immersion method—all day, every day, at the prescribed gain and output settings—but with some initial gradualism on the gain setting for the first few days.

Whatever approach is practiced, it seems to me that the initial fitting of hearing aids is more often a problem to the parents and the professionals than it is to the child. Insecure and fearful clinicians, approaching children in a tentative and uncertain manner, can easily convey their apprehensions to children. Approached in an authoritative and casual manner, most children, particularly the younger ones, will accept hearing aids the same way they accept being fed, changed, bathed, and so on. Involved recipes are usually not necessary in getting a child to accept and wear the hearing aids all day. Approaches that call too much attention to the hearing aids can degenerate into a battle of the wills between the child and the parents. This is not a battle we can afford to lose. We cannot put ourselves in a position in which children have an option of whether to wear the hearing aids. We don't ask children's permission before we put the hearing aids on; what if they say no?

I do not mean to convey the impression that the hearing aids should be put on in a cavalier fashion. The clinician should be observing the child's reactions to sound and be ready to respond appropriately when cued by the child's behavior. However, given properly fitting earmolds, a realistic SSPL 90, pleasant early sound exposures, and parents and professionals convinced of the necessity of amplification, then the adjustment

should go smoothly (Thibodeau, 1994). The following are some specific suggestions:

**1.** Place the hearing aids on the child in the same routine, but definite, manner that one would engage in other nurturing activities. (We don't ask the child for permission before changing diapers, do we?) Make sure the earmolds are completely seated in the ear canals and that the BTE aids (most likely the first type) fit comfortably behind the pinnae. To ensure that the hearing aids are firmly secured behind the ears, I suggest the routine use of "Huggie Aids." These anchor the hearing aids in the postauricular position and also help keep the child from tampering with the volume control (see Figure 12.1).

**2.** Initially, adjust the gain control to a position "somewhat less" than its ultimate setting. We want to achieve some audibility with an average input speech signal but we don't want to suddenly explode from silence to full audibility. This is a personal preference: There is no evidence supporting any specific approach in initially exposing a young child to amplified sounds.

**3.** Once the hearing aids are in, *do not* engage in facial and vocal gyrations ("hi honey, can you hear me?" said with big, animated, and phony smiles). *Do* talk to the child, much as you would with any child. Later (but not too much later), parents should be given specific information on intensive "motherese" linguistic inputs, but for now don't make the hearing aids a specific focus of attention.

**4.** If the child begins to cry or pull at the hearing aids, *first* try to divert the child's attention, and *then,* if the child still apparently objects to the hearing aids, remove them *before* they become a bone of contention. If this occurs, examine the concha and ear canal for pressure points. Put the hearing aids in without turning them on. Still a problem? Check the ears and molds again. If the child accepts the earmolds with the aids turned off, check the SSPL 90. Too high? Turn it down. Run a frequency response curve. Sometimes children object to too many low frequencies, even

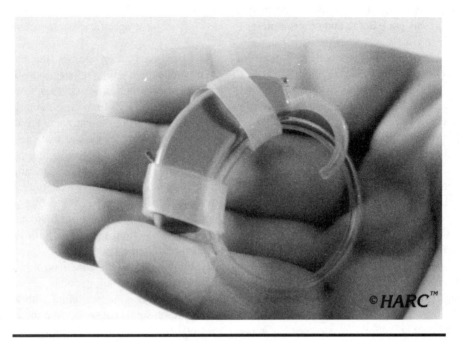

**FIGURE 12.1**    Huggie-Aid hearing aid retainer. This simple device helps secure the hearing aid comfortably behind the ear. (Courtesy of HARC Mercantile)

when correctly "prescribed." Try reducing the lows, temporarily.

**5.** At the conclusion of the first fitting appointment, it is important to leave the child happy with you and the clinic. You are going to see this child again, and again, and again. It is amazing what even infants remember about bad scenes. When the child returns, it is much more pleasant, for all concerned, to have a happy, cooing patient, than one who is throwing a tantrum at the very sight of you and your impressive, and fearful, equipment.

**Follow-Up Appointments**

For young children fit with their first hearing aids, there *will* be a number of follow-up appointments. If possible, the first follow-up appointment should be within the week. Some questions to ask at this time include the following:

**1.** Has the child been wearing the hearing aids all day, every day? Are objections associated with

particular events, like when the older siblings come home from school and turn the TV set full on?

**2.** What have been the child's responses to environmental sounds? To meaningful language? Instruct the parents to keep a log of the child's auditory responses to both sounds and language (Table 12.1). This may be helpful in not only charting auditory development, but also will give the audiologist cues about the aided response of the hearing aids. It will also give parents some concrete evidence of the efficacy of the hearing aids.

**3.** Some parents write much more elaborate logs than is provided for in Table 12.1. The important consideration is to ascertain the relationship between the stimulus evoking auditory responses (environmental or linguistic) and the nature of the child's responses. Some parents may not be aware that, for example, the spontaneous turning to the source of an environmental sound may be very

**TABLE 12.1**   Auditory Responses of Child

| DATE | TIME | CHILD'S OBSERVED REACTIONS | NOTED ELICITED STIMULUS |
|------|------|----------------------------|-------------------------|
| ___ | ___ | _____ | _____ |
| ___ | ___ | _____ | _____ |
| ___ | ___ | _____ | _____ |
| ___ | ___ | _____ | _____ |
| ___ | ___ | _____ | _____ |
| ___ | ___ | _____ | _____ |

significant. Being able to point out the small, but vital steps to auditory development can be quite encouraging to parents who desperately need to see some tangible signs of progress.

**4.** Has the child attempted to imitate speech sounds? It is helpful for the parent to include these observations in the log as well. What is the quality of the child's spontaneous vocalizations? This information will also help us understand what the child is hearing. Skilled clinicians can often predict the changes in the frequency response simply by listening to the child's vocalizations (Brackett, 1994, personal communication).

**5.** Ask the parents to remove and reinsert the hearing aids, and observe them while they do this. Is it done correctly and efficiently? Ask them to troubleshoot the hearing aids in your presence. It is not what you *say* that is important, it is what they *do*.

**6.** Following the questions, ensure that the hearing aids are set to the "use" position. Run the hearing aids in the hearing aid test chamber to ensure that the responses are those that were prescribed. If the SSPL 90 and frequency responses were decreased earlier from the prescribed settings because of fearful or negative reactions from the child, now is the time to begin readjusting them to the appropriate targets.

**7.** Try to get more accurate audiometric information during the follow-up visits. It is unlikely that valid bilateral hearing thresholds were obtained at the time the hearing aids were initially fit. I would add that if so, the child has probably

been detected and fit with hearing aids much later than the optimal readiness period.

**8.** The frequency of follow-up appointments should be "as necessary." This may seem to be rather a loose formulation, but in reality it need not be. *All* young children with hearing loss should be enrolled in a parent–infant program (Atkins, 1994; Luterman, 1979, 1987). Therefore, "somebody" is keeping tabs on the child's status—and working with the parents and the children on an ongoing basis. Whoever this "somebody" is must take the responsibility for keeping the audiologist informed about the child's status (auditory–vocal, maturation, etc.). Either changes in behavior or demonstrated readiness for further testing signal the need for a continuation of the audiologic evaluation process.

**9.** Once the child's situation has been stabilized (measured bilateral hearing thresholds across frequency, appropriate hearing aid settings, enrolled in a parent–infant program), then the follow-up audiologic appointments can be routinely scheduled. Ideally, this schedule should allow for appointments every 3 months for the younger children, moving to 6 months and then every year by age 5 years. Appointments should be more frequent if events signal a need.

## TROUBLESHOOTING THE HEARING AID

Anyone troubleshooting hearing aids should assume that Mr. Murphy is lurking in the background, gleefully observing occasions of his law in action ("anything that can go wrong, will"), The best way to thwart Mr. Murphy is to begin by assuming the existence of one or more problems. The troubleshooter's task, then, is simply to discover them. *Particularly* when the wearers of the hearing aids are children, one can predict the occurrence of the most unpredictable events. I have seen hearing aids buried in sand boxes, drooled on by the family dog (and by a hearing twin), chewed on by the child (sometimes sharing a bite with the dog!), washed in the bathtub, flushed down the toilet, battered by toy hammers, washed and dried in the laundry, and just generally abused. So, as stated above, assume that there is a problem that has to be identified, modifying this orientation only when repeated experiences demonstrate otherwise.

In the beginning, it is the parent who must take the primary responsibility for daily troubleshooting. Before the hearing aids are put on in the morning, they should be checked. If the child goes to a play group, a nursery, or a kindergarten, the hearing aids should be checked by the caregivers and teachers *before* the day's activities begin. When the child returns home, the hearing aids should be checked again. This seems a little obsessive, and it is, but it is necessary. Something can always happen between checks, and if something does happen, the child will not receive the benefits of amplification. It is possible to ease up if repeated checks demonstrate that the hearing aids are functioning properly.

Eventually, it is necessary to transfer the troubleshooting responsibility to the child. At a time when 6-year-old children can already operate complicated electronic games, troubleshooting hearing aids should be, literally, "child's play." I have no doubt that average 6-year-old children can learn to operate and troubleshoot their own hearing aids. The kicker, of course, is that they must *want* to do it; they must perceive the hearing aids as much a part of them as their eyes and hands. When something goes wrong, not only must they *know* it, but they must also *show* the problem to their caregivers. I have often had chil-

dren come to me complaining that one hearing aid was not working, or that one or the other was not quite right. These are children who perceived amplified sound as necessary to their well-being and adjustment to the world. Without the amplified sound provided by the hearing aids, they felt anxious and insecure, as if a part of them was absent (as it was).

## Equipment Needed

**1.** A battery tester (see Figure 12.2). The simplest ones simply read "green" (for good) or "red" (for bad). For the professional, it would be preferable to use a battery tester from which the actual battery voltage can be read.

**2.** A hearing aid "stethoscope." This device permits normal-hearing people to listen to the hearing aid. For BTE hearing aids, there is a rubber cup at the tip that fits over the earmold; for body aids, or FM receivers, the tubing from the stethoscope can be removed and the button receiver snapped in place (see Figure 12.3). Many parents and teachers have elected to obtain a personal earmold for troubleshooting purposes. This is a little more convenient and provides slightly better fidelity than the stethoscope.

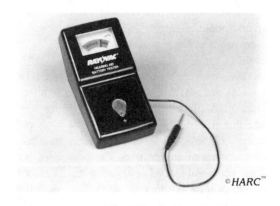

© *HARC*™

**FIGURE 12.2**  An example of a simple hearing aid battery tester. Some testers provide voltage measures rather than a simple "good-bad" indication. (Courtesy of HARC Mercantile)

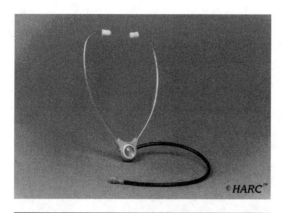

**FIGURE 12.3**   A hearing aid stethoscope. The rubber tip at the end is placed over the tip of an earmold. The tubing can be disconnected and a snag-ring on the stethoscope accepts button-type receivers. (Courtesy of HARC Mercantile)

**3.** Earmold cleanser, air blower, a dehumidifier bag, spare batteries, and devices to remove wax from the earmolds (brushes, wax loops, toothpicks).

Troubleshooting kits are available at a nominal cost from hearing aid dispensers and include all the equipment listed above (see Figure 12.4).

## Visual Inspection

The first step in troubleshooting a hearing aid is to look at it and the earmold carefully.

**1.** Inspect the earmold. Is the surface clean? If not, the wax can build up and abrade the ear. It is a good idea to wash the earmold daily with warm soap and water, ensuring that it is dry and that all water has been removed from the tubing. One of the most common problems with earmolds is wax clogging the sound bore. If wax can be observed, remove it with a pick or with an air blower. This is one of the most common reasons for hearing aid malfunction.

**2.** Examine the tone-hook. This is a plastic connector that fits over the end of the BTE hearing aid and to which the tubing is attached. Does it fit snugly on the hearing aid? If it screws on, does it

rotate continuously, indicating that the threads are stripped? Are there cracks or holes in it? A poorly fitting or cracked tone-hook will permit sound to escape and cause acoustic feedback.

**3.** Examine the tubing leading from the tone-hook to the earmold. Are there any cracks or crimps? Is the tubing still flexible, or extremely stiff and discolored? Any of these conditions require the insertion of a new tubing.

**4.** Examine the case of the hearing aid. Any evidence of maltreatment? While the physical appearance of the case does not, in itself, signify an electroacoustic problem, it does suggest the increased likelihood of such a problem.

**5.** Are the controls in the position recommended by the audiologist? Somehow, the control positions often seem to change between troubleshooting sessions. If the hearing aid is set on the "T" position (necessary when the aid is coupled to an FM neckloop, for example), the hearing aid microphone is deactivated. How about the gain, output, and frequency response controls? Are they where they should be?

**6.** Now look into the battery compartment. Is the battery inserted correctly? Usually the battery compartment has the positive symbol (+), which matches a similar symbol on the battery. *Don't force the battery in the compartment.* If you have to, then it is probable that the battery is in the wrong position or that it is the wrong battery.

**7.** Check the battery voltage with the battery tester, preferably one that displays voltage rather than simply red or green. The battery voltage is normally about 1.4 volts. If the voltage drops to 1.3, the aid should still function adequately, but not if it drops below this point. Sometimes there is a temptation to compensate for a minor drop in voltage with increased rotation of the gain control. This is not a good idea, since voltage drops may be accompanied by increased distortion when the gain is increased.

## Listening Inspection

Use the hearing aid stethoscope (Figure 12.3) or a personal earmold to listen to the hearing aid. A

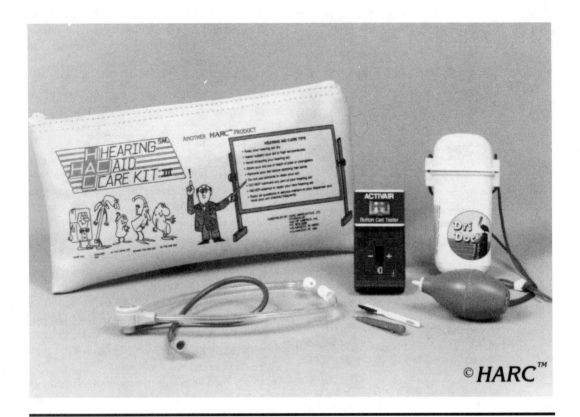

**FIGURE 12.4**    An example of a common hearing aid troubleshooting kit for parents and teachers. (Courtesy of HARC Mercantile)

normal-hearing person will quickly realize that the sound quality is usually not "high fidelity," and sometimes very far from it. Recall, though, that the hearing aid is not designed to be used by someone with normal hearing. Ideally, if the audiologist has done his or her job effectively (see Chapter 11) and depending upon the nature of the child's hearing loss, the hearing aid will ordinarily function in a more or less nonlinear fashion. A normal ear can find this disconcerting, but nevertheless the pattern of amplification may be perfectly appropriate for the child. It is necessary for the troubleshooter to internalize a perceptual norm, derived from the first listening experiences with the hearing aid, at which time one can be assured that what one is hearing is "correct."

**1.** To listen to the hearing aids, the troubleshooter should place the tip of the earmold into the rubber tip of the stethoscope and turn the aid "on." Then, while talking at a normal loudness level, begin the listening check. Rather than simply counting ("one, two three, four"), or saying "hello," it is preferable to first use speech stimuli that sample the entire acoustic range of speech (such as the Ling "six-sound test"—/m/, /a/, /ee/, /oo/, /sh/, and /s/), and then to employ running speech. A perceptual norm should be established for each of the speech stimuli used

**2.** At this time, the volume control should be rotated, from the lowest setting to the highest while listening for static, discontinuances, sudden bursts of loudness, or distortion. The slow rotation of the gain control should produce a smooth and undistorted increase in loudness. What is not acceptable is for the aid to jump to maximum loudness with only a slight turn of the control.

**3.** If the hearing aid is very powerful, the normal hearing listener will not want to be exposed to the full output of the hearing aid for more than a few seconds. Sometimes hearing aids begin to distort at higher sound pressure level outputs and it is necessary that this be checked. However, if a normal-hearing listener finds that the hearing aid output is extremely uncomfortable, perhaps approaching the pain threshold, a listening test at this level is *not* advised. Use a hearing aid test chamber for this analysis.

**4.** After the listening test has been completed for a normal speech level input, try using soft and then loud speech (but keep in mind that the purpose of this exercise is not to create more hearing-impaired audiologists!). Each of the stimuli used will give distinct acoustic impressions. Often when a hearing aid begins to malfunction, it will affect only certain frequencies (such as emphasizing the low frequencies or eliminating the higher frequencies).

**5.** If the troubleshooter detects any perceptual variations from previous tests, then the battery, earmold, tubing, and potentiometer settings should all be rechecked. If the problem persists, then a comprehensive electroacoustic analysis is required. If the source of the problem cannot be identified and corrected, return the hearing aid to the factory for repairs.

**6.** If the hearing aid is being used with a personal FM system, then a listening check is also required through whatever coupling mode is being used (neck loop or direct audio input). A helper is necessary to talk into the FM microphone, while the troubleshooter listens to the output through the hearing aid. This arrangement will detect major problems in the transmission path and significant variations in a hearing aid's "prescribed" electroacoustic responses due to coupler variables. Whenever children use a personal FM system with their personal hearing aids, it is necessary,

because of the probability of these coupler variables, to evaluate the entire system with an electroacoustic analyzer (Seewald and Moodie, 1992; Lewis, 1994).

By the time this book is published. it will probably be impossible to distinguish between FM systems and many hearing aids (Ross, 1986; Yuzon and Ross, 1994). Some BTE model hearing aids will include the capacity for FM reception (two such units are presently on the market). When a child is fit with such a unit, then the troubleshooting process *must* include the FM transmission path separately from the hearing aid circuit.

When troubleshooting the FM transmission in such units, ensure that any FM microphone gain or AGC controls are set where prescribed. Then, set the hearing aid portion to the "use" gain position and turn the receiver to the combined position (FM and HA). As a helper talks into the FM microphone, listen to the FM signal. Ask the helper to continue talking while moving away to the maximum distance at which the FM system will be used. Has the signal broken up, or is it still clear?

While the helper is at the maximum distance, talk into the HA microphone at a normal level. What is the relative loudness between these two inputs? They can be the same, or the FM portion can be slightly louder, depending upon the situation and the opinions of the teachers and the audiologist.

## COMMUNICATING

There is a widespread belief that the auditory needs of children with hearing loss are being met once hearing aids are selected and worn. Nothing could be further from the truth. A child's use of hearing aids is only the beginning of the habilitative process (Thibodeau, 1994). Parents, teachers, and all involved with hearing-impaired children must understand the limitations as well as the advantages of amplification. They must not only accept the need for amplification, but be informed of the situational variables that restrict auditory benefits from amplification. Realistic expectations must be conveyed without, at the same time, appearing to be accentuating the negative. Our stance has to be positive. While no one can predict exactly how much, hearing aids will enhance auditory–verbal development. We can be sure that parents and teachers play a crucial role in maximizing this development.

## Parents and Family

There is no question but that the parents are the key players in the habilitative process. They are the ones who bear the greatest emotional burden, and the ones who have the greatest impact upon a child's overall (not just auditory–verbal) development (Atkins, 1994). While audiologists can select appropriate hearing aids, and clinicians can conduct a parent–infant program, the effectiveness of all these efforts will be constrained by the quality of the parental involvement. As it relates to "post hearing aid selection," (and assuming that they have been instructed in the described troubleshooting procedures outlined earlier), parent communication should include the following points:

**1.** The parents have to be convinced of the necessity, and potential value, of the hearing aids. There *will* be a tendency for the parents to view the hearing aids as a constant reminder of the trauma they experienced in learning that their child was hearing impaired. What clinicians *must* do is work through these feelings with the parents. They have to see the hearing aids as part of the solution and not simply as a reminder of the problem.

**2.** Therefore, the parents must be informed about how the hearing aids can help their particular child. Aided audiograms, however, should be used cautiously (Seewald, Hudson, Gagne, and Zelisko, 1992). They *should not* be explained as equivalent to unaided hearing of the same magnitude (e.g., 20-dB aided thresholds do not mean a child has only a mild hearing loss). It is helpful to explain the "speech banana" (Ross et al., 1991) to assist parents in understanding the potential ca-

pacity of a child to detect various speech features. If, for example, the child has little or no residual hearing past 2000 Hz, then it is not realistic to expect the child to detect some high-frequency phonemes (but it is amazing what some children can perceive in running speech by using secondary and alternative perceptual cues, e.g., formant transitions, durational effects, etc.)

**3.** Dramatic increases in a child's auditory–verbal development do not often occur (except for some older, moderately hearing-impaired children, for whom one often sees almost an "explosion" of linguistic competencies soon after wearing personal amplification). The concept of "hearing age" is sometimes useful. This is the time a child has been using amplification as distinguished from chronological age. The concept can help in developing realistic expectations about a child's auditory–verbal development.

**4.** The necessity to optimize the speech-to-noise (S/N) ratio must be carefully explained to parents. It is sometimes difficult for normal-hearing people to understand just how much more sensitive a person with hearing loss is to poor acoustical conditions than they are. Normal-hearing siblings may be able to do their homework while the stereo or TV is blasting, and engage in a conversation with the parents at the same time with no difficulty. This is an impossible situation for a hearing-impaired child wearing hearing aids. While we cannot always control the level of the ambient sounds in our lives, we must make parents aware of its potential effect upon their child. If the signal (i.e., speech) you want a child to listen to is buried in the noise, or only several dB more intense than the noise, there is no way the child will be able to associate the signal with experience or meaningful events (a prerequisite for auditory language development). The S/N ratio can be increased *either* by decreasing the noise or by increasing the signal (moving closer to the child, or by using an FM system).

**5.** Siblings and grandparents have to be included in the (re)habilitative process (Atkins, 1994). A hearing loss not only impacts upon the child and his or her parents, but has repercussions throughout the entire family. Like it or not, siblings and grandparents are involved, directly and indirectly.

Siblings of hearing-impaired children often tend to get shortchanged. They have their own need for their parent's time and love, and they can understandably resent their parent's focus on their hearing-impaired sibling. They should not have to compete or agitate for their parent's love. A hearing-impaired child cannot help but affect family dynamics; the trick is to include the hearing siblings in the family constellation without making them their "brother's keeper." This is precisely the kind of issue about which some parents can provide valuable advice and information to other parents. Parental suggestions for the siblings of children with hearing loss may be found in Appendix 8.

Professionals often overlook the impact of a child's hearing loss upon the grandparents. Since grandparents do not ordinarily live with the child, their involvement is considered tangential at best. This is not fair to them for a number of emotional and practical reasons. They *are* involved and it is only fair to them to welcome their participation, but often very helpful as well (e.g., who does the baby sitting for the other siblings during all the clinic visits, etc.). This, too, is an issue for which parent groups can provide suggestions and support. In many such groups I know of, and have managed myself, grandparents were welcomed and participated fully in the discussion, to the benefit of all participants.

## Teachers

Separating postselection hearing aid concerns from everything else teachers need in order to effectively manage a hearing-impaired child in their classroom is neither realistic nor recommended. Amplification systems represent only part of the information they need (Johnson, 1994). However, regular classroom teachers cannot develop the requisite skills to manage a hearing-impaired child with only occasional exposures to such children. While an in-service training program will help (Maxon, 1990), it is even more important to assure teachers that there is somebody out there (speech-language pathologist, educational audiologist, teacher of the deaf) who they can call upon when needed. No inservice training program, no matter how comprehensively implemented, is going to make them experts in amplification. They can, and should, be expected to engage in routine troubleshooting and to quickly identify problems beyond their expertise to solve. Beyond this, they need rapid access to an expert resource person.

An in-service training program for teachers is best conducted in the early spring, when the next year's classroom teachers have been identified. The following elements should be included:

**1.** Teachers need general information about the speech, language, academic, and psychosocial consequences of a hearing loss, with *particular reference to how these apply to the classroom management of the specific child in question* (see Chapters 9 and 16 and Conway, 1990). Expectations are a key consideration. Hearing-impaired children represent the same range of potential and intelligence as do normal-hearing children. Teachers should not reduce standards because a child is hard-of-hearing. We do these children no service by pitying them or accepting less than they are capable of. Focusing on the *impact* of the hearing loss, in other words, is only half the picture; the other half has to be their potential for normal achievements.

**2.** The benefits and limitations of hearing aids should be clearly explained. The focus should be on the child's potential receptive capacities, with and without amplification. Video and audiotape demonstrations are very useful.

Many teachers feel understandably insecure about troubleshooting hearing aids, particularly, it seems, when they are required to insert and remove the earmolds. Much of this information cannot be conveyed by a written report, but has to be taught and demonstrated in a hands-on fashion.

However, a personal visit must also not substitute for a well-written and informative report.

**3.** Teachers need to appreciate the relatively greater impact of classroom acoustics upon the speech perception capabilities of hearing-impaired children and how this relates to their ability to learn language through the auditory channel.

I am very sensitive to this particular issue, perhaps because of my own hearing loss. I have been in too many classrooms in which I could barely understand the teacher through my hearing aids, and I have an excellent language base. How on earth can we expect children to learn new language and their classroom lessons in poor acoustical circumstances? "Poor" for those with hearing loss may be S/N ratios of +6 dB, and reverberation times of .6 seconds, conditions quite acceptable for normal-hearing children.

**4.** The importance of enhanced S/N ratios dictates that post hearing aid selection considerations for classroom teachers *must* include evaluation of the need, and the potential advantages of, an FM auditory training system. With all the advances we have lately seen in hearing aid technology, there is still no better device capable of increasing the S/N ratio than an appropriately used FM system (Ross, 1992). In my own view, any audiologist who does not routinely at least *consider* the need for an FM system for every mainstreamed hearing-impaired child is either incompetent or insensitive.

**5.** Educators need to know how to assist the psychosocial acceptance of the hard of hearing child into the life of the classroom (Ross et al., 1991; Schwartz, 1990). A child wearing visible amplification devices in a regular classroom is still an oddity. Teachers can foster acceptance, not by ignoring the presence of the hearing aids and FM systems, which the other children won't do in any event, but by casually and objectively giving a classroom lesson on hearing loss, hearing aids, FM systems, et cetera.

The key to acceptance by the other children—or inclusion to use the current term—is, in my opinion, personal acceptance. Children who accept themselves and their hearing losses, who can deflect or ignore the teasing, or who can effectively retaliate against tormenters, will have few psychosocial adjustment problems in the classroom.

## SUMMARY

In this chapter, I have stressed the purpose of amplification for children, rather than only providing the reader with how-to guidelines. Without a deep gut belief in the efficacy of amplification, procedural guidelines will be useless. With such a belief, the inadequacies of this chapter will be overcome by self-study and sensitive experiences. Even if this chapter presented a comprehensive state of the art regarding pediatric amplification, use and adjustment, the passage of time and new developments would render the current status incomplete and obsolete. Clinicians who are committed to using residual hearing to its fullest will be the ones who keep up, by their own exertions and efforts, with the latest developments.

Audiologists should not take a narrow view of their role. Selecting amplification and ensuring that the selected devices are working properly is the beginning and not the end of the process. Everyone involved in the education of a hearing-impaired child must be informed and convinced of the value of amplified sound. No one else can do this as effectively as the audiologist. Having some understanding of speech and language development and how this can be fostered by appropriate amplification, or hindered by inadequate amplification, makes the audiologist an important part of the rehabilitative team. Audiologists who limit their contributions to the selection and troubleshooting of devices are not only limiting themselves professionally, but losing half the fun of being an audiologist. The profession offers no greater reward than seeing children grow up to be successful adults, based in part on what you have done for them at an early age.

## REFERENCES

Atkins, D. V. (1994). Counseling children with hearing loss and their families. In J. G. Clark and F. N. Martin (eds.), *Effective Counseling in Audiology: Perspectives and Practices* (pp. 116–146). Englewood Cliffs, NJ: Prentice Hall.

Conway, L. (1990). Issues related to classroom management. In M. Ross (ed.), *Hearing-impaired Children in the Mainstream* (pp. 131–158). Parkton, MD: York Press.

Downs, M. P. (1967). The establishment of hearing aid use: A program for parents. *Maico Audiological Series, 4*(5), 13–15.

Fry, D. B. (1978). The role and primacy of the auditory channel in speech and language development. In M. Ross and T. G. Giolas (eds.), *Auditory Management of Hearing-Impaired Children* (pp. 15–43). Baltimore: University Park Press.

Johnson, C. D. (1994). Educational considerations: Talking with parents and school personnel. In J. G. Clark and F. N. Martin (eds.), *Effective Counseling in Audiology: Perspectives and Practices* (pp. 184–209). Englewood Cliffs, NJ: Prentice Hall.

Lewis, D. E. (1994). Assistive devices for classroom listening. *American Journal of Audiology: A Journal of Clinical Practice, 3*(1), 70–83.

Ling, D. (1978). Auditory coding and recoding: An analysis of auditory training procedures for hearing-impaired children. In M. Ross and T. G. Giolas (eds.), *Auditory Management of Hearing-Impaired Children* (pp. 181-218). Baltimore: University Park Press.

Luterman, D. (1979). *Counseling Parents of Hearing-Impaired Children.* Boston: Little, Brown, & Company.

Luterman, D. (1987). *Deafness in the Family.* Boston: Little, Brown, & Company.

Maxon, A. M. (1990). Implementing an in-service training program. In M. Ross (ed.), *Hearing-impaired Children in the Mainstream* (pp. 257–274). Parkton, MD: York Press.

Moodie, K. S., Seewald, R. C., and Sinclair, S. T. (1994). Procedure for predicting real-ear hearing aid performance in young children. *American Journal of Audiology: A Journal of Clinical Practice, 3*(1), 23–31.

Norton, S. J., and Stover, L. J. (1994). Otoacoustic emissions: An emerging clinical tool. In J. Katz (ed.), *Handbook of Clinical Audiology* (4th ed., pp. 448–464). Baltimore: Williams & Wilkins.

Pollack, D., and Downs, M. (1964). A parent's guide in hearing aids for young children. *Volta Review, 66,* 745–749.

Ross, M. (1986). Classroom amplification. In W. R. Hodgson (ed.), *Hearing Aid Assessment and Use in Audiological Habilitation* (pp. 231–265). Baltimore: Williams & Wilkins.

Ross, M. (1992a). Room acoustics and speech perception. In M. Ross (ed.), *FM Auditory Training Systems: Characteristics, Selection, and Use* (pp. 21–44). Timonium, MD: York Press.

Ross, M. (1992b). Implications of audiologic success. *Journal American Academy of Audiology, 3,* 1–4.

Ross, M., and Calvert, D. R. (1967). The semantics of deafness. *Volta Review, 69,* 644-649.

Ross, M., and Tomassetti, C. (1980). Hearing aid selection for preverbal hearing-impaired children. In M. C. Pollack (ed.), *Amplification for the Hearing-impaired* (2nd ed., pp. 213–253). New York: Grune & Stratton.

Ross, M., Brackett, D., and Maxon, A. B. (1991). *Assessment and Management of Mainstreamed Hearing-impaired Children: Principles and Practices.* Austin: Pro-Ed.

Schwartz, S. (1990). Psycho-social aspects of mainstreaming. In M. Ross (ed.), *Hearing-impaired Children in the Mainstream* (pp. 159–180). Parkton, MD: York Press.

Seewald, R. C., Hudson, S. P., Gagne, J. P., and Zelisko, D. L. C. (1992). Comparison of two methods for estimating the sensation level of amplified speech. *Ear and Hearing, 13*(2), 142–149.

Seewald, R. C., and Moodie, K. S. (1992). Electroacoustic considerations. In M. Ross (ed.), *FM Auditory Training Systems: Characteristics, Selection, and Use* (pp. 75–102). Timonium, MD: York Press.

Seewald, R. C., Ramji, K. V., Sinclair, S. T., Moodie, K. S., and Jamieson, D. G. (1993). A computer-assisted training implementation of the desired sensation level method for electroacoustic selection and fitting in children. *The Hearing Health Care Research Unit, Technical Report O2,* University of Western Ontario, London, Ontario, Canada.

Seewald, R. C., and Ross, M. (1988). Amplification for young hearing-impaired children. In M. C. Pollack (ed.), *Amplification for the Hearing-impaired*

(3rd ed., pp. 213–272). New York: Grune & Stratton.

Thibodeau, L. M. (1994). Counselling for pediatric amplification. In J. G. Clark and F. N. Martin (eds.), *Effective Counseling in Audiology: Perspectives and Practices* (pp. 147–183). Englewood Cliffs, NJ: Prentice Hall.

White, K. R., and Behrens, T. R. (1993). The Rhode Island Hearing Assessment Project. *Seminars in Hearing, 14*(1).

Wilson, G. B., Ross, M. and Calvert, D. R. (1974). Experimental study of the semantics of deafness. *Volta Review, 76,* 408–414.

Yuzon, E., and Ross, M. (1994). FM systems for adults: Some ideas for realizing their full potential. *The Hearing Journal, 47*(2), 35–40.

# CHAPTER 13

# CHILDREN AND COCHLEAR IMPLANTS

*DANIELLE M.R. KELSAY AND RICHARD S. TYLER*

In the last 10 years, cochlear implants have dramatically changed our approach to aural (re)habilitation for children with profound hearing impairment. Although clearly not a panacea, many children have been helped dramatically by cochlear implants. With careful selection of recipients, precise device fitting, the support of educators and parents, and a comprehensive aural (re)habilitation program, many more children will be helped. However, we must have accurate means to determine which children will benefit from cochlear implants more than from hearing aids. Long-term results for large numbers of children have not yet been documented. This chapter provides an overview of the important issues pertaining to cochlear implants in children.

## PROFOUNDLY HEARING-IMPAIRED CHILDREN

Profoundly hearing-impaired children are audiologically defined as children with pure-tone averages at 500, 1000, and 2000 Hz of greater than 90 dB HL (Boothroyd, 1993). This definition includes children with a wide variety of auditory, speech production, and language skills. In addition to the amount of residual hearing, several other factors affect a child's development of these skills. Contributing factors include age at onset of hearing loss; age at identification of the profound hearing impairment; the interval of time between the diagnosis of the profound hearing impairment and the initiation of amplification; how consistently appropriate amplification is used; communication mode used; and family involvement in the (re)habilitation process.

The amount of residual hearing profoundly hearing-impaired children have will affect their auditory capabilities. Some children defined as profoundly hearing impaired may have residual hearing at all speech frequencies (250 Hz through 8000 Hz); other children may not have sound detection abilities at any speech frequencies even with powerful hearing aids. As a result, some children cannot even detect suprasegmental cues of speech (e.g., duration and intensity), while those with significant residual hearing are able to detect segmental cues including some vowel and consonant features.

In addition to the degree of residual hearing, age of onset of profound hearing loss has a significant impact on a child's auditory capabilities. Exposure to speech allows a child to develop an auditory representation of language, something that a child might never develop if the child is born with a profound hearing loss or acquires one during the first 2 years of life. These children would be considered **prelinguistically deafened.** It is likely that they will have significant delays in speech production and language development. Children who acquire a profound hearing impairment after the age of 2 years are considered **postlinguistically deafened.** Since these children have had an opportunity to develop an auditory representation of language, their auditory and speech production skills will likely exceed those of prelinguistically deafened children. Some postlinguistically deafened children may even have age-appropriate speech production and language skills.

A timely diagnosis of profound hearing impairment and consistent use of amplification initiated shortly after a diagnosis of deafness are important in the development of auditory skills. Congenitally deafened teenagers and adults who have never used amplification often do not develop auditory skills beyond the sound detection stage. They do not find sound useful, possibly even distracting when communicating. In contrast, children who receive amplification immediately after a timely diagnosis of profound hearing impairment may master more advanced auditory skills such as discrimination, identification, and even comprehension of speech. The communication mode the child uses will affect the development of auditory, speech production, and language skills. One child may be brought up in the Deaf Culture, communicate manually, acquire American Sign Language as a first or only language, and have no use for sound in communicating. Though this child is not likely to develop any spoken language, manual language skills could be highly sophisticated. In contrast, another child with the same degree of hearing loss may be fit with amplification as soon as the hearing loss is identified, acquire English as a first or only language, and use simultaneous (manual and oral/aural) or oral/aural communication to acquire sophisticated speech production and spoken language skills.

Finally, family involvement in the (re)habilitation process will have a significant affect on the development of a child's auditory, speech production, and language skills. How successfully a family uses a chosen communication mode will affect the child's language development. Whether the family plays an active part in the child's rehabilitation process will influence whether the child generalizes auditory, speech production, and language skills learned in therapy into daily life.

In summary, children with profound hearing impairments do not represent a homogeneous group. Some have limited but useful residual hearing, whereas others do not. Many factors will contribute to a child's ability to use what residual hearing he or she has, including whether the child is prelinguistically or postlinguistically deafened, whether amplification is used consistently, the type of communication mode used, and family involvement in (re)habilitation.

## COCHLEAR IMPLANTATION SELECTION CRITERIA AND CONSIDERATIONS

A complete evaluation for a cochlear implant includes medical, audiologic, speech and language, and psychological assessments. The purpose of the medical evaluation is to determine the general health of the child and the status of the child's cochleas. A standard medical exam will determine whether a child is in good health and not at risk for complications during surgery. A high-resolution computerized axial tomography (CT) scan of the temporal bones is obtained to determine if the child's cochleas are anatomically suitable for implantation. The electrode array cannot be successfully implanted in a cochlea that is not at least partially patent.

Meningitis is a disease that can result in bony growth in the cochlear duct. A CT scan will determine if bony growth in the cochlea is so extensive that successful implantation of the electrode array is not possible. If bony growth is present, but not extensive, it may be possible to drill through the bone to place the electrode array (Gantz, McCabe, and Tyler, 1988). The CT scan can also determine if congenital malformations of the cochlea are extensive enough to contraindicate implantation of the electrode array.

The purpose of the speech and language evaluation is to determine a baseline for comparing changes in a child's overall communication skills following receipt of a cochlear implant. Receptive and expressive language skills and speech production skills are assessed. Generally, children are not excluded from candidacy based on their performance on speech production and language tests. However, a cochlear implant may not be recommended for an older child who communicates solely by manual communication and has no oral communication skills.

One purpose of the psychological assessment is to determine the general cognitive functioning of the child. It should be determined that a child is mentally capable of accepting and wearing the device and undergoing surgery and hospitalization. Motivations for pursuing cochlear implantation also need to be ascertained to determine whether the family or the child has unrealistic expectations on how a cochlear implant will impact the child. Counseling may be necessary to discuss unrealistic expectations and establish realistic ones. When this is age-appropriate, the child should be interviewed independently from the rest of the family. This allows children to openly discuss their feelings about cochlear implantation.

For a child to be considered a candidate for a cochlear implant, the child must have a reasonable chance to perform better with a cochlear implant than with any present sensory aid (e.g., hearing aid, frequency modulated (FM) system, and/or tactile aid). Before the assessment process begins, a child must use an appropriate sensory aid for an extended period of time (i.e., greater than 3 months). Then, an audiologic assessment that focuses on speech recognition abilities must be completed to determine whether the child meets criteria for cochlear implantation. If a child meets the audiologic criteria for cochlear implantation, other issues that affect benefit derived from a cochlear implant should be addressed (e.g., educational setting, family support, cognitive skills, and physical handicaps).

## Trial Period

Before considering cochlear implantation, an adequate trial period with appropriate hearing aids is essential for two reasons: (1) to ensure that speech recognition test results, which determine cochlear implant candidacy, are an accurate representation of a child's performance with hearing aids, and (2) to evaluate the child's progress with hearing aids. During the trial period, emphasis should be placed on developing auditory skills, even if the goal is development of rudimentary listening skills (e.g., sound detection). If a child does not show progress in auditory and speech production skills when using hearing aids, the child should be considered for cochlear implantation—provided the lack of progress is due to limited auditory perception.

The length of a trial period will vary depending on the child's experience with appropriately fit hearing aids. Two categories of children do not need to complete a trial period: (1) children, regardless of hearing aid experience, for whom even high-gain hearing aids cannot provide auditory information in the speech range (i.e., children with aided speech detection thresholds greater than 65 dB HL), and (2) children who have been using appropriate hearing aids for greater than 3 months and who clearly meet the audiologic criteria for a cochlear implant. Children with no hearing aid experience or experience with inappropriately fit hearing aids need to complete at least a 3-month trial period. If the child is a borderline candidate for a cochlear implant (see next section) a trial period of greater than 3 months may be recommended even if the child has been using hearing aids for an extended period of time.

To be very conservative, a trial period with a tactile device would be recommended before a child is considered for cochlear implantation (Pickett and McFarland, 1985). One advantage of a trial period with a tactile device may be that the child can master some simple auditory detection and discrimination tasks using it. Mastering these skills with a tactile aid may help a child later when using a cochlear implant. At the University of Iowa Cochlear Implant Program, we do not recommend a trial period with tactile aids because recent studies, although limited in the numbers of subjects included, indicate that children who receive multichannel cochlear implants perform better on measures of speech perception and production than children who use two-channel vibrotactile devices (Hesketh, Fryauf-Bertschy, and Osberger, 1991; Geers and Moog, 1991; Osberger, Robbins, Berry, Todd, Hesketh, and Sedey, 1991; Osberger, Robbins, Miyamoto, Berry, Myres,

Kessler, and Pope, 1991; Miyamoto, Osberger, Robbins, Myres, Kessler, and Pope, 1989).

## Audiologic Assessment

Selection criteria for cochlear implantation vary among implant centers. The criteria presently used at the University of Iowa Cochlear Implant Center will be discussed here. The selection criteria for prelinguistically deafened children and postlinguistically deafened children are identical at this time.

The focus of the audiologic assessment is to evaluate the child's aided speech recognition abilities. Testing should be done in the best aided condition with test stimuli presented at a loud conversational level (65 dB HL). Speech recognition ability can be assessed using a variety of tests including open-set and closed-set speech perception tests. (See Tyler, 1993, for a discussion of speech perception tests available for profoundly hearing-impaired children.) Open-set speech perception tests assess the ability to identify words in sentences or monosyllabic words in isolation. Closed-set speech perception tests assess the ability to identify a stimulus (e.g., monosyllabic word, spondee) from a set number of possible responses. Typically, the audiologist says a word and the child chooses which word was spoken from a set of pictures. Closed-set speech perception tests are not as difficult as open-set speech perception tests because the child has a set of responses from which to choose an answer. Open-set tests, however, more closely represent real life communication situations.

Open-set speech recognition tests are the most desirable measures from which to base a decision on cochlear implant candidacy when evaluating adults who use spoken language. Open-set measures should be attempted with children, however, limited language and/or cognitive skills often preclude using this type of test. In these cases, closed-set measures of speech recognition ability can be used.

Children with limited open-set speech recognition ability and/or children who do not perform significantly above chance on closed-set measures of speech recognition in the best-aided condition are good implant candidates. Appropriate candidates for cochlear implantation include children who score:

1. Less than 4 percent on an open-set measure of word recognition, e.g., a children's monosyllabic word list
2. Less than 10 percent on an open-set measure of sentence recognition, e.g., a children's sentence test
3. Less than or equal to chance on a closed-set measure of word recognition, e.g., less than 36 percent on the Word Intelligibility by Picture Identification (Ross and Lerman, 1971), less than 50 percent on the Early Speech Perception Test—four-choice spondees (Moog and Geers, 1990).

As more long-term data are obtained on how children perform with cochlear implants, these criteria may be modified.

For the profoundly hearing-impaired child 2 to 5 years of age, speech recognition testing may be limited to measures such as the four-choice spondee portion of the Early Speech Perception Test (Moog and Geers, 1990). Some young children (2 to 4 years of age) may not be able to participate in any speech recognition testing. For these children, pure-tone audiometry may be the only information from which to base a decision on cochlear implant candidacy. In these instances, a child might only be considered a candidate if the aided speech detection threshold is greater than 65 dB HL.

Speech perception testing of young deaf children should be performed judiciously, since many of them do not have the language and/or cognitive skills necessary for speech recognition testing. Speech perception tests should not be influenced by limitations imposed by the child's language. Furthermore, children must understand what is required of them, the desired response to the test must be within their physical abilities, and the test should measure perceptual abilities, not ability to concentrate (Boothroyd, 1991). If these criteria cannot be met for a particular child, speech recognition testing cannot be used to determine cochlear implant candidacy for that child.

In order to ensure that a test is within a child's capabilities, the audiologist could have the child say or sign words shown in the pictures of a closed-set monosyllabic word identification test. If the child does not know the words, they should not be used on the test. Alternatively, the audiologist could present the test items visually. The test items could be signed or the child could be shown objects representing the test items (e.g., the child is shown a ball and required to point to the picture of the ball). Children who cannot complete the test visually should not be tested.

## Additional Considerations

If a child meets criteria for cochlear implantation, family support and the child's educational setting should be discussed with the family, since both affect benefit derived from a cochlear implant. Children should be in educational programs that foster the use of listening skills and the use of voice when communicating (Moog and Geers, 1991; Robbins, 1990), regardless of whether signing is also used. Total Communication settings should include auditory training as an integral part of their programs. Parents and other family members need to understand that family involvement is crucial for their child to generalize the language, speech production, and auditory skills learned in therapy into daily life activities. Parents should be motivated to incorporate language and auditory skills development into their child's daily routines and play time (Kelsay, Tye-Murray, Kirk, and Schum, 1993; Kelsay and Tye-Murray, 1993; Tye-Murray, 1992).

Certain physical and cognitive characteristics can also affect the benefit derived from a cochlear implant and should be discussed with the family, if relevant. It may take additional training for a child with lower cognitive functioning to make progress with a cochlear implant as compared to a child with normal cognitive functioning. Certain

physical handicaps such as cerebral palsy should not affect a child's performance, since they do not affect the auditory system. Blindness may be a reason to consider a child more aggressively for a cochlear implant (Fryauf-Bertschy, Kirk, and Weiss, 1993; Martin, Burnett, Himelick, Phillips, and Over, 1988). Auditory input may be especially crucial for blind children since visual input from lipreading and sign language is not available. Finally, children with malformations of the head and neck (e.g., Goldenhar syndrome) need to be considered with caution. This includes children with malformed cochleas. The electrode array cannot be successfully implanted in a cochlea that is not at least partially patent. Even when the electrode array can be implanted, electrical stimulation may cause facial stimulation in a child with abnormal anatomy. In these cases, it may be impossible when programming the child's processor to determine whether the child is responding to an auditory sensation or to a tactile sensation. Even when this distinction can be made, facial stimulation often prevents the use of sufficient current for audition to occur.

## COCHLEAR IMPLANT HARDWARE AND PROGRAMMING

Cochlear implants consist of internal and external components (Figures 13.1 and 13.2). The internal components consist of a receiver/stimulator attached to an electrode array. The electrode array, consisting of several electrodes, is inserted into the cochlea surgically. The receiver/stimulator is seated in a small trough made in the skull directly behind the patient's ear. It contains a receiver coil, stimulator circuits, and a small magnet. The internal components are completely implanted beneath the skin within the hair line. In smaller children, it may be possible to feel and/or see the outline of the internal component under the skin.

The external components consist of a headset, speech processor, and connecting cables. The patient is fit with the external components approximately 6 weeks following surgical implantation

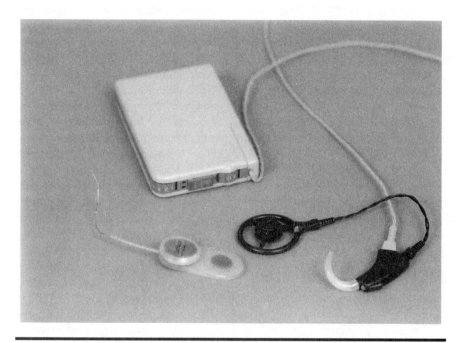

**FIGURE 13.1**   Internal and external components of the Cochlear Corporation Nucleus 22-Channel cochlear implant. (Courtesy of Cochlear Corporation)

of the internal components. The speech processor must be programmed specifically for each individual user. For young children, this requires several fitting sessions within the first several months of cochlear implant use. The speech processor is worn in a harness, on a belt, or in a fanny pack, in a similar fashion to how a body style hearing aid is worn (Figure 13.3). It is approximately the size of a deck of cards and is powered with a rechargeable battery. The headset contains a microphone and a transmitting coil and is connected to the speech processor by a cord. It is worn behind the ear and is held to the head by a magnet in the headset that attracts the magnet in the internal receiver (Figure 13.4).

**Signal Processing**

Acoustic signals are picked up by the ear-level microphone and sent to the speech processor via a cable. The speech processor codes the signal and

sends the information to the transmitter coil via the same connecting cable. The electric code of the acoustic signal is then transmitted transcutaneously via a frequency modulated (FM) signal to the internal receiver. This code is sent to the electrode array. Electrical impulses generated by the electrodes stimulate the remaining nerve fibers in the cochlea.

**Setting the Processor**

Four to six weeks following cochlear implant surgery, the child is fitted with the external components of the cochlear implant. This waiting period allows the surgical incision to heal properly before the headset is worn. The initial appointment is typically made for 2 days, allowing ample time for programming the speech processor and for trying the initial program. For children 8 years of age and older, all channels (i.e., electrodes) may be activated at the initial session. For children 2 to 7

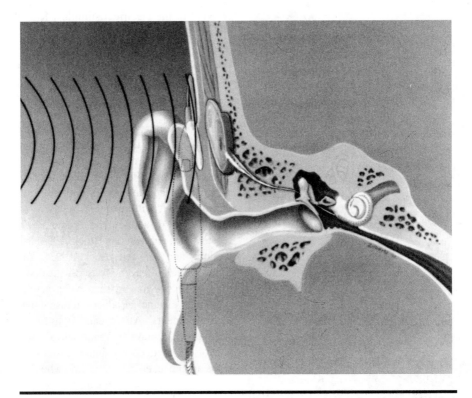

**FIGURE 13.2**   Schematic of cochlear implantation of multielectrode array (Courtesy of Cochlear Corporation.)

years of age, several appointments may be necessary to activate all channels during the first 6 months of cochlear implant use.

During programming, the child's processor is interfaced with a computer using customized software. The child wears his or her headset connected to the speech processor and receives signals generated by the computer. The computer generates pulses of electrical current sent to individual channels chosen by the clinician. To program the speech processor, threshold levels and maximum comfort levels (loud, but not uncomfortably loud) need to be determined for each channel. Channels that cause pain, facial stimulation, or an aberrant loudness growth (e.g., stimuli are always soft or always loud) when activated are eliminated from the program.

When programming children 2 to 8 years of age, it is often helpful to have two audiologists. Young children need to be conditioned to respond behaviorally to the stimuli using play audiometry. A variety of toys such as board games, puzzles, peg boards, and blocks help to keep the child's attention, since programming sessions can last 2 to 4 hours.

Initially, many young prelinguistically deafened children do not show an overt behavioral response to the electrical stimulus even though they can hear it. This makes it difficult for the audiologist to find an appropriate stimulus level for conditioning the child to respond. Since young children have a limited attention span, it is crucial to find this level as efficiently as possible. Information obtained from electrical auditory brain

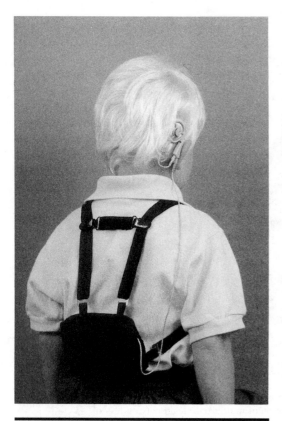

**FIGURE 13.3**    Example of how the speech processor can be worn.

stem response testing can be very useful for determining this level (Brown, Abbas, Fryauf-Bertschy, Kelsay, and Gantz, 1994; Kileny, 1991; Shallop, Van Dyke, Goin, and Mischke, 1991; Shallop, Beiter, Goin, and Mischke, 1990). Electrically evoked auditory brainstem response (ABR) thresholds are the auditory brain stem responses to electrical signals produced by the cochlear implant. ABR thresholds can be obtained at the end of the cochlear implant surgery or postoperatively. Brown and colleagues report that the ABR threshold recorded intraoperatively for a particular channel is typically audible and rarely exceeds the behavioral comfort level for that channel. This stimulus level is therefore generally an appropriate level for conditioning the child to

respond to the electrical stimulus. Knowledge of EABR thresholds can greatly facilitate the programming process, however, it may still only be possible to activate a small number of channels during a young child's initial appointment.

Surface electrodes and the equipment used to measure the ABR can also be used to record the average electrical voltage (AEU). This electrical potential is not a neural response, but rather a recording of the current pulses produced by the internal hardware of the cochlear implant. In cases in which the electrodes being stimulated are malfunctioning, AEUs will be absent or have an abnormal morphology (Mahoney and Proctor, 1994; Mens, Oostendorp, and van den Broek, 1994; Mens, Oostendorp, and van den Broek, 1993). Young children, unlike older, more sophisticated children, may be unable to verbalize when activation of a particular channel produces unusual auditory or tactile percepts. AEUs can be used to identify channels that may be abnormal. These channels can be avoided during initial programming sessions and checked at a later time when the child is more adept at communicating problems with a particular channel.

For young children, follow-up appointments may need to be scheduled every 2 or 3 weeks for the first 4 months of cochlear implant use in order to program all channels. For children 8 years of age and older, typically only two follow-up appointments are needed in the first 4 months. At each follow-up appointment, threshold and comfort levels need to be checked for all previously programmed channels. It is likely that these levels will shift in either direction during the initial months of cochlear implant use. In addition, as the children's experience with sound increases they will be better able to reliably respond at their true thresholds and comfort levels. Young children may learn to label soft versus loud sounds after some cochlear implant experience that will facilitate establishing accurate dynamic ranges. Once the child's program includes all available channels and the threshold and comfort levels are stable, follow-up appointments are needed at 6-month or

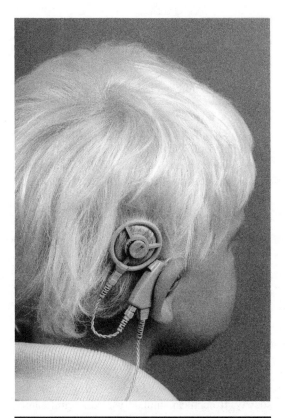

**FIGURE 13.4** Illustration of how the Cochlear Corporation Nucleus 22-Channel cochlear implant headset is worn.

12-month intervals, similar to the follow-up schedule of a child using hearing aids.

### Fostering Acceptance of the Cochlear Implant

The first year of cochlear implant use can be very important in determining whether a child accepts and bonds to the cochlear implant. Initially, some children, particularly prelinguistically deafened children, are not motivated to wear the cochlear implant. Since progress is slow and often not evident during the first year of use, parents may lack the motivation for ensuring that their child wears the cochlear implant on a regular basis. During this time, audiologists need to inform parents that

their child has the ability to perceive sounds even though parents may not notice an overt response to sound. Parents need to be aware that children need to be taught to respond to sounds. Parents can help teach their child to respond to sound by (1) requiring their child to wear the cochlear implant consistently at home as well as at school and (2) incorporating listening into their child's daily routines and play time. Parents can make listening a part of their child's daily life by playing listening games (e.g., peek-a-boo) and bringing their child's attention to sounds around the home (e.g., the microwave alarm that signals when snacks are ready to eat). Once a child begins to use sound in daily life, the child will be more motivated to wear the cochlear implant.

Teenagers may also be reluctant to accept wearing the device. Making listening part of a teenager's recreational activities (e.g., listening for the referee's whistle while playing sports) and daily routines (e.g., listening for the doorbell to signal that a friend has arrived) is the most effective way to motivate a teenager to consistently use a cochlear implant. In addition, classroom presentations including hearing and cochlear implants may help the child feel more comfortable wearing the device because classmates have an understanding of what it is and why it is being worn. Finally, creative ways of wearing the device (e.g., in a fanny pack) may be helpful in encouraging the child to wear the cochlear implant hardware.

## PERFORMANCE WITH COCHLEAR IMPLANTS

### Speech Perception

Initial speech perception results from prelingually deafened children show a large range in performance following receipt of a cochlear implant. While speech perception abilities generally improve following cochlear implantation, it often takes 2 years of experience using the cochlear implant before measurable gains are noted. Vowel recognition improves over time for all children. While some children may show great improvements during the first 12 months of cochlear implant use, most will show substantial increases in vowel recognition after 2 or 3 years of use.

Measures of combined audiovisual consonant perception reveal enhanced performance over the vision-only and audition-only conditions, demonstrating that the children with cochlear implants who were assessed were able to intergrate information from the two modalities. However, the consonant feature information that is perceived when listening with the cochlear implant without lipreading, even after 3 years of cochlear implant experience, remains low for these children.

Monosyllabic word recognition is typically poor in the first year or two of cochlear implant use. Many prelinguistically deaf children have shown that high levels of word recognition can be obtained; however, a number of prelinguistically deaf children show only limited word understanding, even after 4 years of cochlear implant use.

## Speech Production

The speech of children with profound hearing impairment is often characterized by numerous suprasegmental errors (e.g., deviations in duration, intensity and pitch) as well as segmental errors (i.e., misarticulations of vowels and consonants), resulting in speech that is unintelligible (Osberger and McGarr, 1982; Smith, 1975). Cochlear implants facilitate the ability of children with profound hearing impairments to hear their own speech as well as the speech of others. Therefore, an improvement in speech production skills following cochlear implantation is expected. Research assessing the impact of multichannel cochlear implants on speech production skills of profoundly hearing-impaired children demonstrates that the improvements observed exceed what would be expected based on maturation and training alone (Tye-Murray and Spencer (in press); Tye-Murray and Kirk, 1993; Osberger, Robbins, Miyamoto, et al., 1991).

Improvements of speech production skills of pediatric cochlear implant users include improvements in suprasegmental production, phoneme production, and intelligibility (Tye-Murray, and Kirk, 1993; Osberger, Maso, and Sam, 1993). These improvements tend to follow improvements in speech perception of the produced features. Similar to speech perception skills, the development of speech production skills is slow. Most often, changes in speech production are not noted until 1 or 2 years postimplantation in prelinguistically deafened children. While the speech production abilities of prelinguistically deafened children improve after receipt of a cochlear implant, numerous segmental and nonsegmental error patterns still exist in the speech of many of these children. Speech production skills would be expected to improve at a faster rate following receipt of a cochlear implant for postlinguistically deafened children. Some postlinguistically deafened children may even regain age-appropriate speech production skills following receipt of cochlear implant.

## Language

Language is fundamental to interacting within our society. If cochlear implant use can significantly and meaningfully improve speech perception in children, we could expect to see improvements in language. Much of the information available on how a child's language system is affected by cochlear implant use focuses on phonological development and subsequent speech production. However, to have a complete view of how a child's communicative competence is affected by cochlear implant use, pragmatic, semantic, syntactic, and morphological skills should also be assessed. Since numerous factors can affect all areas of a child's language development, it is difficult to determine to what extent changes in language skills are a result of cochlear implant use. We expect that a normal-hearing child's language development is affected by the child's age, life experiences, and geographic location (Hasenstab and Tobey, 1991). In addition to these factors, the language development of a child who is profoundly hearing impaired is affected by the age of onset of profound deafness, prior language ability, communication mode used, and language system used. Language skills in children who use cochlear implants are as varied as they are in the deaf population in general. Language skills can be expected to range from being age-appropriate to significantly delayed.

Improvements in expressive and receptive language skills following cochlear implantation have been documented for children who are profoundly hearing impaired who communicate using only spoken language as well as for those who use simultaneous communication, even when expected maturational changes are factored out (Kirk and Hill-Brown, 1985; Robbins, Osberger, Miyamoto, and Kessler, 1994). These data are only preliminary, however. Researchers who have studied language development in children with cochlear implants have all stated that further long-term research is necessary on larger numbers of children (Kirk and Hill-Brown, 1985; Hasenstab and Tobey, 1991; Robbins et al., 1994; Geers and Moog, 1991).

In the absence of further data on language development and cochlear implant use, a few hypotheses can be considered. We might expect that a child who acquires a profound hearing loss during the teenage years would be more similar to an adventitiously deafened adult than to a congenitally deaf child of the same age. If a postlinguistically deafened teenager receives a cochlear implant shortly after acquiring a hearing loss, minimal regression in the child's language skills, if any, would be expected. Language skills (primarily vocabulary development) would be expected to progress at a near normal or normal rate following receipt of a cochlear implant. This child may require minimal language therapy to acquire the subtleties of language, such as jargon, slang, and idioms.

In contrast, a postlinguistically deafened 3- to 5-year old may be expected to continue to require intense language therapy following cochlear implantation. The benefits of cochlear implantation have the potential to include a cessation of the regression of language skills that will likely occur following the onset of the profound hearing impairment. The potential exists for such children to achieve age-appropriate language skills, especially if cochlear implantation is pursued shortly after the onset of the hearing loss. For this to be the case, however, intense language therapy along with full-time cochlear implant use and strong familial support are necessary.

Prelinguistically deafened children would also require intense language therapy and family support following cochlear implantation. However, even with intense therapy, a congenitally deafened child who received a cochlear implant during the teenage years is likely to maintain current delays in language skills. It would be expected that a cochlear implant would have less of an impact for this teenager than for a congenitally deafened preschooler who receives a cochlear implant at age 2 years. For the preschooler, intense therapy, consistent use of the cochlear implant, and strong family support provide the potential for substantial growth in language skills, perhaps even the potential for the development of spoken language. Some prelinguistically deafened children may even be able to approximate age-appropriate language skills, or in some cases, achieve age-appropriate language abilities.

## Education

Changes in a child's speech perception, speech production, and language skills following cochlear implantation could certainly affect a child's academic achievement and hence educational placement options. (See Chapter 16 on educational options for children with hearing loss.) However, limited information on changes in academic achievement has been reported for children who use cochlear implants. This is likely due to the difficulty in controlling for the numerous compounding factors, other than cochlear implant use, that affect educational performance.

Available information indicates that a child who obtains a cochlear implant may have increased educational placement options (Selmi, 1985). It might be expected that use of a cochlear implant may allow postlinguistically deafened children to remain in mainstream classrooms with limited support services. Furthermore, some prelinguistically deafened children in self-contained classrooms may progress to the point that a change to mainstream classrooms would be recommended. Children not previously progressing in aural/oral educational programs, for whom a switch to a total communication program has been recommended, may show renewed progress in the aural/oral program following cochlear implantation (Selmi, 1985). Finally, it may be expected that a small number of children in total communication programs may progress to the point that a change to aural/oral programs is appropriate.

## SUMMARY

Children with profound hearing losses represent a heterogeneous group of individuals who display a vast range of auditory, speech production, and language skills. Cochlear implant technology provides the potential for benefiting profoundly hearing-impaired children in each of these areas. Careful selection of patients for cochlear implantation, a comprehensive aural rehabilitation program, and family support are essential components for successful cochlear implant use.

While cochlear implants can be very beneficial for some young deaf individuals, they are clearly not the choice for all deaf children. Some members of the Deaf Culture strongly believe that the best language system for a profoundly deaf child is American Sign Language, and the best educational placement is in a school for the deaf. They do not place importance on use of residual hearing and strongly oppose the use of cochlear implants in deaf children (Lane, 1990; Tyler, 1993). Audiologists play a major role in the selection of appropriate candidates for cochlear implantation. They need to have a clear understanding of the issues surrounding cochlear implants, including the differing philosophies on the appropriate language for and education of deaf children.

## REFERENCES

Boothroyd, A. (1991). Assessment of speech perception capacity in profoundly deaf children. *American Journal of Otolaryngology, 12,* 67–72.

Boothroyd, A. (1993). Profound deafness. In R. S. Tyler (ed.), *Cochlear Implants: Audiological Foundations* (pp. 1–34). San Diego: Singular Publishing Group.

Brown, C. J., Abbas, P. J., Fryauf-Bertschy, H., Kelsay, D., and Gantz, B. J. (1994). Intraoperative and postoperative electrically evoked auditory brain stem responses in Nucleus cochlear implant users: Implications for the fitting process. *Ear and Hearing, 15,* 168–176.

Fryauf-Bertschy, H., Kirk, K. I., and Weiss, A. L. (1993). Cochlear implant use by a child who is deaf and blind: A case study. *American Journal of Audiology,* March, 38–47.

Gantz, B. J., McCabe, B. F., and Tyler, R. S. (1988). Use of multichannel cochlear implants in obstructed cochleas. *Otolaryngology Head and Neck Surgery, 98, (1),* 72–81.

Geers, A. E., and Moog, J. S. (1991). Evaluating the benefits of cochlear implants in an education setting. *The American Journal of Otology, 12, (Suppl.),* 116–125

Hasenstab, M. S., and Tobey, E. A. (1991). Language development in children receiving Nucleus multichannel cochlear implants. *Ear and Hearing, 12,* 55S–65S.

Hesketh, L. J., Fryauf-Bertschy, H., and Osberger, M. J. (1991). Evaluation of a tactile aid and a cochlear implant in one child. *The American Journal of Otology,* March, 182–186.

Kelsay, D. and Tye-Murray, N. (1993). *Stepping Out: Specific Activities to Do at Home.* Iowa City: University of Iowa Press.

Kelsay, D. M. R., Tye-Murray, N., Kirk, K. I. and Schum, L. K. (1993). *Five Steps to Improving Your Child's Use of a Cochlear Implant.* Iowa City: University of Iowa Press.

Kileny, P. R. (1991). Use of electrophysiologic measures in the management of children with cochlear implants: Brain stem, middle latency, and cognitive (P300) responses.. *American Journal of Otology, 12,* 37–42.

Kirk, K. I., and Hill-Brown, C. (1985). Speech and language results in children with a cochlear implant. *Ear and Hearing, 6,* 36S–47S

Lane, H. (1990). Cultural and infirmity models of deaf Americans. *Journal of the Academy of Rehabilitative Audiology, 23,* 11–26.

Mahoney, M. J., and Proctor, L. A. R. (1994). The use of averaged electrode voltages to assess the function of Nucleus internal cochlear implant devices in children. *Ear and Hearing, 15,* 177–183.

Martin, E. L., Burnett, P. A., Himelick, T. E., Phillips, M. A., and Over, S. K. (1988). Speech recognition by a deaf-blind multichannel cochlear implant patient. *Ear and Hearing, 9,* 70–74.

Mens, L. H. M., Oostendorp, T., and van den Broek, P. (1994). Cochlear implant generated surface potentials: Current spread and side effects. *Ear and Hearing, 15,* 339–345.

Mens, L. H., Oostendorp, T., and van den Broek, P. (1993). Electrode-by-electrode mapping of cochlear implant generated surface potentials: (Partial) device failures. In B. Fraysse and O. Deguine (eds.), *Cochlear Implants: New Perspectives. Advances in Otorhinolaryngology, 48,* 475–478. Basel, Switzerland: Karger.

Miyamoto, R. T., Osberger, M. J., Robbins, A. M., Myres, W. A., Kessler, K., and Pope, M. L. (1989). Comparison of sensory aids in deaf children. *Annals of Otology, Rhinology, and Laryngology, 98,* 2–7.

Moog, J. S., and Geers, A. E. (1990). *Early Speech Perception Test.* St. Louis: Central Institute for the Deaf.

Moog, J. S., and Geers, A. E. (1991). Educational Management of children with cochlear implants. *AAD/ Reference, 136,* 69–76

Osberger, M. J., Maso, M., and Sam, L. K. (1993). Speech intelligibility of children with cochlear implants, tactile aids, or hearing aids. *Journal of Speech and Hearing Research, 36,* 186–203.

Osberger, M. J., and McGarr, N. S. (1982). Speech production characteristics of the hearing-impaired. In N. Lass (ed.), *Speech and Language: Advances in Basic Science and Research* (pp. 221–283). New York: Academic Press.

Osberger, M. J., Robbins, A. M., Berry, S. W., Todd, S. L., Hesketh, L. J., and Sedey, A. (1991). Analysis of the spontaneous speech samples of children with cochlear implants or tactile aids. *American Journal of Otolaryngology, 12,* 151–164.

Osberger, M. J., Robbins, A. M., Miyamoto, R. T., Berry, S. W., Myres, W. A., Kessler, K. S., and Pope, M. L. (1991). Speech perception abilities of children with cochlear implants, tactile aids, or hearing aids. *American Journal of Otolaryngology, 12,* 105–115.

Pickett, J. M., and McFarland, W. (1985). Auditory implants and tactile aids for the profoundly deaf. *Journal of Speech and Hearing Research, 28,* 134–150

Robbins, A. M. (1990). Developing meaningful auditory integration in children with cochlear implants. *Volta Review, 92,* 361–370.

Robbins, A. M., Osberger, M. J., Miyamoto, R. T., and Kessler, K. S. (1994). Language development in young children with cochlear implants. Paper presented at the Second European Symposium on Paediatric Cochlear Implantation, Montellier, France, May 26–28, 1994.

Ross, M., and Lerman, J. (1971). *Word Intelligibility by Picture Identification.* Pittsburgh: Stanwix House.

Selmi, A. (1985). Monitoring and evaluating the educational effects of the cochlear implant. *Ear and Hearing, 6,* 52S–59S.

Shallop, J. K., Beiter, A. L., Goin, D. W., and Mischke, R. E. (1990). Electrically evoked auditory brain stem responses (EABR) and middle latency responses (EMLR) obtained from patients with the Nucleus multichannel cochlear implant. *Ear and Hearing, 11,* 5–15.

Shallop, J. K., VanDyke, L., Goin, D. W., and Mischke, R. E. (1991). Prediction of behavioral threshold and comfort values for Nucleus 22-channel implant patients from electrical auditory brain stem response test results. *Annals of Otology, Rhinology and Laryngology, 100,* 896–898.

Smith, C. R. (1975). Residual hearing and speech production in deaf children. *Journal of Speech and Hearing Research, 18,* 795–811.

Tobey, E. A., and Hasenstab, M. S. (1991). Effects of a Nucleus multichannel cochlear implant upon speech production in children. *Ear and Hearing, 12,* 48S–54S.

Tye-Murray, N. (1992). *Cochlear Implants and Children: A Handbook for Parents, Teachers and Speech and Hearing Professionals.* Washington D.C: Alexander Graham Bell Association for the Deaf.

Tye-Murray, N., and Kirk, K. I. (1993). Vowel and diphthong production by young users of cochlear implants and the relationship between the phonetic level evaluation and spontaneous speech. *Journal of Speech and Hearing Research, 36,* 488–502.

Tye-Murray, N., and Spencer, L. (in press). Acquisition of speech by children who have prolonged cochlear implant experience. *Journal of Speech and Hearing Research.*

Tyler, R. S. (1993). Speech perception by children. In R. S. Tyler (ed.), *Cochlear Implants: Audiological Foundations* (pp. 191–256). San Diego: Singular Publishing Group.

# CHAPTER 14

# ASSISTIVE LISTENING
# AND ALERTING DEVICES

*LINDA M. THIBODEAU*

## INTRODUCTION

In determining the appropriate assistive listening device(s) for a child, there are many issues to consider, including the environment in which the communication occurs, the degree of the hearing loss, the possibility of interfacing with personal amplification, and who is responsible for providing the device. This chapter is designed to assist the audiologist in providing information and recommendations on these issues to parents and children with hearing loss. Suggestions are provided on ideal arrangements with respect to electroacoustic characteristics and multipurpose functioning rather than cosmetic appeal. The use of assistive devices can be hindered by the notion that the hearing loss is something to be hidden. After children are educated about the devices that are available and how they can be of benefit, they must learn to be advocates for the provision of such devices. Although many parents will want to provide these assistive devices in the home, the child with hearing loss will encounter many of them, such as phone amplifiers and flashing smoke alarms, outside of their homes. Therefore, before they are to consider that such devices are necessary to their communication, they must feel comfortable about acknowledging their hearing loss by using devices that are more visible than the personal hearing aid.

## OPTIONS

Because children with hearing loss do not always listen in quiet situations in which they are close to the signal source, there is a need for assistive devices. In some situations, these devices may be used in conjunction with the personal hearing aid. In other cases, they provide nonauditory signals such as a vibrating alarm clock or flashing smoke alarm. When considering the use of assistive devices by children, they may be classified by the communication demands. One significant area in which an optimal signal-to-noise (S/N) ratio is most important is the learning environment, including the educational classroom, preschool programs, and parent–infant home intervention. As children enter the elementary grades, the need for other assistive devices increases as they become involved in phone communication, television reception, and alarm recognition. The following section includes descriptions of some of the more common devices in each of these categories.

### Devices Used in the Learning Environment

The learning environment in this discussion is any situation in which the purpose of auditory communication is to teach. In addition to classroom settings, the learning environment includes the mother or father at home with an infant when oral language development is the focus through daily discussion of household routines. Given that portability is desirable in most learning situations, the use of frequency modulated (FM) systems will be described first, followed by the more restrictive, but more cost effective, induction loop (IL) systems.

### FM Systems

The basic FM arrangement consists of two main components, a transmitter and a receiver (Figure 14.1). The signal is delivered to the transmitter via a microphone worn by the speaker. The signal is frequency modulated and broadcast on a specific frequency band. The FM receiver that is tuned to that band demodulates the signal, amplifies it, and delivers it to the user through a variety of coupling methods. As explained by Boothroyd (1992), signals can be broadcast on one of thirty-two narrow-band channels or one of 7 broadband channels within the frequency range of 72 to 76 MHz. The main considerations in selecting the transmitters and receivers will be reviewed in the next sections. A more complete description of FM options may be found in several sources (e.g., Thibodeau, 1992; Hammond, 1991; Lewis, 1991).

**FM Transmitters.** One of the most important variables in selecting a transmitter is the type of microphone. Microphone options for the transmitter are illustrated in Figure 14.2. The most common types are lapel microphones that are worn about 6 inches from the mouth on the chest. These can either be omnidirectional (sensitive to sound from all around) or directional (most sensitive to sound entering the top). Another type is a boom microphone that is worn approximately 2 inches from the lips via a headband or clip-on eyeglasses. Thibodeau, Mayfield, and Champlin (1994) reported a significant improvement in speech recognition for adults with normal hearing when a boom microphone was used compared to a directional or omnidirectional microphone and the FM-plus-environmental microphones were active. Finally, a conference microphone may be used during group discussions. Other features on the transmitter that are important to consider include a user-selected transmission channel, an input jack for another signal source such as a video player, and malfunction lights such as "No FM" and "Low Battery" lights.

## BASIC FM SYSTEM

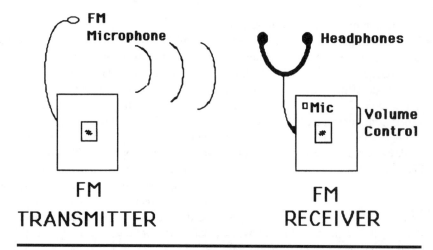

**FIGURE 14.1** Basic FM system. The receiver worn by the student is on the right and the transmitter worn by the parent/teacher is on the left.

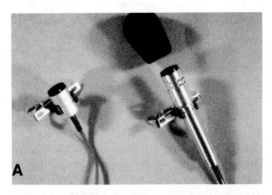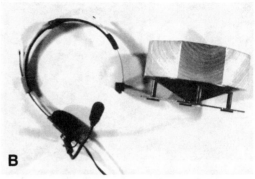

**FIGURE 14.2**  Transmitter microphone options. *(A)* The omnidirectional microphone is on the left and the directional microphone is on the right. *(B)* The boom is on the left and the conference microphone is on the right. (Courtesy of Phonic Ear, Inc., and York Press, Inc.)

**FM Receivers.**  The FM receiver, which is worn by the child, also has several options to be considered. First, it is important to have a microphone on the receiver unless the system is being used with children who have normal hearing. The options, illustrated in Figure 14.3, include a self-contained, a plug-in, and an ear-level microphone. These are often referred to as the environmental microphone as opposed to the FM microphone used with the transmitter. They may be omnidirectional or directional. Which type is chosen will depend to some extent on the gain requirements. The higher gain receivers are more likely to have the self-contained or ear-level microphones. Thibodeau and colleagues (1994) did not find a significant difference between speech recognition performance with a self-contained microphone worn on the chest and an ear-level microphone. However, this was in normal-hearing listeners in a stationary listening situation with both the FM and environmental microphones active. Children with hearing loss should receive some localization benefit with ear-level microphones. Related to the issue of receiver microphone are the switch options for activating the microphone. Ideally, the child should have the option to deactivate the environmental microphone so that only the FM signal is received for

maximum reception of the signal from the FM transmitters.

Another feature of importance is the option to change the receiving frequency by removing the color-coded or numbered oscillator or selecting a general frequency that is housed within the receiver. This is most important for children in educational settings where they are instructed by more than one teacher throughout the day, each of whom would be transmitting on a different frequency.

Depending on the degree of hearing loss, a receiver with the option to adjust gain, maximum output, or tone may be desirable. An output jack is useful for sending the FM signal to a tape recorder or assistive device such as a cochlear implant. Luduena and Thibodeau (1993) reported substantial improvements in auditory–visual speech recognition for patients with cochlear implants when the FM system was used in conjunction with the implant.

Probably the most difficult choice with respect to FM systems is the method of coupling the signal to the ear. For mild losses, a simple earphone or earbud is the most convenient. In educational situations where several children could benefit from the improved S/N ratio, the delivery

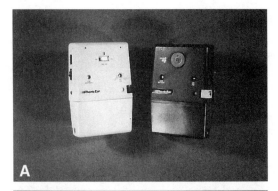

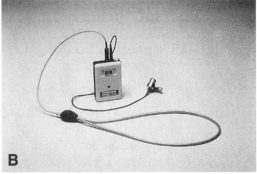

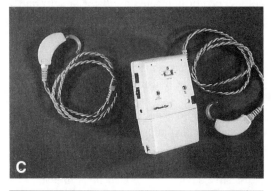

**FIGURE 14.3** Receiver microphone options. *(A)* The microphone on the FM receiver, *(B)* A plug-in microphone to the FM receiver *(C)* Ear-level microphones. (Courtesy of Comtek, Inc., York Press, Inc. and Phonic Ear, Inc.)

of the signal via speakers may be advocated (Flexer, Milin, and Brown, 1990). Although this restricts the portability of the system, no one child is identified as needing assistance.

If the child uses a hearing aid, the first consideration should be whether the output from the

FM receiver can be coupled to the hearing aid via a direct-input connection. The signal from the FM receiver is delivered to the hearing aid via a boot or shoe that fits over the lower portion of the hearing aid as shown in Figure 14.4A. The direct-input capability of the hearing aid and the resulting signal options may be difficult to determine because such information is not always provided in manufacturer specifications. Thibodeau and Watson (1993) reported that 74 percent of direct-input hearing aids were capable of receiving only the combined FM and environmental signals. Hawkins (1984) found that most of the FM advantage was lost when the environmental microphone was used. Therefore, if the hearing aid will not allow receipt of the FM signal only, then direct-input coupling is not recommended. Advantages and disadvantages of this coupling over others are discussed by Thibodeau and McCaffrey (1992).

Another coupling option for personal hearing aids with telecoils is a neck loop as shown in Figure 14.4B. The signal from the FM receiver is delivered to a loop worn around the neck in which an electromagnetic field is created. When the hearing aid is set to the "T" position, the electromagnetic signal is received. In this arrangement, the signal options are more straightforward because "T" position results in receiving only the FM signal (assuming the environmental microphones on the FM receiver are deactivated), and the "M/T" position results in receiving the FM signal through the neck loop and the environmental signal via the microphone on the hearing aid. Although the neck loop may be more desirable cosmetically because there is no cord to the hearing aid, there are disadvantages including variations in signal strength with head movement, higher internal noise, and reductions in low-frequency gain (Thibodeau, McCaffrey, and Abrahamson, 1988). Another option in which the problem of signal strength variation is avoided is the use of a silhouette. The silhouette is a wafer-like case containing a coil that is worn between the head and the hearing aid and plugged into the FM receiver. This option results in a stronger electromagnetic field that is constant with head movement.

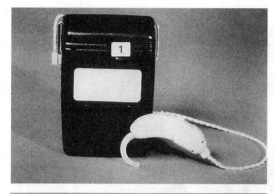

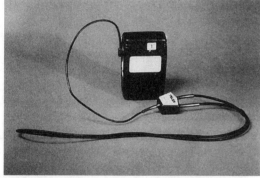

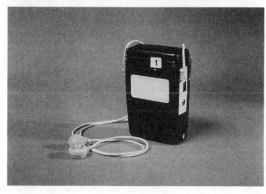

**FIGURE 14.4** Options for coupling the signal from the FM receiver to the ear. *(A)* Direct-input. *(B)* Neckloop. *(C)* Ear-level earphones. (Courtesy of Telex Communications, Inc.)

Another option that involves a personal hearing aid is the ear-level FM receiver as shown in Figure 14.5. The receiver is similar to those worn at the chest or on one's belt in that it demodulates the FM signal and has an environmental micro-

phone. There is the option to receive the FM-only signal, the environmental-only signal, or both. Because it also has an amplifier, this unit may serve as the personal hearing aid. The main difference between the ear-level and body-worn receivers is the transmitting range, which is reduced about one-third (40 feet for the ear-level receivers). Although in one model there is the ability to change the receiving frequency by changing the oscillators on the inside curve of the case, there are no output jacks, malfunctioning indicator lights, or telecoils. In addition, there is no option to operate on rechargeable batteries. In other words, the options to interface with other systems are exchanged for the compact size and the convenience of having a single unit.

Coupling options for the FM receiver that do not require the personal hearing aid include a button receiver with custom snap-ring earmold. In this common arrangement, the child must remove the personal hearing aid daily to wear the FM receiver. The potential for different electroacoustic characteristics between the hearing aid and the FM receiver has been a concern with this arrangement; however, the greater probability of having functioning amplification each day often outweighs this concern (Thibodeau and McCaffrey, 1992).

### Induction Loop Systems

The basic induction loop (IL) system is illustrated in Figure 14.6. The main components are a microphone, an amplifier, and a loop of wire. The signal is picked up through a microphone worn by the talker and delivered to the listener through the electromagnetic field created in the loop of wire. The listener must be in the near vicinity (approximately 1 foot) of the loop to receive the signal via the telecoil on the hearing aid. Unlike the case with FM systems, there are specifications, IEC 118-4 (International Electrotechnical Commission, 1981), which include optimal characteristics of induction loops with respect to field strength and frequency response. The size of the amplifier and the gauge of the wire are important variables in IL systems. For a typical classroom, 20 × 30

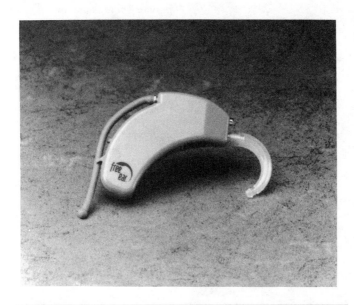

**FIGURE 14.5** Behind-the-ear FM receiver. (Courtesy of Phonic Ear, Inc.)

feet, an amplifier with 15 watts and No. 14 gauge wire are minimally adequate. The problems discussed earlier with neck loops are also applicable to room loops. Because the telecoil of the personal hearing aid is involved, there can be signal variations with head movement, increased internal noise, and reductions of low-frequency gain. Another problem is spillover in which signals from adjacent rooms with IL systems are received. A new design referred to as the 3-D loop overcomes the problem of spillover and signal-strength variation by having several loops within a floormat that carry the signal at different phase relationships (Gilmore and Lederman, 1989; Gilmore and Monte, 1994). This 3-D system is most applicable to situations in which instruction is confined to a specific location such as the story corner at a library or lecture auditorium.

Although IL systems are not used as often as FM systems in classroom settings, there are certain activities that are ideally suited for their use in the home. One area that is particularly amenable to an IL system is the television room. The loop may be installed under the carpet in the viewing area, and the child would simply need to switch the hearing aid to the "T" position to hear the signal. Because the child is relatively stationary while watching, the problems of variable signal strength would be minimal. Another area of significant communication is the dinner table at which not only meals but also homework are often completed. A loop could be placed under the table with multiple microphone inputs. Some loop manufacturers have units that would be small enough to be attached by Velcro under the table.

*Summary*

Ideally the child with a hearing loss would receive auditory information in learning situations with the best S/N ratio possible. Given that much learning occurs outside of a classroom, it is recommended that children with hearing loss have an FM system. Ideally, this system could be used at home as well as in extracurricular activities

# INDUCTION LOOP SYSTEM

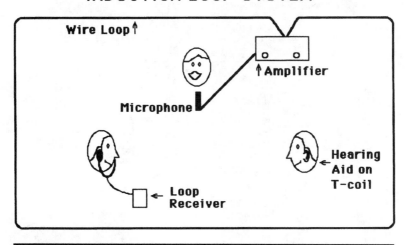

**FIGURE 14.6**   Basic induction loop system. The listener on the left is using an induction loop receiver and the person on the right is using the t-coil of the personal hearing aid.

such as scouts, church, and sports. Children should become accustomed to asking their teachers and leaders to wear the FM transmitter and microphone. The use of IL systems should be considered in instances in which instruction/communication is provided in a localized area. To have access to both of these options, a child's hearing aid should have a telecoil and a direct-input connection. Whether functioning with an FM system or an IL system, one should have the option to receive the signal from the speaker alone, the environmental signal alone, or the speaker plus the environmental signal. An overview of signal options on hearing aids when interfaced with an FM system is provided by Thibodeau (1992) and Thibodeau and Watson (1993).

## Devices Used for Telephone Communication

### Amplifiers

Many people benefit from amplification of the telephone signal. Of the many amplification devices, there are some that interface with hearing aids and some which do not. The devices reviewed in this section are appropriate for those children without hearing aids or for those whose hearing aids do not have telecoils. One consideration in selecting a phone amplifier is whether portability is required. When amplification on only one phone is desired, the options include a replacement handset with an amplifier or an in-line amplifier as shown in Figures 14.7A and 14.7B. A self-contained acoustic amplifier that requires a battery and attaches over the earpiece of the handset provides a portable solution (Figure 14.7C). This is preferable for older children who may need to use the phone during after-school activities. To avoid acoustic feedback with each of these amplifier devices, the child must learn how to properly position the phone handset near the microphone of the hearing aid. One other option is to use a speakerphone in which the signal is amplified by a small loudspeaker. This is most beneficial when another person can assist to provide speechreading cues and/or sign language. Finally, there are specialized phones with volume controls built into the base and increased high-

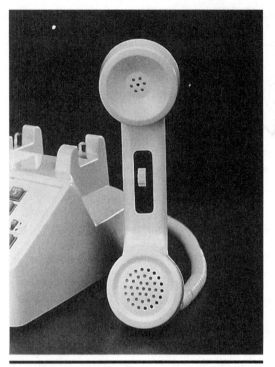

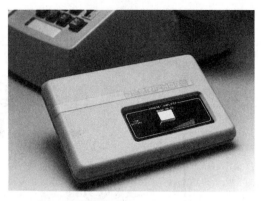

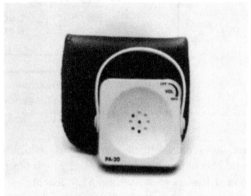

**FIGURE 14.7**    Amplifiers for phones. *(A)* Handset. *(B)* In-line. *(C)* Self-contained. (Courtesy of Ameri-phone, Inc.)

frequency emphasis designed for persons with hearing loss. A disadvantage of all of these amplifiers arises as the signal is sent to the child acoustically. Because the microphone of the hearing aid is still active, background noise is amplified and may result in an unfavorable S/N ratio.

### Use of a T-coil
When a child has a hearing aid with a telecoil and the phone emits an adequately strong electromagnetic signal, the telephone signal may be received through inductive coupling. After switching the hearing aid to the "T" position, the child may place the handset near the aid and vary the position until the strongest signal is received. When the hearing aid is set to the "T" position, only the electromagnetic signal is received and back-

ground noise is not amplified. Because the orientation of the telecoils in different hearing aids varies, the best position for the handset must be determined by the user. When the phone does not emit a strong enough electromagnetic signal, one may use a portable electromagnetic amplifier that attaches over the earpiece of the receiver in the same way as the portable acoustic amplifier. The Hearing Aid Compatibility Act (Public Law 100-394) requires that as of August 16, 1988, all telephones manufactured or imported for use in the United States must be compatible with hearing aids. Feedback is not a problem with this arrangement because the signal is electromagnetic rather than acoustic. However, the problems mentioned earlier with increased internal noise and reduced low-frequency gain are applicable.

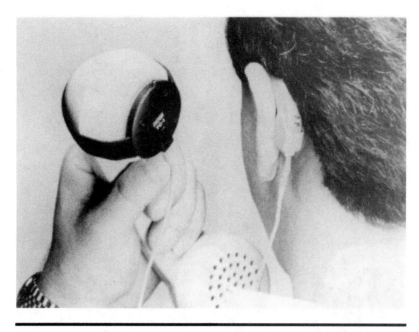

**FIGURE 14.8**   Direct-input connection to phone. (Courtesy of Phonak, Inc.)

### Direct-Input Connection

A microphone may be attached to the handset that delivers the signal to the user through a direct electrical connection to the hearing aid as shown in Figure 14.8. The connection is made via a boot or shoe that is also used for the direct-input connection to an FM receiver. Placement of the handset relative to the hearing aid is not an issue as long as the mouthpiece is close to the user's mouth. Although this is very portable and the hearing aid would provide the frequency shaping, it may be inconvenient to be hardwired to the phone.

### Caller ID

One option that facilitates communication over the phone by providing a visual display of the phone number of the caller is referred to as Caller ID. Many times older children with hearing loss are faced with taking a message for someone to return a call. A way to verify that the correct phone number was recorded is to view the number

on a display unit. The unit displays the number of the caller within the first two rings and it is stored in memory until erased by the user. This is also useful for the child with hearing loss to anticipate the conversation when a familiar phone number is recognized. For example, knowing that the person they will speak with when answering the phone is a grandparent may define a more limited set of conversation topics than if it is an unfamiliar phone number from a salesperson.

### Teletype Machine

Teletype machines (TTY), also referred to as Telecommunication Devices for the Deaf (TDD) or Text Telephone machines (TT), include a keyboard and visual display. By calling another person with a TTY, an exchange of typed messages may occur. These are now being provided on public phones in airports and convention centers as shown in Figure 14.9. In addition, they have become more portable so that individuals may

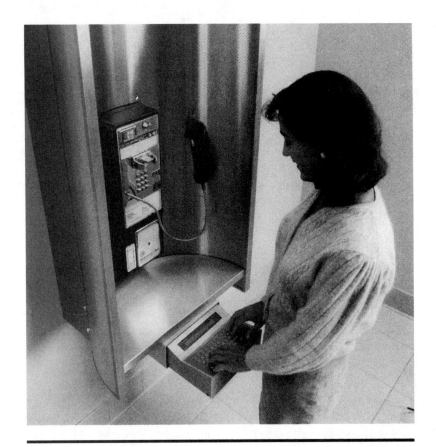

**FIGURE 14.9**    Public Phone Telecommunication Device for the Deaf. (Courtesy of Ultratec, Inc.)

easily carry them. It is not necessary to dedicate a phone line to the TTY, but simply to place the handset on the cups when the high-pitched signal is heard. The restriction of calling another person with a TTY is overcome by what is called a Relay Service. If the person with a TTY must call someone without a TTY, they may call the Relay Service and an operator will make the appropriate translation.

*Summary*

There are numerous options for enhancing the telephone signal. The selection of a device depends on the degree of the hearing loss, options on the personal hearing aid, and need for portability. Because a child's first phone experience is typically in the home, a simple acoustic amplifier may be the first option of choice for those with mild to severe hearing losses. As a child gets older, the need for a greater variety of options increases, and the telecoil on the hearing aid may provide the greatest flexibility. Other types of amplifiers may be necessary for optimum performance. For persons with profound losses the visual display provided by the TDD will probably be necessary, in which case independent phone conversations will depend on the user's command of written language.

## Devices Used for Television Reception

### Devices to Improve Signal Reception

**FM System.** The most common problems with television reception for those with hearing loss is the volume level and the background noise picked up by the hearing aid microphone. Use of an FM system described earlier reduces these detrimental effects because the microphone of the FM transmitter is placed near the speaker of the television. Another option is to provide an electrical connection between the television output jack and an input jack on the FM transmitter. The child with a hearing loss wears the FM receiver and receives the signal through one of the coupling methods described earlier.

**Infrared System.** An infrared system for television reception operates in the same way as the FM system except that the signal from the television is transmitted to the receiver via infrared light rays. This transmitter is usually placed on the top of the television and the person receiving the signal must be in a clear sight path. Any obstructions between the transmitter and the receiver will disrupt the signal. For this reason, this device may be restricted to primarily seated activities, whereas the FM system is more portable and may be used in a variety of situations.

**Induction Loop System.** As described earlier, the IL system involves a microphone or direct electrical connection to the signal being transmitted. The electrical representation of the auditory signal is then amplified and delivered through a loop of wire around the television seating area or a loop worn around one's neck. The child must have a telecoil on the hearing aids to receive the electromagnetic signal created around the loop. Although it is an inexpensive alternative to the FM system, it is not portable.

**Direct Audio Input.** Some hearing aids are equipped to receive the television signal directly through a wire from the television output to the hearing aid boot. This may be referred to as a hard-wire connection and also shares the problems of portability.

**TV Band Radio.** Perhaps the least expensive solution for children with mild to moderate hearing loss is to provide a radio that is tuned to the TV station. They may receive the signal by sitting near the radio or by using an earphone or direct-input connection to the radio. A disadvantage of this alternative is the inability to pick up many of the cable stations.

### Closed-Captioned Decoders

Closed-captioned decoders allow the verbal communication of a television program to be printed on the lower portion of the television screen. Unfortunately, not all programs have captioning. The captioning is referred to as "closed" because only televisions equipped with special circuitry are capable of producing the captioning. The first units available were the size of video players that were external to the television. As of October 15, 1990, the Television Decoder Circuitry Act (Public Law 101-431) requires televisions with 13-inch screens or larger to be equipped with decoders internally. The captioning is provided only when the decoding circuitry is activated. The captioning may also facilitate development of language and reading skills in children with hearing loss.

When captioning is provided for a live program, it is referred to as real-time captioning. As with the closed captioning, the printed words do not occur simultaneously with the spoken word. Therefore, in some cases, the benefits derived from captioning may not be immediately apparent but may occur over an adjustment period.

### Summary

Because television can be a significant source of language input, audiologists should regularly consult with parents about their child's interest in and reception of the television. To facilitate television viewing, one must choose among enhanced auditory input or visual input or a combination of these. Given that captioning provides an opportunity to reinforce reading skills, this option could prove to be very valuable. Because all newer televisions are equipped to receive the captioning, it is recommended that parents start directing their children to captioned programs whenever possible. If the child has some residual hearing, then adding the auditory signal via an FM, infrared, induction loop, direct-input, or radio system would also be of benefit. Regarding these choices, parents should consider the flexibility that the FM system provides for use in the classroom as well as for television viewing and other general communication such as after-school activities and riding in the car.

## Alerting Devices

### Wake-Up Alarms

Because most alarm clocks now have an electrical beeping signal that is of relatively weak intensity, a child with hearing loss will often require a non-auditory signal. There are several types of vibrating alarms, which range from a small device placed under the pillow to larger devices that shake the bed. Visual systems include flashing lamps or flashing the time in large numbers on the ceiling. One system involves creating an air stream by activating a fan at the designated time. Obviously, this selection requires a personalized decision, which may require trial periods with more than one system.

### Doorbell and Telephone

The most common type of system for the doorbell and phone involves flashing lamps. These are designed so that a lamp will flash on and off whether it is normally on or normally off. If both the door and the phone are being monitored, different lamps or different flash patterns would be necessary to signal the different signals. Another solution for persons with mild to moderate hearing loss is to have ringers with increased intensity or ringers in a frequency range that is more audible.

### Smoke

As with the doorbell and phone alerting systems, a visual alternative is most common as a smoke alarm. A high-intensity flashing strobe light may be easily distinguished from other flashing signals.

### Hearing Ear Dogs

Dogs that are trained to alert the person with hearing loss to specific signals are available to persons who have limited contact with other individuals with normal hearing. Although this may not be an option for children with a hearing loss until they move away from home, parents may want to consider this possibility early in order to place a request for a dog. The dogs are usually selected from humane societies and are trained for several weeks before being placed in a home. When a placement is made, the trainer accompanies the dog and provides onsite training to the specific sounds for that location. For example, people may need a dog to alert them to the doorbell, phone, smoke detector, and a crying baby. These dogs should be accepted and treated by the general public as are the more familiar seeing eye dogs.

### Summary

Parents should be advised to consider alerting devices as soon as the child is able to understand the significance of the signal. Although the use of an alarm clock may vary with parental preference, all parents should be encouraged to place visual smoke alarms in the home. Children should be taught safety procedures as early as language comprehension permits. Regarding the recognition of the doorbell and phone, there are complete systems with several sensors that can be placed near the signals of interest. The person with hearing loss can wear a wristband with visual/tactile indicators that correspond to the various signals. As with the hearing ear dog, this more complicated system may be more appropriate as the child approaches independent living. For children with residual hearing, it is recommended that the visual/tactile alerting systems not completely replace the auditory signal. It is important to help the child learn to recognize the auditory signal in the event that the visual/tactile system fails or that the child is in a new environment without such accommodations.

## PREPARING STUDENTS FOR ASSISTIVE LISTENING DEVICES SELECTION

Because the use of assistive devices is often considered an "option," it is important that children are taught to become their own advocates. It is unfortunate that some students with hearing loss may complete two years of college before they reach a level of frustration that leads them to consult with student services about assistive devices in the classroom. Early education on the benefit of these devices should begin with the initial fitting of amplification. In addition to the visual alerting systems in the home to facilitate safety and environmental awareness, the use of an FM system in the home can greatly enhance communication learning (Madell, 1992).

One reason for the lack of emphasis on the use of such devices is related to the fact that these systems are not regulated by the Food and Drug Administration or state licensure laws in the same way that hearing aids are. Persons may purchase many of these devices through mail order and local electronic stores. Only recently have these devices been manufactured by some of the major hearing aid companies. Thus, there have not been intense marketing efforts to educate the professionals who serve persons with hearing loss on the options to interface assistive devices with amplification. There is a committee of audiologic engineers, hearing aid manufacturers, and university professors who are currently developing a standard for the American National Standards Institute on the electroacoustic evaluation of assistive listening devices. Although visual/tactile alerting devices are not addressed in the standard, electroacoustic measurements that are similar to those required for hearing aids are described. This

should result in more attention from audiologists who are familiar with the purposes of such measurements and how they may relate to performance predictions.

### Providing Information

Once the audiologist is more accustomed to routinely incorporating assistive listening devices into the hearing aid evaluation process, various options for educating the family must be considered. This should include demonstration of the devices and preferably some group sharing of their benefits. Another important aspect of the education is to provide information on the process by which these devices may be obtained.

In addition to general lectures regarding the various options that may be provided during office appointments or parent meetings, there are several materials that may be used by parents at home (Appendix 12). In addition to these materials for parent education, a program for children, entitled KIP—Knowledge Is Power, was designed to help students learn about their hearing loss (Mississippi Bend Area Education Agency, 1992). Along with pretests and posttests, there are instructional worksheets for students on an elementary and intermediate level, goals and objectives, and parent letters. The topics included in KIP are anatomy, causes of hearing loss, hearing measurement, hearing aids, coping with a hearing loss, assistive listening devices, and resources. The section on assistive listening devices provides an overview of systems to assist the child in the classroom, in communicating on the telephone, in viewing television, and in recognizing alerting signals such as alarm clocks and doorbells. There is also a reference to a program known as Places with Assistive Listening Systems (PALS), which is a service that provides a listing of accessible facilities around the country for the traveler.

### Providing Experience

To facilitate the education of parents and children on assistive devices, a display of the various options should be readily available. Whether this is put together for a special lecture or set up on a permanent basis, the devices should be in working order for demonstration. The initial cost of such a demonstration center was determined to be $2,546 by Palmer (1992). If possible devices should be available for checkout on a trial basis.

Another useful way to provide experience is to demonstrate the devices during support group meetings. During a parent discussion group, for example, a loop may be set up and a listening device passed around during the speaker's presentation. In addition, group discussion on the benefits of such devices adds validity to the information the audiologist provides. Knowing that someone else has had a positive experience in solving a problem with an assistive device may make it easier for someone to try one that they may have previously thought was unacceptable, either cosmetically or financially.

## Responsibility for Providing Systems

The responsibility for providing assistive listening devices lies primarily with the dispensing audiologist. The evaluation for amplification should include an assessment of communication activities followed by demonstrations and recommendations of appropriate devices. During annual evaluations, the need for assistive listening devices should be reassessed. When the dispensing of products was approved by the American Speech-Language-Hearing Association (ASHA, 1979), it was mandated that dispensing should be part of a comprehensive habilitative care program. A comprehensive program must include consideration of the need for assistive listening devices.

Consider the possibility that a 9-year-old child receives a hearing aid and then is injured in a fire at home because despite having the amplification, the child was not able to hear the smoke alarm. Is the audiologist liable for not recommending that the family acquire a smoke alarm with increased intensity or a visual signal? Certainly the entire communication functioning of the child must be maximized. Depending on the age of the child, the comprehensive rehabilitation program may include a recommendation for a hearing aid and assistive devices for large group and telephone communication, television reception, telephone and doorbell signal recognition, sleep alarm, and smoke detector awareness.

The responsibility for providing assistive listening devices has increased to include the public sector with the passage of the Americans with Disabilities Act (1990). Places that provide public access such as theaters, restaurants, and airports are now required to provide these devices. The most common accommodations provided for persons with hearing loss by businesses include some type of amplifier for receiving auditory signals in large groups (e.g., movie theaters) and amplifiers for public phones.

Parents must consider their child's use of assistive devices at school when discussing the individualized educational plan. If a group amplification system is not provided, a parent may request this as part of the plan that is formulated in conjunction with school personnel. The school is responsible for providing the device for use during school activities. However, some parents may want the child to have access to the improved S/N ratio during extracurricular activities. In the case of an FM system, the parents may purchase a transmitter and receiver and ask the school to provide another transmitter for use during school activities. The child's transmitter may be used as a backup and for after school functions.

The responsibility for providing assistive devices also lies with the consumer. There are many instances in which devices may be of benefit but lack of experience precludes installation. Individuals with hearing loss must be assertive and ask businesses about the availability of devices. Children should be given opportunities to practice making requests for such devices with the understanding that many businesses may not be aware of the need and will gladly provide the accommodation when requested to do so.

## Summary

Because of the Americans with Disabilities Act, there is more attention by business owners and the general public about accommodations for persons with disabilities. Therefore, it is most important that audiologists assume a lead role in educating others about the devices available to assist persons with hearing loss. Fortunately, materials have recently become available for instructing adults as well as children on the benefits of assistive devices. However, the audiologist cannot always ensure that the child has access to such devices. Therefore, it is important that the parent, and eventually the child, become advocates for assistive devices whether they are requested for use in school or in a public facility. Many locations have organized advocacy groups that can provide information on access for persons with disabilities. To find out more about these groups, one may contact the National Association of Protection and Advocacy Systems, 900 Second Street NE #211, Washington, DC 20002 (Phone: 202-408-9514).

## EVALUATION OF ASSISTIVE LISTENING DEVICES

Once an assistive device is received, there must be some evaluation of the device on the user unless it has been provided by a public entity for general use. In this case it is incumbent upon the professionals who dispensed the device to determine the appropriateness of the devices they provide. Although families may order some personal devices directly from a distributor, whenever presentation of an auditory signal is involved, an audiologist should be consulted to evaluate the electroacoustic characteristics in relation to the user's residual hearing. Although there are few procedures for the evaluation of assistive listening devices described in the literature (Hawkins, 1987; Grimes and Mueller, 1991a, 1991b; Lewis, Feigin, Karasek, and Stelmachowicz, 1989; Mueller, Hawkins, and Northern, 1992), some of these (e.g., evaluation of FM systems) may be applied

across a group of devices. The following discussion addresses only those devices with auditory signal presentation. Devices with visual or vibratory signal presentation still require behavioral evaluation in conjunction with the audiologist/dispenser to ensure proper functioning, but the audiologist is not equipped to evaluate the quality of the operational characteristics of such devices.

There are four components of the evaluation of assistive listening devices. The first component, the behavioral evaluation, can be applied to all types of assistive listening and alerting devices. Electroacoustic and probe–microphone evaluations are applicable to those devices designed to improve personal communication via an auditory signal. The final step, applicable to all devices, is the personal evaluation by the child/family during a loaner period. As Palmer (1992) suggests, conducting an evaluation implies that some action will take place if the evaluation does not meet one's standards. In some cases in which there are no internal controls, such as with a loud-ring indicator for a phone, the action may be to return the device to the manufacturer. Procedures for each of the four evaluation components are provided in the following sections.

### Behavioral Evaluation

Devices obtained through an audiologist should, at a minimum, be set up and demonstrated before the child leaves the clinic. This would not only allow for evaluation of the functioning of the device but also facilitate the orientation to its care and use while its operation is demonstrated. This type of behavioral evaluation would involve a demonstration center that is equipped with a television, phone, radio, lamp, cassette player, and speakers. In some cases, the most benefit from a device must be determined through some process of moving the orientation of the hearing aid and/or moving a microphone relative to the sound. During this initial behavioral evaluation, the preferred volume control may also be determined. In some cases with small children, the behavioral evaluation may be conducted by the audiologist and/or the parents.

The behavioral evaluation does not consist of determining aided thresholds while wearing devices that deliver an audio signal. There are too many variables regarding the spectrum and level of the input to the microphone and the location of the microphone when used in the real-world situation that cannot adequately be replicated in a threshold testing situation (Thibodeau, Roberts, and Barr, 1990). During threshold testing the level of the signal may not cause the system to go into compression as it would during a real-world situation, and thus testing may not validly reflect the gain that is realized in the real world.

## Electroacoustic Evaluation

As mentioned earlier, at this time, there is no standard for the electroacoustic evaluation of assistive listening devices. Therefore, the purpose of the evaluation is not to compare results with manufacturer standards, but to establish baseline performance to use in future monitoring. If the device can be coupled to the widely available 2-cc coupler, several of the tests used for the evaluation of hearing aids may be performed. Because of the various placements of microphones on these devices, the actual input to the real ear is difficult to predict from the electroacoustic measures. Perhaps the most extensive evaluation of assistive devices electroacoustically has been performed with FM systems.

Guidelines for the evaluation of FM systems recently were published (ASHA, 1994). In the testing arrangement shown in Figure 14.10, the microphone of the system is placed in the test box in the calibrated position near the sound. The receiver of the FM system is placed outside the test box and connected to the 2-cc coupler via a button receiver or a direct-input/neck loop connection to the hearing aid. First, a 90-dB SPL input is delivered to the FM microphone while the receiver is set to full on to evaluate maximum output. Next, the input to the FM transmitter microphone is 80 dB SPL while the FM receiver is set to user

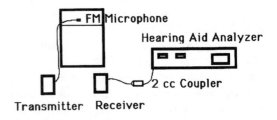

## TYPICAL ARRANGEMENT FOR ELECTROACOUSTIC MEASURES

**FIGURE 14.10**  Electroacoustic test arrangement for an FM system.

settings to simulate the input level to the FM microphone when it is worn in the typical position, 6 inches from the mouth. Harmonic distortion and equivalent input noise may be measured using the procedures recommended in the standard for evaluation of hearing aids (ANSI, 1987).

When the coupling device does not attach reliably to the 2-cc coupler (e.g., earbuds), then KEMAR (Knowles Electronic Manikan for Acoustic Research) and a Zwislocki coupler may be used to simulate user conditions. However, these components are expensive and not readily available. The use of probe–microphone measurements is probably the best way to monitor performance of devices that do not conveniently fit on a coupler.

## Probe–Microphone Evaluation

The evaluation of assistive listening devices that deliver an acoustic signal to the user via probe–microphone measurement techniques requires alteration from the automated procedure that is often used with hearing aids. The minimum requirement for the probe–microphone measurement system is that the input levels can be user adjusted and that the reference microphone can be deactivated and separated from the primary measuring microphone. The goal is to select an assistive device that allows the desired signal (e.g., speech or a doorbell) to be comfortably audible. Therefore the level of the signal in the ear canal without the assistive device must be compared with the level when the device is used to deter-mine the gain. This gain must be added to the typ-ical level of the signal to be amplified and compared to the unaided thresholds and uncom-fortable loudness levels. In some cases in which the desired output level in the ear canal has al-ready been determined in the process of fitting personal hearing aids, the output of the assistive device may be matched to the output of the hear-ing aids. The main differences in evaluating an as-sistive device compared to a hearing aid with a probe–microphone system are the microphone's input level and placement.

An example of this process will be provided for an FM system. For more specific measure-ment details, the reader is referred to Hawkins (1987), Lewis (1991), and Seewald and Moodie (1992). Because many children who use an FM system also have personal hearing aids that pre-sumably are fit appropriately, the goal of the probe–microphone evaluation with the FM sys-tem is to match the output in the ear canal while using the FM system to the output in the ear canal while using the personal hearing aid. As shown in Figure 14.11, for an FM system, the input is typi-cally 80-dB SPL compared to the typical 60-dB SPL input to the hearing aid. Therefore, the output of the FM system is measured with an 80-dB SPL input and compared to the output of the hearing aid that is measured with a 60-dB SPL input. To achieve the same output in the ear canal (e.g., 110 dB) less gain will be needed for the FM sys-tem (e.g., 30 dB) than for the hearing aid (e.g., 50 dB). Less gain is needed for the FM system be-cause some of the increase in signal level is ac-complished simply by moving the microphone closer to the sound source.

If a hearing aid has already been fit appropri-ately, the first step, as shown in Figure 14.12A, is to determine the output in the ear canal with the hearing aid in the typical probe–microphone ar-rangement while using a 60-dB SPL input. To evaluate maximum output level, an output curve with 90-dB SPL signal is obtained. Next, the hear-ing aid is removed and the FM microphone is placed at the location of the reference micro-phone. The output of the FM receiver is coupled to the ear while the probe tube remains in the ear canal in the same position as for testing of the hearing aid as shown in Figure 14.12B. Then an 80-dB SPL signal is presented and the output is compared to that obtained with the hearing aid. Adjustments to volume and/or tone controls may be necessary to obtain as close a match as possi-ble. Finally, a 90-dB SPL input is used to adjust the settings so that maximum output does not ex-ceed that obtained with the hearing aids.

This basic procedure may be altered for a va-riety of assistive devices that are used to enhance personal communication with the following con-siderations. First, the microphone of the assistive device must be placed as close as possible to the reference microphone. The reference microphone may be placed at a location other than the head, particularly if feedback is a problem. Second, the input level must resemble that which arrives at the microphone of the assistive device when used. For example, if the device is to be used for television listening, ideally the evaluation could be made at the child's home or on a television at the clinic that is used for video demonstrations. The level at the microphone of the assistive device when

## COMPARISON OF INPUT LEVEL TO MICROPHONES

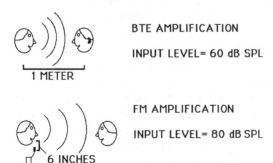

BTE AMPLIFICATION

INPUT LEVEL= 60 dB SPL

1 METER

FM AMPLIFICATION

INPUT LEVEL= 80 dB SPL

6 INCHES

**FIGURE 14.11**  Typical input levels to the hearing aid and to the FM microphone.

**(A) Real Ear Aided Response**
**(REAR)**
**Measures**

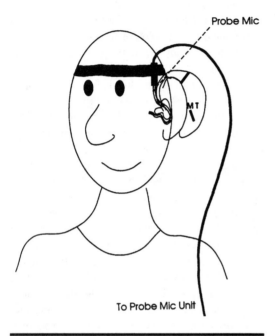

Probe Mic

To Probe Mic Unit

**(B) Real Ear Aided Response**
**(REAR)**
**Measures**
**with Neckloop**

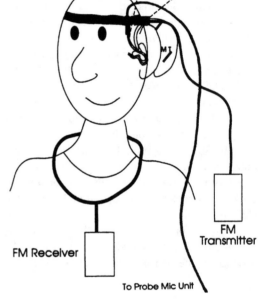

.Probe Mic

FM Microphone

FM Receiver

FM Transmitter

To Probe Mic Unit

**FIGURE 14.12** Real-ear measurement with an FM system. *(A)* Setup for evaluation of the hearing aid only. *(B)* Setup for evaluation of the FM system when used with a neckloop arrangement.

placed on the television speaker during normal operation must be determined. This may be done by placing the probe microphone at the television speaker and reading the output on the probe–microphone system. This is the level that should be delivered to the assistive device microphone that is near the reference microphone during the probe–microphone evaluation.

### Trial Period

Perhaps the most significant aspect of the selection of an assistive listening device is the trial by the child and family. The purpose of the trial period is to complete the validation of the fitting procedure. The procedures described above are based on theoretical principles that may not be applicable in every case. For example, the 60- and 80-dB SPL inputs used to evaluate the FM systems may not result in a particular teacher being audible if that teacher has an unusually weak voice. During the trial period, this may be noted and a visit to the school may be necessary to actually measure the level of the teacher's voice arriving at the child's hearing aid microphone compared to that arriving at the FM microphone. The ultimate goal of the trial period is to document the benefit of the recommended device for the child during daily activities.

During the trial period, which is ideally at least 30 days, the child/family should be instructed each week to focus on noting behavior changes in specific situations. In addition, they should be contacted once a week about device operation and troubleshooting. If the device is used by other persons (e.g., classroom teacher), they should be consulted at least twice during the trial period. Simply asking if the family has any questions about the device is not sufficient. The parents/child should be asked specific questions on the operation such as, "How would you know if the battery is weak?" During this time, procedures to ensure consistent operation should be put in place. Teachers should have spare parts (e.g., batteries, cords, and headphones) provided by the school program or parents, depending on how the system was acquired.

## Summary

The steps involved in ensuring adequate function and use of an assistive listening device include behavioral, electroacoustic, and probe–microphone evaluations as well as the personal trial period. Because of problems associated with threshold testing, the behavioral evaluation is primarily a listening check or trial demonstration of a device. Although there are no standards by which to collect electroacoustic information, the information is valuable as a baseline measurement to monitor future performance. The most useful evaluation is with the use of the probe–microphone system, particularly if it can be conducted in the real-world environment. During the final validation step, the 30-day trial period, it is very important to maintain close contact with the family/child to ensure that the benefits observed in the clinical setting carry over to the real world.

## SUMMARY

The use of assistive listening devices maximizes a child's auditory capabilities. For children with hearing loss to benefit from these devices they must be introduced as early as possible. Parents may choose to use an FM system in the home as the primary means of amplification. Such a system may be taken with the preschooler to various activities including nursery school, ballet, and/or Sunday school. Use of the FM system while riding in the car may add substantial language input opportunities. While the children are learning the meanings of environmental sounds, it is important to allow visual as well as auditory access to important ones including the smoke alarm, doorbell, and telephone. An amplifier or other assistive device should be considered as phone communication skills develop.

The audiologist's responsibility goes beyond providing recommendations on the use of assistive devices. Audiologists must provide education for the child and family on the types and suppliers of the devices as well as the basis upon which they may be requested. The audiologist must also recommend systematic evaluation of any device that provides amplification through an earphone of some sort. It is certainly unfair to the child to receive a hearing aid that was selected after careful analysis of threshold and loudness discomfort test results only to have it removed upon arrival at school in order to use a group amplification system with an arbitrarily set volume control. It seems unethical for an audiologist to carefully fit one amplification device and then ignore the evaluation of other devices that the child might wear.

In view of the lack of standards that require manufacturers to provide electroacoustic information, audiologists must create their own protocols to obtain baseline information for comparison when monitoring the device's performance over time. The evaluation of assistive devices that are coupled to the ear, whether by behavioral, electroacoustic, or probe–microphone measures, is of utmost importance to ensure that devices are of benefit and do not result in damage to residual hearing. Because there is no regulation of manufacturers of assistive listening devices, it is incumbent upon the audiologist to educate the family and insist upon being involved in the selection process of those devices that are coupled to the ear.

# REFERENCES

Americans with Disabilities Act (1990). §302(a), 102(b) (5) (A).

American National Standards Institute. (1987). American national standard for the specification of hearing aid characteristics (ANSI S3.22-1987). New York: ANSI.

American Speech-Language-Hearing Association. (1979). Ethical practice board interpretations of principles governing the dispensing of products to persons with communicative disorders. *Asha, 16,* 237–240.

American Speech-Language-Hearing Association. (1994). Guidelines for fitting and monitoring FM systems. *Asha,* 12 (Suppl.), 1–9.

Boothroyd, A. (1992). The FM wireless link: An invisible microphone cable. In M. Ross (ed.) *FM Auditory Training Systems: Characteristics, Selection, and Use* (pp. 1–19). Timonium, MD: York Press.

Flexer, C., Milin, J., and Brown, L. (1990). Children with developmental disabilities: The effect of soundfield amplification on word identification. *Language, Speech and Hearing Services in Schools, 21,* 177–182.

Gilmore, R., and Lederman, N. (1989). Induction loop assistive listening systems: Back to the future? *Hearing Instruments, 40,* 14–20.

Gilmore, R., and Monte, D. (1994). Innovative classroom amplification: The 3-D loop option. *Educational Audiology Monograph, 3,* 35–37.

Grimes, A., and Mueller, G. (1991a). Using probe-microphone measures to assess telecoils and ALDs. *The Hearing Journal, 44,* 16–21.

Grimes, A., and Mueller, G. (1991b). Using probe-microphone measures to assess telecoils and ALDs: Part II. *The Hearing Journal, 44,* 21–29.

Hawkins, D. (1984). Comparisons of speech recognition in noise by mildly-to-moderately hearing-impaired children using hearing aids and FM systems. *Journal of Speech and Hearing Disorders, 49,* 409–418.

Hawkins, D. (1987). Assessment of FM systems with an ear canal probe tube microphone system. *Ear and Hearing, 8,* 301–303.

Hammond, L. (1991). *FM Auditory Trainers: A Winning Choice for Students, Teachers, and Parents.* Minneapolis: Gopher State Litho.

International Electrotechnical Commission. (1981). IEC Standard 118-4: Methods of measurement of electro-acoustical characteristics of hearing aids, Part 4: Magnetic field strength in audio frequency induction loops for hearing aid purposes. New York: Engineering Societies Library.

Lewis, D. (1991). FM systems and assistive devices: Selection and evaluation. Vanderbilt Conference on Pediatric Amplification. Omaha, NB: Boys Town National Research Hospital.

Lewis, D., Feigin, J., Karasek, A., and Stelmachowicz, P. (1989). Evaluation and assessment of FM systems. *Ear and Hearing, 12,* 268–280.

Luduena, L., and Thibodeau, L. (1993). Evaluation of the benefits of FM systems with cochlear implant users. Paper presented at the American Speech, Language, and Hearing Association, Anaheim, CA.

Madell, J. (1992). FM systems as primary amplification for children with profound hearing loss. *Ear and Hearing, 13,* 102–107.

Mississippi Bend Area Education Agency (1992). *KIP— Knowledge Is Power.* Iowa: Mississippi Bend Area Education Agency.

Mueller, H. G., Hawkins, D. B., and Northern, J. L. (1992). *Probe Microphone Measurements: Hearing Aid Selection and Assessment.* San Diego: Singular Publishing Group.

Palmer, C. (1992). Assistive devices in the audiology practice. *American Journal of Audiology,* March, 37–57.

Public Law 101-431 47 United States Code sec 303 and note to 303, 330 and note, and note to sec 609.

Public Law 100-394. 47 United States Code, sec 609 note, 610 and note.

Seewald, R., and Moodie, K. (1992). Electroacoustic considerations. In M. Ross (ed.), *FM Auditory Training Systems: Characteristics, Selection, and Use* (pp. 45–73). Timonium: York Press.

Thibodeau, L. (1992). Physical components and features of FM systems. In M. Ross (ed.), *FM Auditory Training Systems: Characteristics, Selection, and Use* (pp. 45–73). Timonium, MD: York Press, Inc.

Thibodeau, L., Mayfield, M, Champlin, C. (1994). Comparison of FM transmitter microphones. Paper presented at the American Academy of Rehabilitative Audiology, Snowbird, UT.

Thibodeau, L., McCaffrey, H., and Abrahamson, J. (1988). Effects of coupling hearing aids to FM systems via neckloops. *Journal of Academy of Rehabilitative Audiology, 21,* 49–56.

Thibodeau, L., and McCaffrey, H. (1992). The complexities of using direct-input hearing aids with FM systems. *Volta Review, 95,* 189–193.

Thibodeau, L., Roberts, M, and Barr, M. (1990, March). Using a probe mic system to evaluate FM amplification. Paper presented at the Texas Speech, Language, and Hearing Assn, Dallas, TX.

Thibodeau, L., and Watson, K. (1993). Hearing aids and personal FM systems. Paper presented at the American Speech, Language, and Hearing Association, Anaheim, CA.

# PART FIVE

# INTERVENTION/EDUCATION FOR CHILDREN WITH HEARING LOSS

# CHAPTER 15

# EARLY INTERVENTION

*DONALD M. GOLDBERG*

*A parent is worth 10,000 schoolmasters.*

—*A Chinese Proverb*

## INTRODUCTION

There is a critical need for the *early* detection, identification, and management of infants, toddlers, and children with hearing disorders. To maximize intellectual growth and speech and language development, intervention must begin during the first 3 years of life. Research suggests that the number of neurons infants keep and the synapses between them, are influenced by the child's environment and early sensory experiences (Sharpe, 1994). In order to benefit from the "critical periods" of neurological and linguistic development, the identification of hearing disorders, use of appropriate amplification and medical technology, and stimulation of hearing must occur as early as possible (Clopton and Winfield, 1976; Johnson and Newport, 1989; Lennenberg, 1967; Marler, 1970; Newport, 1990).

Even the earliest intervention does not, however, guarantee "success." The magnitude of the role of parental influence is great as well. Parents of these youngsters embark on a journey, often completely foreign, as more than 90 percent (Moores, 1987) have normal hearing. The parents of children with hearing disorders will typically become part of a team composed of numerous professionals, which might include an audiologist, speech-language pathologist, teacher of the hearing impaired, social worker, otolaryngologist, and other physicians, teachers, among others.

The purpose of this chapter is to describe issues in the area of early intervention for children with hearing disorders in which parents should become "experts" so that they are returned to their rightful place as parents, albeit parents with a wealth of knowledge, so that they can be their child's best advocate.

## VARIABLES OF HEARING IMPAIRMENT

Children with hearing disorders are a heterogeneous population. A number of variables (including type and degree of hearing loss, age of onset, consistency of amplification, intervention provided, etc.) make comparisons among these children difficult and inherently inappropriate. No one variable is categorically more important than another, but instead, it is the unique combination of several of these factors that result in a wide variety of outcomes.

It is not uncommon for parents to try to compare children with the same degree of hearing loss. Difficulty exists, however, in categorizing hearing disorders into discrete levels due to the fact that the degree of hearing loss exists on a continuum. Two children, even with the same audiogram, most likely will have different communication abilities due to the variety of factors noted above. Although patterns do exist—for example, children with prelingual, severe to profound hearing disorders will not learn spoken language unless intervention occurs (Ling, 1989)—predictions of how children with hearing disorders *will be* when they grow up is not advisable. Generalizations from an audiogram alone are inappropriate due to myriad factors influencing the behavior of children with hearing disorders.

## DIAGNOSIS OF HEARING DISORDER

According to the National Institutes of Health (1993), there is a clear need in the United States for improved methods and models for the early identification of hearing impairment in infants and young children. The average age of identification of hearing loss in children is presently 2.5 years with some children unidentified until 6 years of age. There is an inverse relationship between the average age of identification and the degree of hearing loss, with more severe hearing disorders being diagnosed earlier in life (Pappas and McDowell, 1983). The earlier a hearing disorder is identified, the sooner medical, audiologic, and amplification intervention can be initiated.

Chapter 5 presents a detailed discussion of the screening of children's hearing. Because not all hearing impairments are present at birth, the significant number of infants and children who develop hearing disorders during the first years of life must be detected via hearing screening programs through day-care and head-start programs; education programs of parents, primary caretakers, medical and nursing personnel; and all other professionals who have opportunity to observe the child and recognize factors that place the child at high risk for hearing impairment. School entry will also provide an additional opportunity for universal identification of children with significant hearing impairment (NIH, 1993).

The profession is currently embroiled in the controversy on the appropriateness of universal newborn screening (see Bess and Paradise, 1994; Northern and Hayes, 1994). However, all would agree that intervention should be initiated as early as possible via universal screenings, use of high-risk registers, and/or professional responsiveness to parental concerns regarding infants, toddlers and children with suspected hearing disorders. Identification and intervention will ideally transpire at earlier ages in the future.

## AMPLIFICATION AND AUDIOLOGIC MANAGEMENT

For children with hearing disorders, hearing aids, FM systems, cochlear implants, and/or other sensory aids are their "ears." The consistent use of appropriately fitted and functioning equipment, including earmolds, cannot be overemphasized as

the most critical component of any auditory-based early intervention program.

In response to the need to delineate recommended components of a comprehensive audiologic and amplification management program for children with hearing disorders, Auditory-Verbal International (AVI) (1991a) developed a suggested protocol. Its use is recommended, regardless of the communication methodology in which a child might be enrolled.

As discussed in Chapter 3, the aggressive medical and audiologic management of middle ear problems is critical for children with sensorineural hearing loss. The addition of the conductive hearing loss on top of the existing sensorineural hearing loss leads to an increased communicative deficit and, therefore, must be attended to quickly and proactively.

In view of the fact that for school-age children, hearing aids and FM systems often do not function (e.g., Potts and Greenwood, 1983), an aggressive amplification management program is required in the overall intervention program. Personal experience has revealed in many cases less than regular audiologic evaluations, inadequate assessment components (e.g., limited speech perception measurements and missing real-ear measurement data), poorly fitting earmolds, inappropriate amplification systems and settings, and an overall lack of case management in the areas of audiologic and amplification assessment and management. If the child's earmolds, hearing aids, FM system, and/or cochlear implant are their "ears," it is imperative that children have well-fitted and functioning amplification systems. The ideal intervention program will pay significant attention to, and be respectful of, the issues involved in pediatric amplification and audiologic management.

## FAMILY COUNSELING

As discussed in Chapter 9, the members of the team of individuals working *with* the family of a child with a hearing disorder must be cognizant of the role family counseling should play in early intervention. The feelings and reactions of *all* members of the child's family need attention and must be addressed.

## Parents

Although today's changing times have modified the "typical" mother role as primary caregiver, the child's mother is often the individual who still transports and participates with the child in lessons in center-based early intervention programs. Feelings of being overwhelmed with the responsibilities of raising a child with a hearing disorder should be acknowledged. The interplay between parents and the feeling that one parent is doing more for the child and the resentment that may develop, for example, due to the other parent feeling neglected, are not uncommon.

The formation of regular parent support groups or at least "connecting" two families is strongly recommended during early intervention. Professionals might assist in facilitating the gathering of the parents and *not* participate, because the dynamics of the group will often change in the presence of a professional. I have found myself saying to parents, "Not being the parent of a child with a hearing loss, I cannot truly know how you might be feeling." Because of this, parent-to-parent support is invaluable.

## Siblings

Similar to the situation for the parents, the feelings of the siblings of a child with a hearing disorder must also be acknowledged and addressed. It is recommended that siblings be encouraged to participate in lessons. One of my special memories is a lesson with Joey, his twin brother Tony, their younger sister Gina, and their mom. The opportunity to observe how the three young children interact, including one with a significant hearing loss, was informative and educational in the assessment of family dynamics, in addition to evaluating the child's auditory, speech, and language abilities.

Support groups and/or "rap" sessions among siblings might be scheduled. It is important to keep in mind that siblings often have numerous questions about their brother or sister with a hearing disorder. Time and attention to, as well as an understanding of, the siblings' situation, is critically important.

## Grandparents

Atkins (1987, 1994a, 1994b) has poignantly written and spoken about the needs of grandparents when their child's child has a hearing disorder. Tables 15.1 and 15.2 outline several of Atkins' recommendations to enhance the relationship between grandparents and their grandchild, as well as the grandparents and their adult children. They are all in need and are each in a position to be supportive of each other's needs. With attention to the whole family, the positive and negative experiences of rearing a child with a hearing disorder can be dealt with so that early intervention can grow with the family unit.

## COMMUNICATION METHODOLOGIES

Perhaps the most emotionally laden and vitriolic area in the arena of audiologic (re)habilitation for

**TABLE 15.1**  What Grandparents Can Do

---

Educate yourself about hearing loss in children and the different options for their education:
- Subscribe to journals.
- Join national organizations and local support groups.
- Talk to professionals.

Ask you children for specific suggestions so you can help in ways that would benefit everyone.

Be supportive of your children—even if you do not fully understand or agree with their decisions.

Visit your grandchild's school.

Tell your family history with photos and maps.

Take day trips with your grandchild.

Remember your other grandchildren.

---

Adapted from Atkins, 1994b.

**TABLE 15.2**   What Parents Can Do (for *Their* Parents)

Make and send videotapes and photos of children engaged in their favorite activities.

Provide printed information (in their language and printed in large type, if necessary). Send copies of articles you have found helpful.

Compile a glossary of terms for easy reference.

Explain—in writing or on audiotape—the philosophy behind your child's educational program.

Make appointments for them to talk to audiologists, teachers, and other professionals.

Help them connect with national organizations and local support groups.

Offer specific ideas of how they can be involved.

Adapted from Atkins, 1994a

children with hearing disorders is that of communication methodologies. Anecdotal accounts of the communicative abilities of individuals with hearing impairments abound, regardless of the intervention methodology. Indeed, there are many intervention options, each one distinct in philosophy, methodology, programming, expectations, and assumptions (Goldberg and Flexer, 1993).

The following quote creatively describes the "methodological controversy": "Debates in the past have centered on the issue of oralism versus manualism. Today, issues are more complex. Present controversy pits morphosyntactic approaches against semantic/pragmatic approaches, ASL/ESL against various manually coded forms of English as philosophies, and naturalistic pedagogy against metacognition, among others." (Easterbrooks, 1987, p. 188). Certainly, it is far too simplistic to categorize the longstanding debate as merely oral versus manual.

There appears to be a positive movement towards evaluating each child with a hearing disorder individually to determine a program of intervention. However, the controversy is not yet quiescent and many families are still not provided with nonbiased information on the range or cascade of *options* that exist.

It is not my purpose to categorically state that one particular philosophy, method or outcome of intervention is superior to any other. That is not our role to decide, even though many professionals have formed particular biases. The role of the audiologist is, however, to inform, guide, and counsel the parents of children with hearing disorders. Parents do need to be informed about the host of options available and guided to materials and resources about each method (including other families with a child who is hearing impaired). It is most important that the audiologist be nonjudgmental about the programming selected. *No choice regarding methodologies is the right or wrong choice.* Parents make decisions that are right for them and their family. The inherent biases that professionals possess are not appropriate in the counseling of a parental choice. Audiologists are, however, in a position to provide learned counsel based on objective information. The greatest danger is when a professional directs parents to one methodology, without informing them of the fact that choices exist. For each of the approaches to be described, the reader is directed to Appendix 7 for referral to major organizations formed, in part, to disseminate information about their particular intervention method.

## Auditory–Verbal Philosophy

The auditory–verbal philosophy (formerly referred to as unisensory or Acoupedics) is a model of intervention that incorporates the principles outlined in Table 15.3 (adapted from Pollack, 1970, 1985). These principles outline the essential requirements needed to realize the expectation that young children with hearing impairments can be educated to use even minimal amounts of amplified residual hearing. The auditory–verbal philosophy states that the use of amplified residual hearing, in turn, permits children with hearing impairments to learn to listen, to process verbal language, and to speak. The goal of auditory–verbal practice is that children with hearing impairments can grow up in typical learning and living environments that enable them to become indepen-

**TABLE 15.3**  Auditory–Verbal Principles (AVI, 1991b)

1. Support and promote programs for the early detection and identification of hearing impairment and the auditory management of infants, toddlers, and children so identified.

2. Provide the earliest and most appropriate use of medical and amplification technology to achieve the maximum benefits available.

3. Instruct primary caregivers in ways to provide maximal acoustic stimulation within meaningful contexts and support the developing of the most favorable auditory learning environments for the acquisition of spoken language.

4. Seek to integrate listening into the child's total personality in response to the environment.

5. Support the view that communication is a social act and seek to improve spoken communication interaction within the typical social dyad of infant/child with hearing impairment and the primary caregiver(s), including the use of the parents as primary models for spoken language development, and implementing one-to-one teaching.

6. Seek to establish the child's integrated auditory system for the self-monitoring of emerging speech.

7. Use natural sequential patterns of auditory, perceptual, linguistic, and cognitive stimulation to encourage the emergence of listening, speech, and language abilities.

8. Make ongoing evaluation and prognosis of the development of listening skills an integral part of the (re)habilitative process.

9. Support the concepts of mainstreaming and integration of children with hearing impairments into typical education classes with appropriate support services and to the fullest extent possible.

From Auditory–Verbal International (1991b). Auditory–verbal position statement. *The Auricle, 4*(4), 11, 15.

dent, participating, and contributing citizens in mainstream society (AVI, 1991b).

The auditory–verbal method is not merely a "technique" to be delivered 2 hours per week, but rather a way of life to be practiced on a daily basis. Comprehensive audiologic management is the foundation of the auditory–verbal approach (Marlowe, 1993). Professionals, who are now eligible for certification as a "certified auditory–verbal therapist," work intimately with the parents in an auditory–verbal program.

## Cued Speech

Developed by Cornet (1967, 1972), cued speech is a system of eight hand configurations and four hand positions on or near the face (base, chin, mouth, throat, and larynx) that allow the child to identify those speech sounds that are difficult to differentiate by sight alone. The cues are used to reduce the redundancy of the homophenous nature of numerous speech sounds. The cues are

provided following natural English spoken language production (Cornet, 1967).

Cued speech was originally purported to be a compromise system that would end the "oralism versus manualism" controversy. Northern and Downs (1984) stated that the greatest advantage of cued speech is that it facilitates the acquisition of vocabulary and the syllabic-phonemic-rhythmic patterns of spoken language, without interrupting the natural process of communication. For a hearing person to acquire fairly fluent "cueing," cued speech is reportedly learned in about 30 hours through training available on videotapes.

## Oral Approach

In the oral approach, spoken language is perceived by the recipient through the speech reading or lipreading cues provided. The child is asked to look at the way the speaker is forming a sound. The child may look directly at the speaker's mouth or simultaneously may look at the speaker and their own productions through a mirror. Pictures of the correct phonetic placement of the articulators may be used as well (Easterbrooks, 1987). In the oral approach, various written representations of the graphemes corresponding to the speech phonemes have been utilized. A goal of oral programs is the development of intelligible speech (Paul and Quigley, 1987).

## Rochester Method

The Rochester Method, also known as "Visible Speech" was developed at the New York School for the Deaf and is defined as the simultaneous use of speech and fingerspelling. This "writing in air" technique is superimposed on normal speech (Scouten, 1964).

## Total Communication

The Conference of Executives of American Schools for the Deaf defined total communication as "a philosophy requiring the incorporation of appropriate aural, manual, and oral modes of communication in order to insure effective communication with and among hearing-impaired persons" (Brill, 1976). In total communication, every and all means to communicate are utilized. Natural gestures, signs, fingerspelling, facial expression, body language, and the like, accompanied by the simultaneous use of speech through hearing aids, are all provided as a means to convey information.

## Verbotonal

In 1952, Guberina in Yugoslavia began developing a method to improve foreign language teaching through emphasis on the spoken rhythm of the language to be learned. Guberina later applied his theory and methods in teaching deaf children and adults (Northern and Downs, 1984). Craig and Craig (1972) characterized the Verbotonal approach as (1) emphasizing low frequencies (below 500 Hz) and vibratory clues in perception of spoken language; (2) matching a special amplification device to the person's optimum "field of hearing"; (3) using body movements to assist in speech production and perception; (4) emphasizing acoustic memory for language patterns aided by body movements and by articulatory movements from the production of speech; (5) providing speech and language work in active play type situations in order to increase spoken language instruction time; and (6) emphasizing language in natural and meaningful contexts. In the Verbotonal method, wrist vibrators typically are provided for the reception of tactile cues to emphasize the suprasegmental features of spoken language.

## American Sign Language

American Sign Language (ASL or Ameslan) is, in the United States, the native language of many deaf people who have deaf parents and is the language of many deaf adults (Wilbur, 1987). The signs created with the hands allow for faster communication than finger spelling.

## Manually Coded English Systems

A variety of Manually Coded English (MCE) systems have been developed, each based on the general premise of representing the structure of written standard English. Some of the more common MCE systems include Seeing Essential English (SEE I) (Anthony, 1966); Signing Exact English (SEE II) (Gustason, 1983; Gustason, Pfetzing, and Zawolkow, 1980); and Signed English (Bornstein, 1973; Bornstein and Saulnier, 1981; Bornstein, Saulnier, and Hamilton, 1980).

## DETERMINATION OF COMMUNICATION METHODOLOGY

As was discussed in the previous section on communication methodologies, parents should be provided with information on the cascade of intervention options available. In an effort to provide unbiased information to families so that they might make informed decisions about rearing a child with a hearing disorder, Beginnings for Parents of Hearing Impaired Children (see Appendix 7) developed an open-captioned videotape describing the assorted communication approaches, *Beginnings: For Parents of Hearing Impaired Infants and Toddlers.*

## Variables Affecting Choice

Assorted variables play a role in the initial determination of the communication methodology a family chooses for their child. Where a family resides may unfortunately limit choices for consideration, as not all approaches are conveniently located near the child. It is not uncommon, however, for families to relocate in order to access their chosen methodology.

Another factor is the hearing status of the parents. Parents tend to be influenced by their own backgrounds. For example, if one or both parents are deaf or hard-of-hearing themselves and communicate in American Sign Language (ASL), they may see only one option for their child—ASL. Hearing parents with no prior experience or contact with individuals who sign may have a preference towards an oral or aural methodology.

A third variable that might effect methodological choice is the degree of hearing loss. The selection of a manual approach may be influenced by the child presenting with a greater severity of hearing loss. Conversely, an oral or aural approach might be chosen for individuals with less significant hearing disorders. It should be pointed out, however, that *all* options should be initially offered because, degree of hearing disorder alone, does not predispose a child for one method.

### *Formulas to Determine Methodology*

Past research has suggested several formulas that might be used to determine *the* communication approach to employ with a given child. Downs (1974) described the Deafness Management Quotient (DMQ) in which five areas are rated as a way to direct families to an auditory–oral or a total communication program. Similarly, the Feasibility Scale for Language Acquisition Routing for Hearing-Impaired Children (Rupp, Smith, Briggs, Litvin, Banachowski, and Williams, 1977) evaluated seven prognostic factors to compute a score,

resulting in the recommendation for the oral/aural approach, total communication, or continued study of the child, that is, a further diagnostic period before a placement decision was made. The Spoken Language Predictor Index (Geers and Moog, 1987) was developed to rate five predictor factors: hearing, language, nonverbal intelligence, family support, and speech communication attitude. The resulting point values computed result in one of three educational recommendations, specifically, speech emphasis, provisional speech instruction, or sign language emphasis.

Each of the above-noted formulas have merits in that they address a variety of factors that play a significant role in the determination of a communication methodology to follow. However, these formulas' inherent flaw is that this most significant decision *cannot* be reduced to the calculation of weighted rating values alone. Even with the best diagnostic evaluation regarding methodologies, ultimately the family must commit to the chosen approach.

The Diagnostic Early Intervention Project, a cooperative program of the Omaha Public Schools and Boys Town National Research Hospital provides a more comprehensive approach to methodology selection. This multifaceted review of fourteen factors, monitored by a team of professionals in conjunction with the family, assists in the determination of communication methodology as well as in recommendations if a change in programming is warranted (Table 15.4).

## Diagnostic Intervention

A key recommendation for all communication methodological approaches is that there be ongoing diagnostic therapy, qualitative intervention, and ongoing parent guidance. Prognosis regarding the development of auditory, speech, language, reading, thinking skills, and so forth, must be routinely assessed with a battery of standardized tests and informal observations as well as an evaluation of frustration levels and family dynamics.

Parents may demonstrate signs that their commitment to a particular approach is waning, for ex-

**TABLE 15.4** Factors Monitored in Omaha Public Schools and Boys Town National Research Hospital Diagnostic Early Intervention Project

| FACTOR | METHOD OF MONITORING |
|---|---|
| 1. Family support | Social work evaluation<br>Psychological interview |
| 2. Parent–child interaction | Caregiver-child interactive behaviors<br>Home observation for measurement of the environment<br>Teaching scale<br>Family sign program analysis |
| 3. Parental compliance and preferences | Attendance records<br>Brown Parent Attitude Inventory<br>Interviewer Rating of Family and Child Adjustment |
| 4. Etiology | Medical/genetic evaluation<br>CT scan<br>Lab studies |
| 5. Developmental status | Developmental psychology evaluation<br>Minnesota Infant/Child Developmental Inventory |
| 6. Medical status | Pediatric examination and management<br>ENT examination and management |
| 7. Audiologic factors | Auditory brainstem response evaluation<br>Behavioral audiological evaluation |
| 8. Age of identification versus age of amplification | Audiologic records<br>Hearing aid evaluation records |
| 9. Documentation of secondary disabilities | Psychological evaluation<br>Neurologic evaluation<br>Ophthalmology evaluation<br>OT/PT evaluation<br>Other medical specialist evaluations<br>Learning rates data |
| 10. Motor development | Vestibular evaluation<br>OT/PT evaluation<br>Speech physiology evaluation<br>Documentation of gross motor and phonological landmarks and learning rates |
| 11. Interpersonal/social skills | Clinical observation<br>Westby Play Scales |
| 12. Learning rates in receptive and expressive communication | Assessing linguistic behaviors<br>Sensorimotor Communication Profile<br>Pragmatic/semantic analysis<br>SKI*HI Language Development Scale<br>Sequenced Inventory of Communication Development<br>Reynell Developmental Language Scale<br>Systematic analysis of language transcripts<br>Multiple baselines of learning skills |

**TABLE 15.4**  *Continued*

| FACTOR | METHOD OF MONITORING |
|---|---|
| 13. Phonological development | Assessing linguistic behaviors |
|  | Phonological sampling |
|  | Ling Phonetic Level Speech Evaluation |
|  | Goldman-Fristoe Test of Articulation |
|  | Frequency/intentionality of vocalization |
| 14. Auditory learning | Functional auditory checklist |
|  | Hearing aid use charts |
|  | Probe microphone results |
|  | Multiple baselines of auditory learning |
|  | Vibrotactile/electrotactile trial |

Adapted from: Moeller, M. P. and Condon, M. C. (1994). D.E.I.P.: A collaborative problem-solving approach to early intervention. In J. Roush and N. D. Matkin (eds.), *Infants and Toddlers with Hearing Loss: Family Centered Assessment and Intervention*. Baltimore: York Press 163–192.

ample, by attendance problems and nonverbal communication signs of unhappiness. Honest and open communication in a trusting environment between therapist/teacher and parents, in addition to objective appraisals of the child's progress, will ultimately lead to appropriate management, which in some cases might result in the recommendation to change communication methodologies.

## COMMUNICATION ASSESSMENT AND INTERVENTION

Regardless of the communication methodology chosen, intervention should focus on goals and objectives in the major areas of audition, speech, and language. These areas, however, are not the only issues that need to be addressed as the child grows older and enters school. Additional information on the multitude of services to be considered in intervention programs for school children are discussed in Chapter 16.

As would be expected from the variety of services that might be needed for a child with a hearing disorder, rarely would *one* professional have the academic and practicum background necessary to provide all intervention services. Therefore, a team of professionals, working in conjunction with the parents, will typically address the stipulated service needs.

The areas of auditory learning, speech, and language services are the major focus of communication intervention and will therefore be discussed. For each of these areas, to be described below, a sample of evaluation tests and protocols will be recommended, along with intervention references. No "cookbook" or packaged communication programs can possibly address all of the service needs for children with hearing disorders; however, references will be provided so that the new professional can "get started" and hopefully for the more seasoned professional, suggest insights so that one can evolve and learn about new areas, materials, activities, and insights.

### Auditory Learning

Standard audiometric information such as the unaided and aided audiograms serve as the basic information for children with hearing disorders. Cumulative data sheets with numeric audiometric results from serial assessments of unaided and aided thresholds are especially helpful in evaluating auditory functioning.

Thresholds on the audiogram, however, only demonstrate an auditory response at the level of detection (presence or absence of sound). It is important to ascertain how the child functions at the levels of discrimination (perception of same versus different), identification (recognition), and comprehension (Erber, 1982).

The Ling six sound test should be routinely used to determine the child's detection or identification/recognition of the sounds /a/, /u/, /i/, /ʃ/, /s/, and /m/. These sounds span across the frequency range and allow the clinician to judge basic auditory abilities. The six sounds can be easily presented in a quick fashion in order to obtain a baseline of auditory-only responses. Once the baseline has been established, should subsequent measures indicate a change in responses, the clinician must investigate if middle ear or amplification status is negatively influencing the child's auditory abilities. Responses to the Ling sounds should be noted at varying distances, as well as threshold data, measured via monitored live voice in the test booth.

A variety of additional speech audiometric tests and speech perception protocols exist that also can be administered to measure auditory functioning (see Table 15.5). Which measures to be administered will depend upon the child's auditory skills, age, and receptive vocabulary, among other factors.

It is not possible to provide a complete auditory learning curriculum within a single chapter; however, a variety of references and materials have been developed to address the auditory learning of children with hearing disorders. Some examples of texts, videotapes, and programs on auditory learning include: Auditory Skills Instructional Planning System, 1986; Beebe, 1953; Berg, 1987; Cole and Gregory, 1986; Erber, 1982; Estabrooks, 1992; Estabrooks and Edwards, 1986; Flexer, 1994; Goldberg, 1987, 1993; Ling, 1989; Maxon and Brackett, 1992; Pollack, 1985; Ross, Brackett, and Maxon, 1982; Stout and Windle, 1992; Vaughan, 1981.

## Speech

Speech production training for children with hearing disorders has been greatly influenced by the work of Daniel Ling (1976). Included in Ling's (1976) text on speech is an assessment tool, the Phonetic Level Evaluation (PLE), which evaluates speech at both the suprasegmental and segmental level. The PLE addresses analytic speech production skills at the single phoneme and sylla-

**TABLE 15.5**   Auditory and Other Speech Audiometric/Perception Measurements to Assess Auditory Functioning

| | |
|---|---|
| Threshold data with Ling six sounds (/a/, /u/, /i/, /ʃ/, /s/, /m/) | |
| Ling six sounds at varying distances | |
| Early Speech Perception Battery | Moog and Geers, 1990 |
| Auditory Numbers Test | Erber, 1980 |
| Children's Auditory Test | Erber and Alencewicz, 1976 |
| Glendonald Auditory Screening Procedure | Erber, 1982 |
| Sound Effects Recognition Test | Finitzo-Hieber, Matkin, Cherow-Skalka, and Gerling, 1977 |
| Auditory Perception of Alphabet Letters Test | Ross and Randolph, 1988 |
| Word Intelligibility by Picture Identification | Ross and Lerman, 1971 |
| Northwestern University Children's Perception of Speech | Elliott and Katz, 1980 |
| Test of Auditory Comprehension | Trammell, 1981 |
| Minimal Auditory Capabilities Battery | Owens, Kessler, Raggio, and Schubert, 1985; Owens, Kessler, Telleen, and Schubert, 1981 |

ble level. Speech remediation targets can be determined by the PLE for immediate attention.

Speech evaluation at the word level can be addressed with articulation measures routinely used with children with normal hearing, such as the Goldman-Fristoe Test of Articulation. In addition, the intelligibility of a child's speech production skills can be evaluated by the Central Institute for the Deaf's Picture Speech Production Evaluation (SPINE) (Monsen, Moog, and Geers, 1988).

A thorough assessment of the child's speech production will ideally address some of the common speech characteristics in Table 15.6. Remediation should be systematic, taking into consideration the developmental sequence of sounds in conjunction with the acoustic features of the target errors (more audible sounds taught before less audible targets). Short teaching sessions, provided several times per day, will ideally result in intelligible speech that reflects automaticity of production.

## Language

Both the receptive and expressive language skills of children with hearing disorders will often be delayed. Yet the assessment of language skills may be compromised by the existence of the hearing disorder. The limited number of standardized tests to assess the unique language problems of these children; inadequate measures of pragmatic skills, question comprehension, and important discourse skills; and the unknown effects of speech reading, short-term memory for signs, and/or the auditory confusions on the child's test-taking performance (Moeller, McConkey, and Osberger, 1983), all influence language evaluation.

The child's amplification or sensory aid system should be in appropriate operating order at the time of evaluation and tested before assessment. In addition, the optimal test environment should be provided, free of noise interference and with adequate lighting. The evaluation report should provide information on the child's chronological age, in addition to listening (hearing) age, in the

**TABLE 15.6**    Common Speech Characteristics of Individuals with Hearing Disorders

**RESPIRATION, PHONATION, AND RATE**

Expend more breath during speech production

Duration of phonation may be about three times greater than other speakers

**SPEECH RHYTHM**

Slow and labored

**VOWEL PRODUCTION**

Substitutions

Neutralization

Diphthongization

Nasalization

Amplitude is weak

Excessive aspiration

**ARTICULATION OF CONSONANTS**

Voiced/voiceless errors

Omission or distortion of initial consonants

Omission of consonant blends/clusters

Omission or distortion of final consonants

Nasalization

Substitution of one consonant for another

Intrusive voicing between abutting consonants

Least visible sounds tend to be misarticulated most frequently

Adapted from Ling, D. (1976). *Speech in the Hearing-impaired Child: Theory and Practice.* Washington, DC: Alexander Graham Bell Association for the Deaf.

test interpretation. Each of the assessment protocols used should be briefly described, including whether the test was standardized on children with normal hearing or on those with hearing disorders. The use of both measurement categories should be considered. Finally, it would be helpful if the test-taking behaviors of the child were described.

A test battery approach including receptive and expressive language measures and formal and informal observations should be planned; with the goal of evaluating the form, content, and use of language and highlighting the areas of vocabulary and concepts. In addition to the host of standardized assessment tools for children with normal hearing, a variety of measures have been developed specifically for students with hearing disorders (Table 15.7). The battery of tests selected should be reflective of the child's age, in conjunction with the diagnostic questions in need of investigation.

Language intervention programs for children with hearing disorders may be structured, natural/communicative, or some combination of these approaches. Regardless of the design of the program, the importance of the integration of effective communication and thinking skills cannot be overemphasized. Similarly, the therapy lesson one might conduct in teaching a child with a hearing disorder can easily integrate auditory and speech training in the context of a *functional* language activity. In contrast, a few minutes working on the /s/, followed by 10 minutes of listening to environmental sounds and noisemakers, and then a section on the prepositions in and out, *will not* result in a natural "communicator," able to integrate the critical areas of audition, speech, and language.

## Communication Programs

A variety of communication programs have been developed for use with children with hearing disorders. Most address the areas of amplification and its management, along with discussion or the areas of auditory, speech, and language intervention. The programs provide information on a variety of topics and include suggestions for intervention goals and objectives that can be individualized for children with hearing disorders. The use of communication programs as a supplement to qualitative programming in auditory learning, speech, and language intervention is recommended.

## INSTRUCTIONAL SETTINGS

A variety of service delivery models exists for children with hearing disorders, most commonly the family-centered model and the medical model. As described by Flexer (1992), the focus of attention and the responsibilities vary within each model. Similar to comments on communication methodologies, no one service delivery model is necessarily better than another. The selection of a model may be dictated by choices available in a particular locale, the work schedules of the parents, and the degree of disability, among other factors.

**TABLE 15.7**    Sample of Assessment Measurements Developed for Children with Hearing Disorders

| TEST | REFERENCE |
| --- | --- |
| SKI*HI Language Development Scale | Tonelson and Watkins, 1979 |
| Grammatical Analysis of Elicited Language—Presentence Level | Moog, Kozak, and Geers, 1983 |
| Grammatical Analysis of Elicited Language—Simple Sentence Level | Moog and Geers, 1979 |
| Grammatical Analysis of Elicited Language—Complex Sentence Level | Moog and Geers, 1980 |
| Carolina Picture Vocabulary Test | Layton and Holmes, 1985 |
| Total Communication Receptive Vocabulary Test | Scherer, 1981 |
| Test of Syntactic Ability | Quigley, Steinkamp, Power, and Jones, 1978 |

Note: Tests and protocols for children with normal hearing *should* be used in addition to the consideration of the above-noted measures.

## Family-Centered Model

Federal funding under the Individuals with Disabilities Education Act (IDEA) and Public Law 99-457, specifically mandated the family-centered approach of service delivery in infant and toddler programs. Flexer (1992) delineated the following as features that a family-centered model is designed to accomplish:

- Empower and enable the family as a system
- Promote independence, not dependence
- Support and strengthen the family's competence in negotiating its own course of development

## Medical Model

Programming in the medical model is typically child-centered, whereby the professional is responsible for directing the intervention program. Families are tangential participants, often observing lessons rather than taking an active role.

## Collaboration among Team Members

The service providers in either of the models described should be team players; collaboratively involved in planning and monitoring educational goals and procedures. The Joint Committee on Infant Hearing (ASHA, 1991) noted that team members can be considered as sharing ownership and responsibility for intervention objectives. Provided that the team includes the parents as an integral part of the (re)habilitative program, intervention should be poised for positive changes.

## COCHLEAR IMPLANTS

Cochlear implants in children with hearing disorders are one of the most exciting and dynamic developments in the fields of medicine, engineering, audiology, speech-language pathology, and education today (see Chapter 13). Provided candidacy issues are comprehensively evaluated and qualitative follow-up programming is implemented, children with hearing disorders who receive cochlear implants are then in a position to listen and learn (or continue to learn) speech and language.

For children who present with profound degrees of hearing impairment, who do not obtain significant benefit from conventional amplification, a whole new world of sound becomes available through the implant. The key, however, is to then tap into the rich perceptual bounty that the cochlear implant can provide.

Candidacy issues and management concerns with exceptional implications for early intervention programs for children with hearing disorders are clearly articulated in a position statement developed by participants from the Network of Educators of Children with Cochlear Implants (NECCI) (1994). The NECCI position statement strongly recommends that parents considering an implant for their child seek out centers and educational settings that include an educator knowledgeable about appropriate (re)habilitation with the implant.

Zara and Brackett (1994) provided recommendations for the evaluation and rehabilitation of children with cochlear implants, stating that there was "no need to reinvent the wheel." For children with cochlear implants, Zara and Brackett noted in the area of *evaluation components,* the need to (1) begin assessment at basic levels of auditory, speech, and language functioning; (2) sample skills daily to determine if a map (speech processor programming) adjustment is needed; (3) complete full evaluations frequently, due to the rapid emergence of skills; and (4) expect auditory function changes to occur more rapidly than speech and/or language. Specific *rehabilitation components* for children with cochlear implants, outlined by Zara and Brackett (1994) included: (1) increase expectation for use of audition; (2) make listening "functional"; (3) rapidly move from detection to discrimination/identification; and (4) take advantage of the device-specific characteristics, specifically high-frequency sounds, among others.

I believe that a variety of areas for continued research on intervention with cochlear implants are important, including candidacy, prediction of remaining auditory nerve fibers, follow-up intervention components, and the different coding strategies.

## SUMMARY

Early identification of hearing loss coupled with early and aggressive intervention to offset its effects are the only hope for developing oral/aural communication skills for children who have impaired hearing. Following diagnosis, audiologists must stand ready to serve as unbiased guides while parents explore available communication options and select the best suited early intervention for their children. An ongoing assessment of the child's communication will then help the (re)habilitation team determine when alterations of the original plans and goals may be advisable.

## REFERENCES

American Speech-Language-Hearing Association (1991). Joint Committee on Infant Hearing Position Statement. *Asha, 33* (Suppl. 5), 3–6.

Anthony, D. (1966). *Seeing Essential English.* Unpublished master's thesis, Eastern Michigan University, Ypsilanti, Michigan.

Atkins, D. (1987). Families and their hearing-impaired children. *The Volta Review, 89,* 1–146.

Atkins, D. (1994a). Counseling children with hearing loss and their families. In J. G. Clark and F. N. Martin (eds.), *Effective Counseling in Audiology: Principles and Practice.* Englewood Cliffs: Prentice Hall, 116–146.

Atkins, D. (1994b). Grandparents: Impact and role. Presentation at the Alexander Graham Bell Association for the Deaf Convention, Rochester, NY.

Auditory Skills Instructional Planning System. (1986). Portland, OR: Foreworks.

Auditory-Verbal International (1991a). *Suggested Protocol for Audiological and Hearing Aid Evaluation.* Easton, PA.

Auditory-Verbal International (1991b). Auditory-verbal position statement. *The Auricle, 4* (4), 11, 15.

Beebe, H. (1953). *A Guide to Help the Severely Hard of Hearing Child.* Basel/New York: Karger.

Berg, F. (1987). *Facilitating Classroom Listening: A Handbook for Teachers of Normal and Hard of Hearing Students.* Boston: College-Hill Press/Little Brown.

Bess, F., and Paradise, J. (1994). Commentaries: Universal screening for infant hearing impairment: Not simple, not risk-free, not necessarily beneficial, and not presently justified. *Pediatrics, 98* (2), 330–334.

Bornstein, H. (1973). A description of some current sign systems designed to represent English. *American Annals of the Deaf, 118,* 454–463.

Bornstein, H., and Saulnier, K. (1981). Signed English: A brief follow-up to the first evaluation. *American Annals of the Deaf, 126,* 69–72.

Bornstein, H., Saulnier, K., and Hamilton, L. (1980). Signed English: A first evaluation. *American Annals of the Deaf, 125,* 467–481.

Brill, R. (1976). Definition of total communication. *American Annals of the Deaf, 121,* 358.

Clopton, B., and Winfield, J. (1976). Effect of early exposure to patterned sound on unit activity in rat inferior colliculus. *Journal of Neurophysiology, 39,* 1081–1089.

Cole, E., and Gregory, H. (eds.), (1986). Auditory learning. *The Volta Review, 88,* 1–122.

Cornet, R. O. (1967). Oralism vs. manualism: Cued speech may be the answer. *Hearing and Speech News, 35,* 6–9.

Cornet, R. O. (1972). Cued speech. In G. Fant (ed.), *International Symposium on Speech Communication Ability and Profound Deafness.* Washington, DC: Alexander Graham Bell Association for the Deaf.

Craig, W. and Craig, H. (1972). *Verbotonal Instruction for Young Deaf Children: Questions and Replies.* Pamphlet from Western Pennsylvania School for the Deaf.

Downs, M. (1974). The deafness management quotient. *Hearing and Speech News, 42,* 8, 28.

Easterbrooks, S. (1987). Speech/language assessment and intervention with school-age hearing-impaired children. In J. Alpiner and P. McCarthy (eds.), *Rehabilitative Audiology: Children and Adults* (1st ed., pp. 188–240). Baltimore: Williams and Wilkins.

Elliott, L., and Katz, D. (1980). *Northwestern University—Children's Perception of Speech.* St. Louis: Auditec.

Erber, N. (1980). Use of the Auditory Numbers Test to evaluate speech perception abilities of hearing-impaired children. *Journal of Speech and Hearing Disorders, 45* (4), 527–532.

Erber, N. (1982). *Auditory Training.* Washington, DC: Alexander Graham Bell Association for the Deaf.

Erber, N., and Alencewicz, C. (1976). Audiologic evaluation of deaf children. *Journal of Speech and Hearing Disorders, 41* (2), 256–267.

Estabrooks, W. (1992). *Do You Hear That?* [videotape]. Toronto: VOICE for Hearing-Impaired Children.

Estabrooks, W., and Edwards, C. (1986). *Sure we can hear* [videotape]. Toronto: VOICE for Hearing-Impaired Children.

Finitzo-Hieber, T., Matkin, N., Cherow-Skalka, E., and Gerling, I. (1977). *Sound Effects Recognition Test* (SERT). St. Louis: Auditec.

Flexer, C. (1992). *Listening and Hearing: A Supplement to Technology in the Classroom.* Rockville, MD: American Speech-Language-Hearing Association.

Flexer, C. (1994). *Facilitating Hearing and Listening in Young Children.* San Diego: Singular Publishing Group.

Geers, A., and Moog, J. (1987). Predicting spoken language acquisition of profoundly hearing-impaired children. *Journal of Speech and Hearing Disorders, 52* (1), 84–94.

Goldberg, D. (1987). Auditory assessment and management of school-aged hearing-impaired students. *Texas Journal of Audiology and Speech Pathology, 13,* 13–18.

Goldberg, D. (ed.), (1993). Special focus section: Auditory-verbal philosophy: A tutorial. *The Volta Review, 95* (3), 181–263.

Goldberg, D., and Flexer, C. (1993). Outcome survey of auditory–verbal graduates: Study of clinical efficacy. *Journal of the American Academy of Audiology, 4,* 189–200.

Gustason, G. (1983). *Teaching and Learning Signing Exact English.* Los Alamitos, CA: Modern Signs Press.

Gustason, G., Pfetzing, D., and Zawolkow, E. (1980). *Signing Exact English: The 1980 Edition.* Los Alamitos, CA: Modern Signs Press.

Johnson, J., and Newport, E. (1989). Critical period effects in second language learning: The influence of maturational state on the acquisition of English as a second language. *Cognitive Psychology, 21,* 60–90.

Lane, H. (1990). Cultural and infirmity models of Deaf Americans. *Journal of the Academy of Rehabilitative Audiology. 23,* 11–26.

Layton, T., and Holmes, D. (1985). *Carolina Picture Vocabulary Test.* Tulsa, OK: Modern Education Corporation.

Lennenberg, E. (1967). *Biologic Foundations of Language.* New York: Wiley.

Ling, D. (1976). *Speech in the Hearing-impaired Child: Theory and Practice.* Washington, DC: Alexander Graham Bell Association for the Deaf.

Ling, D. (1989). *Foundations of Spoken Language for Hearing-impaired Children.* Washington, DC: Alexander Graham Bell Association for the Deaf.

Marler, P. (1970). A comparative approach to vocal learning: Song development in white-crowned sparrows. *Journal of Comparative and Physiological Psychology Monographs, 71* (No. 2, Part 2), 1–25.

Marlowe, J. (1993). Audiological assessment and management in the auditory–verbal approach. *The Volta Review, 95* (3), 205–215.

Maxon, A., and Brackett, D. (1992). *The Hearing Impaired Child: Infancy through High School Years.* Boston: Andover Medical Publishers.

Moeller, M. P., McConkey, A., and Osberger, M. J. (1983). Evaluation of the communicative skills of hearing-impaired children. *Audiology, 8,* 113–127.

Monsen, R., Moog, J., and Geers, A. (1988). *CID Picture Speech Intelligibility Evaluation (SPINE).* St. Louis: Central Institute for the Deaf.

Moog, J., and Geers, A. (1980). *Grammatical Analysis of Elicited Language—Complex Sentence Level.* St. Louis: Central Institute for the Deaf Press.

Moog, J., and Geers, A. (1990). *Early Speech Perception Test.* St. Louis: Central Institute for the Deaf.

Moog, J., Kozak, V. J., and Geers, A. (1983). *Grammatical Analysisof Elicited Language—Presentence Level.* St. Louis: Central Institute for the Deaf Press.

Moores, D. (1987). *Educating the Deaf: Psychology, Principles, and Practices* (3rd ed.). Boston: Houghton Mifflin Company.

National Institutes of Health (1993). *NIH Consensus Statement—Early Identification of Hearing Impairment in Infants and Young Children. 11* (1) March 1–3, 1–24, 1993.

Network of Educators of Children with Cochlear Implants. (1994). *Position Statement.* New York, NY.

Newport, R. (1990). Maturational constraints on language learning. *Cognitive Science, 14,* 11–28.

Northern, J., and Downs, M. (1984). *Hearing in Children* (3rd ed.). Baltimore: Williams and Wilkins.

Northern, J., and Hayes, D. (1994). Universal screening for infant hearing impairment: Necessary, beneficial, and justifiable. *Audiology Today, 6* (3), 10–13.

Owens, E., Kessler, D., Raggio, M., and Schubert, E. (1985). Analysis and revision of the Minimal Auditory Capabilities (MAC) Battery. *Ear and Hearing, 6* (6), 280–290.

Owens, E., Kessler, D., Telleen, C., and Schubert, E. (1981). The Minimal Auditory Capabilities (MAC) Battery. *Ear and Hearing, 34,* 9, 32, and 34.

Pappas, D., and McDowell, C. (1983). The sooner, the better: Identification and rehabilitation of the child with bilateral sensorineural hearing impairment. *Journal of the Medical Association of the State of Alabama, 52,* 34–37.

Paul, P., and Quigley, S. (1987). Some effects of early hearing impairment on English language development. In F. Martin (ed.), *Hearing Disorders in Children* (pp. 49–80). Austin: Pro-Ed.

Pollack, D. (1970). *Educational Audiology for the Limited-hearing Infant.* Springfield, IL: Charles C. Thomas.

Pollack, D. (1985). *Educational Audiology for the Limited-hearing Infant and Preschooler,* (2nd ed.). Springfield, IL: Charles C. Thomas.

Potts, P., and Greenwood, J. (1983). Hearing aid monitoring: Are looking and listening enough? *Language, Speech and Hearing Services in School, 14* (3), 157–163.

Quigley, S., Steinkamp, M., Power, D., and Jones, B. (1978). *Test of Syntactic Abilities.* Beaverton, OR: Dormac.

Ross, M., Brackett, D., and Maxon, A. (1982). *Hard of Hearing Children in Regular Schools.* Englewood Cliffs, NJ: Prentice Hall.

Ross, M., and Lerman, J. (1971). *Word Intelligibility by Picture Identification* (WIPI). Pittsburgh: Stanwix House.

Ross, M., and Randolph, K. (1988). *The Auditory Perception of Alphabet Letters Test* (APAL). St. Louis: Auditec.

Rupp, R., Smith, M., Briggs, P., Litvin, K., Vanachowski, S., and Williams, R. (1977). Feasibility scale for language acquisition routing for young hearing impaired children. *Language, Speech, and Hearing Services in Schools, 8,* 222–233.

Scherer, P. (1981). *Total Communication Receptive Vocabulary Test.* Northbrook, IL: Mental Health and Deafness Resources.

Scouten, E. (1964). *The Place of the Rochester Method in American Education of the Deaf.* Report of the Proceedings of the International Congress on the Education of the Deaf, pp. 429–433.

Sharpe, R. (1994, April 12). To boost IQs, aid is needed in first 3 years. *The Wall Street Journal.*

Stout, G. and Windle, J. (1992). *Developmental Approach to Successful Listening (DASL-II).* Englewood, CO: Resource Point.

Tonelson, S., and Watkins, S. (1979). *The SKI*HI Language Development Scale.* Logan, UT: SKI*HI Institute.

Trammell, J. (1981). *Test of Auditory Comprehension.* Portland, OR: Foreworks.

Vaughan, P. (ed.), (1981). *Learning to Listen.* New York: Bequfort Books.

Wilbur, R. (1987). *American Sign Language: Linguistic and Applied Dimensions* (2nd ed.). Boston: College-Hill Publication/Little, Brown and Company.

Zara, C., and Brackett, D. (1994). *Cochlear Implant Rehabilitation: No Need to Reinvent the Wheel.* Presentation at the Alexander Graham Bell Association for the Deaf Convention, Rochester, NY.

# CHAPTER 16

# EDUCATIONAL MANAGEMENT OF CHILDREN WITH HEARING LOSS

*CAROLYN EDWARDS*

## INTRODUCTION

In order for clinical audiologists to provide comprehensive auditory management for children with hearing loss, they must understand the educational systems in which the children are enrolled. Knowledge of the range of educational settings, the psychosocial implications of various settings, and the support personnel to which the children may have access is essential to counsel parents and children with hearing loss. With this information, the clinical audiologist can also modify current practices to enhance the relevance of clinical information to the educational system.

It is not hearing loss, per se, that creates the need for specialized services for many children with hearing loss. It is the limitations in the development of cognition and language resulting from the effects of reduced intensity and distortion of speech, or a fluctuating signal when recurrent otitis media is present, that affect academic performance. Modifications of room acoustics, use of technological aids, and changes in teaching strategies within the regular classroom can improve access to the teacher's speech signal. These changes alone will be sufficient for some children to progress satisfactorily within a regular school system. Other children with hearing loss, however, will need additional support in the form of tutorial or small group teaching as a result of language capabilities that are below grade level. The purpose of this chapter is to review the educational placement options and support personnel available to children with hearing loss and the important role that clinical audiologists may play in the educational success of these children.

## EDUCATIONAL OPTIONS

The choice of educational systems provided for children with hearing loss within a geographical region is limited by the low prevalence of sensorineural hearing loss. The student population of the average elementary school ranges from a few hundred children to a thousand children while the average secondary school population is typically one to two thousand students. It is therefore unlikely that a school or a small school district will contain sufficient numbers of children with hearing loss of similar age and similar communication needs to offer a wide range of educational options. Only large metropolitan areas or a group of adjacent school districts can offer a range of options from mainstream placement to schools for the deaf. Although children with recurrent otitis media account for a much larger number of children with hearing loss, these children do not require a variety of educational placements. They typically function satisfactorily within the regular classroom environment with provision of various acoustic modifications, possible amplification, and in-school support services.

Most boards of education or school districts offer some educational options for identified children with hearing loss at the preschool level, ranging from parent-centered home visiting programs to child-centered nursery schools. Various communication methodologies may be available within each of these options. When children reach school at age 4 or 5, parents must examine the new educational options available to their children (Table 16.1).

**TABLE 16.1** Educational Options

| TYPE OF SCHOOL SYSTEM | AMOUNT OF INTEGRATION |
|---|---|
| Public | Regular class |
| Private | Segregated class |
| Regular | |
| Segregated | |

| TYPE OF COMMUNICATION | TECHNOLOGY OPTIONS |
|---|---|
| Oral | Classroom amplification |
| Cued speech | Assistive listening or visual devices |
| Oral sign language | |
| Sign language | |

| EDUCATIONAL SERVICES | SUPPORT SERVICES |
|---|---|
| Itinerant teacher | Speech-language pathologist |
| Part-time or full-time teacher of the hearing impaired (school-based) | Educational audiologist |
| | Special education consultant |
| Notetakers | Hearing aid technician |
| Educational interpreters | Educational psychologist |
| Teacher's aide | Social worker |
| Resource teacher | |

Parents will often have to make choices about the best combination of options available to their children. Since clinical audiologists are often the first (re)habilitative professionals that parents meet following diagnosis of hearing loss in their child, audiologists need to be prepared for the many questions that parents may ask about the educational services that their children will need. *Audiologists new to a community should arrange a meeting with local school staff to acquaint themselves with the services for children with hearing loss in the local school district and the districts of surrounding regions.*

## Types of Educational Placements

The topic of educational placement has generated more controversy in the education of children who are hard-of-hearing and deaf than any issue in curriculum, speech, language, auditory skills training, or amplification practices. Although the educational options for children who are hard-of-hearing has received less attention and dispute, there are basic philosophical differences concerning education of deaf children. At issue is the desire of many hearing parents to have their deaf children grow up in the hearing community in an integrated setting. In contrast, the Deaf community wishes to have deaf children grow up using sign language in a Deaf culture within a school for the deaf. Both groups want deaf children to experience their respective cultures. The hearing community regards hearing loss as a sensory deficit and promotes early identification and fitting of hearing aids or cochlear implants. The Deaf community regards hearing impairment as a difference, not a deficit, and supports the use of sign language from birth.

Although the basic dichotomy between the two philosophies continues to exist, the divisions are no longer clear-cut. There are now overlapping options such as students in oral main-streamed programs learning sign language as a credit course and schools for the deaf jointly sharing facilities with schools for hearing children. As sign language becomes more visible on children's television shows, newscasts, and parliamentary/congressional proceedings, societal acceptance of sign language has changed. Conferences for adults with hearing loss offer both oral and sign language interpreters to ensure accessibility of information to all participants.

There is no single setting that is ideal, nor one setting that provides an emotionally secure learning environment for all children with hearing loss. Each educational setting has its benefits and limitations and presents different social and emotional issues for children with hearing loss. *It is not the educational setting itself that is potentially positive or negative; it is a mismatch between the child's communicative, academic, social, and/or emotional needs and an educational setting that will create difficulties.* Children's need for identification with other children with a hearing loss is often dependent on their perception of similarities and differences between themselves and others. The greater the perceived difference, the more impetus to seek out a group of children who are more similar to themselves. That is often why some integrated children with hearing loss have playmates from lower grades, whose language levels are more similar. Other children with hearing loss identify first with their hearing peers and may have no interest in associating with social clubs involving other children with hearing loss.

Although children with mild, moderate, and severe hearing loss with hearing parents are typically placed in the mainstream at the outset, degree of hearing loss is not a sufficient predictor of academic performance (Maxon and Brackett, 1987). Additional factors include the age of diagnosis and fitting of hearing aids, the appropriateness and amount of early intervention, family and community involvement, the child's personality, and the child's innate capabilities. It is the interaction of many factors that results in a broad range

of speech, language, and academic skills in students with hearing loss in regular education settings (Brackett and Maxon, 1986; Maxon and Brackett, 1987).

When U.S. Public Law 94-142 from the Education for All Handicapped Children Act was first published in 1975, its requirement that children be educated in the "least possible restrictive environment" was interpreted as supporting mainstreaming for all children. In fact, mainstreaming is not appropriate for all children. The fact that one out of every three children with sensorineural hearing loss has at least one additional developmental disability must also be considered (Karchmer and Kirwin, 1977). Ross, Brackett, and Maxon (1991) suggest that restrictive environments be redefined as those settings that limit the child's potential in a given classroom and that the least restrictive environment is the one that is most appropriate for the child.

### Regular School System: Mainstream Placement
Integration or mainstreaming in a regular classroom may foster growth in academic, linguistic, social, and/or emotional development. The ability to develop within all four of these areas depends on children's innate capabilities, the support personnel within the schools, and family support.

Children placed in the mainstream setting participate in most or all activities within a regular class with their peers. Children are most appropriately placed in a regular class when they have the receptive language skills to comprehend classroom material and conversations among peers and the expressive language skills to participate in class discussions and communicate with teacher and peers. The provision of a list of classroom management suggestions to the teacher can facilitate successful experiences in the mainstream (Appendix 9). The development of self-worth depends on children's ability to share experiences with peers (Davis, Shepard, Stelmachowicz, and Gorga, 1981; Gibson and Edwards 1994).

The advantage of regular class placement for children with hearing loss is the opportunity to be with their hearing peers of similar age, to experience the speech, language, and socialization models of hearing peers throughout the day, and to participate in the regular curriculum. Attending the school in their community also permits children to become involved in extracurricular activities with schoolmates from their neighborhood. For some children with hearing loss, however, the mainstreamed environment may enhance their feelings of difference from hearing children. This can occur if children with hearing loss are unable to communicate satisfactorily with their classmates or are unable to participate in the sharing of daily experiences. Davis and her associates (1981) reported that the children who were hard-of-hearing in their study had a much more difficult time making friends than their hearing counterparts. Given the low prevalence of hearing loss, mainstreamed children may not encounter any other children or adults with hearing loss. Introduction to children with hearing loss from other schools and to adults with hearing loss can reduce the sense of difference experienced by some children.

**Support Personnel.** Although discussion of support personnel within this chapter will focus on the services offered by school personnel, there is no substitute for family support in a child's de-velopment of self-worth and school progress. *It is important that in our counseling as audiologists, we acknowledge the role of parents and siblings and support family involvement throughout the school years.*

The extent of the support provided by the school depends on the child's needs and the nature of the support services in a particular school district. Table 16.2 provides examples of support personnel available for children in the mainstream. *There is considerable disparity in levels of support service from one region to the next. The clinical audiologist must be cognizant of the services offered through various school boards in the area. Knowledge of support personnel available to children with hearing loss permits the clinical audiologist to make appropriate referrals and assists in decision making about appropriate placements.*

**Communication Issues.**   Communication is the ability to send and receive messages among two or more people. In school, communication occurs:

- Between the child with hearing loss and the classroom teacher
- Between the child and teacher's assistant, where available

**TABLE 16.2**   Types of Support in the Mainstream Setting

| IN-SCHOOL SUPPORT | CLASSROOM SERVICES |
|---|---|
| Classroom teacher | Educational interpreter |
| Teacher's aide | Notetaker |
| Resource teacher | |
| Principal | |

| CONSULTING SERVICES | SCHOOL COLLABORATIVE TEAM |
|---|---|
| Teacher of the hearing impaired | Special education consultant |
| Educational audiologist | Psychologist |
| Speech-language pathologist | Social worker |
| | Other professionals on request (e.g., occupational therapist, pediatrician, psychiatrist, neuropsychologist) |

- Between the child and interpreter where available
- Among classmates
- Among children from other classes in the hallways or cafeteria
- Between the child and other teachers supervising extracurricular activities
- Between the child and administrative staff, such as school secretaries
- Among children on the playground

The ease of comprehension of speech for children with hearing loss depends on the clarity of articulation, the rate of speech and availability of speechreading cues of the speaker; the room reverberation, background noise, and distance from the speaker; and the auditory visual capabilities of the listener. The greater the hearing loss, the greater the challenges for everyday communication. A simulation of hearing loss using earplugs is a particularly effective way of increasing the classroom teacher's and classmates' awareness of the importance of clear articulation and speech reading. Optimizing the acoustic environment, however, has been sadly ignored in many mainstreamed programs and seriously limits children's ability to maximize their auditory capabilities (Montgomery and Matkin, 1992). Audiologists have rarely been involved in advising on acoustic design of regular schools; in fact, an acoustical engineer is not a mandatory member of the architectural team. *The clinical audiologist's advocacy for an optimal acoustical environment for children with normal hearing and children with hearing loss can provide support for the advocacy efforts of speech and hearing professionals in the school district.*

As discussed in Chapter 14, technology can greatly assist children in improving the speech signal delivered to their ears. However, certain situations continue to present auditory difficulties:

- Understanding announcements through public address systems (distortion in speech signal and reduced high-frequency response in the amplification system)

- Participating in conversations within the cafeteria (high noise levels, poor speech-to-noise ratio)
- Understanding instructions in the gymnasium (long reverberation times)
- Understanding school plays with a number of speakers (distance listening in highly reverberant rooms)
- Understanding conversations at lockers or in hallways (high noise levels and long reverberation times)

Buddy systems, in which a member of the class is asked to act as a "buddy" by repeating requested information, are particularly important during these situations. Note that the buddy may require some role-playing and demonstration to acquire the skills to assist children with hearing loss. *The clinical audiologist may wish to discuss some of these issues with parents and children during the counseling session.*

Although intelligible speech is not essential, children's abilities to communicate orally with peers and teacher will facilitate their integration in a regular school placement. Children who use sign language to communicate in the mainstream and require interpreters in the classroom can often feel isolated from the everyday camaraderie of school life. To improve communication, the teacher of the deaf and hard-of-hearing can create a sign language club that meets regularly to learn signs. At the high school level, American Sign Language may be taught for course credit, which can further increase the student's opportunities to talk with other students. More than in any other setting, children must learn to advocate for their communication needs in the mainstreamed environment.

### Regular School: Self-Contained Class
Children who are unable to follow the regular curriculum and need more than a few hours of tutorial support per week, may be placed in a self-contained class in a regular school. Typically children will be bussed from their own neighborhood to the designated school containing the self-

contained class(es) for children with hearing loss. Children will spend 25 percent or more of their time in a self-contained class of four to eight children, taught by a teacher of the hearing impaired.

The amount of integration into regular programs varies with the child's capabilities. However, the obvious reason to locate the self-contained class within a regular school is to take advantage of integration opportunities. Integration may occur for selected academic subjects, or only for subjects such as art, music, and physical education that have a lower linguistic load. Reverse integration, where hearing students are brought into the self-contained class, may also occur in these settings. Finally, team teaching with a regular teacher and the teacher of the hearing impaired occurs in some settings.

The small number of children results in a decrease in noise levels and speaker-listener distance and an increased ease of learning. The ability to monitor childrens' learning more closely to pinpoint where communication breakdowns are occurring, and the presence of a teacher of the hearing impaired who understands the learning problems faced by children with hearing loss, are advantages enjoyed in this setting. For the first time, the children may experience peers who also have hearing loss. This may decrease the sense of isolation sometimes experienced by children in mainstreamed settings.

The potential difficulty with self-contained classes is often the range of ages and abilities of children in the program. Because of the bussing arrangements, children in self-contained classes usually do not have the flexibility to participate in extracurricular activities scheduled after school. Surprisingly enough, the amount of one-to-one time with the teacher of the hearing impaired may not actually increase in a self-contained class versus a comprehensive itinerant service within a mainstreamed setting. Children may still experience the isolation between themselves and other students unless school staff are receptive to the class for children with hearing loss. It is necessary to create activities that bring children with hearing loss and the hearing children in the school together. In one school, children from the self-contained class created a "Hearing Day" for the rest of the school. A series of booth activities demonstrated different aspects of hearing loss through an earplug simulation of hearing loss, a captioned movie of an operation on the ear, a pseudo "sound suite" in which students could have their hearing tested, a technology booth, and a hearing ear dog demonstration.

**Support Personnel.** The key difference between the self-contained class and a fully integrated placement is the presence of the teacher of the hearing impaired as a full-time advocate for the needs of the child with hearing loss within the school. An educational interpreter would not be provided for the small self-contained class; any interpreting necessary would be done by the teacher of the hearing impaired. The resource teacher would function more as a coordinator for meetings than for programming assistance.

**Communication Issues.** As in the fully integrated setting, children in the self-contained class may use oral communication or some combination of oral and manual communication. Children relying on manual communication alone would be more likely to enroll in a school for the deaf.

Acoustic enhancement and accessibility of the educational setting is essential in any oral program. As in mainstreamed settings, these modifications would include acoustic treatment of the classroom, use of a variety of assistive listening devices, and arrangements for school announcements to be typed daily and posted in a central location. Where sign language is used by the children, the teacher and children may wish to conduct some inservice for school staff and schoolmates.

### School for the Deaf

The earliest educational settings for children with hearing loss were schools for the deaf. It is only with the advent of modern technology and wearable hearing aids that mainstreamed settings have become possible for children with hearing loss. Establishment of a school for the deaf necessitates a large population base from which children with hearing loss are drawn. Brill, Merrill, and Frisina (1973) suggested that a minimum of 40 children at the elementary level and 150 children at the secondary level is necessary to establish a local specialized program, although certainly smaller schools exist. Schools for the deaf can be oral, combined oral–sign language, or sign language only. They can be day schools in which all students are bussed to and from their homes daily, a situation typical in large metropolitan areas. Alternatively, the school may be a day-residential school where some students living too far away for a daily ride commute home on weekends only. Students at schools for the deaf typically have a profound hearing loss or are hard-of-hearing with additional learning difficulties that have not been addressed in the mainstream.

Due to the much higher numbers of children with hearing loss within a school for the deaf, there are more homogeneous groupings and programming geared specifically for the needs of children with hearing loss. There are greater opportunities for children to experience deaf and hard-of-hearing role models since a number of the staff are often deaf or hard-of-hearing, and there are more opportunities for exposure to Deaf culture. Since competition for leadership within school activities such as student council is only among students with hearing loss, there may be more opportunities for children with hearing loss to assume leadership positions. Although the students may be comfortable within the school community, they may have little contact with hearing peers and are usually quite isolated from children in their neighborhood. Their school friends are often in different cities or suburbs, limiting social contacts after school. Because of all of the time spent away from home, residential students often have a more limited relationship with their families than do day students.

*Many schools for the deaf operate resource centers providing outreach services to students with hearing loss enrolled in regular school programs. Clinical audiologists may find the resource staff's specific expertise with children with hearing loss helpful in monitoring children in the mainstream.*

**Support Personnel.**    Students with hearing loss in regular school programs have to stand in line with all other children with special needs when support services are requested. In the schools for the deaf, all services are dedicated to students with hearing loss, and support staff have specific expertise in providing services to children with hearing loss. In addition to the other professionals mentioned earlier in the chapter, some schools for the deaf may also employ a sign language specialist as a resource to signing programs.

**Communication Issues.**    For children in oral schools for the deaf, all of the teaching staff will be highly trained in clear oral communication. For children enrolled in schools for the deaf using sign systems, all of the teachers will have signing competencies and a number of the teachers themselves will be deaf and/or native signers. Some institutions also insist that administrative, clerical, and custodial staff acquire a minimum level of signing proficiency. This may be the only totally accessible environment that children in these schools will experience in their lives.

In addition to all of the acoustic and technological modifications available in other settings that are also essential in schools for the deaf, there are other communication options possible due to the large number of children with hearing loss in one location. In Canada, the most recently built school for the deaf in Burnaby, British Columbia, a joint project with a regular school for hearing students, includes television monitors in every classroom and all corridors so that the principal and others signing announcements in the front office are visible in real time, and two-way communication with students in the classroom is possible. Videophones may also be within the realm of possibility in the next few years.

### Combined Regular School and School for the Deaf

The combined schools are seen more frequently as a means to provide some integration between hearing and deaf students and to reduce the administrative costs of running two separate schools. Obviously the number of children within a school for the deaf is considerably less than the number of hearing students enrolled in an adjacent school. Therefore one of the key issues in shared schools is ensuring adequate representation of the interests of children with hearing loss, despite considerably lower enrollment. This can be addressed through a joint administration with equal voting power by the principal of the school for the deaf and the principal for the regular school.

Some integration may occur for selected students with hearing loss who are able to master the curriculum offered in the regular school. Some of the combined schools share sports teams and extracurricular activities, which creates more avenues for developing interaction among students. One joint school that I am familiar with creates a musical each year. The actual creation of the production prompts some hearing students to learn sign language, and deaf students to attempt to communicate with hearing peers. The final production is a play totally accessible to both student populations with a signing actor or actress for every voice part.

**Support Personnel.**   As with other educational settings, support personnel remain crucial to the students' success. Like the schools for the deaf, the combined schools employ support staff dedicated to the needs of students with hearing loss.

**Communication Issues.**   When facilities such as the cafeteria, the auditorium, and the school corridors are shared jointly by deaf students and hearing students, the deaf students again feel their differences on a daily basis. However, it does provide them with opportunities to experience the hearing community and to develop strategies for coping with communication breakdown in a supportive environment. It is essential to provide ongoing inservice for hearing students on the effects of hearing loss and ways to communicate successfully with students who have hearing loss.

## CHANGING NEEDS THROUGH THE YEARS

### Choice of Communication Methodologies

As discussed in the previous chapter, considerable evaluation and diagnostic teaching occurs in the preschool years to help parents select appropriate communication modes for their child. Regardless of the initial communication mode selected during preschool years, acknowledgement of the child's continual growth demands an ongoing review of the child's communication needs with teacher and peers throughout a child's academic career.

As part of the decision-making process for educational placement, review of communication needs of the child must be evaluated and discussed at least annually. Recommendations to change communication mode may necessitate a change in schools in some jurisdictions and may simply necessitate a change in personnel in other school districts. *The clinical audiologist's information about the child's ability to comprehend speech under a variety of conditions can contribute vital data to decisions about communication methodology.*

### Decision-Making Process for Educational Placement

Most school boards use a collaborative approach to determine the initial and subsequent educational placements for children with hearing loss. Parents should be informed of all of the available educational options and communication methodologies, and children should be involved in the decision making when they are ready. In addition to the assessment information provided by the collaborative team, the parents and child need an opportunity to visit various programs and to meet with the director/principal, the teacher, and various support personnel before making a decision on placement. Although academic and linguistic needs of children with hearing loss are often the foremost considerations in the selection of school setting or programs, sensitivity to the social and emotional needs of children with hearing loss is equally important. Parents and children are the final arbiters, for they are the ones who must live with their choices, not the educators.

Once a child has been placed in a particular program, the child's progress will be reviewed on a regular basis. The frequency of review is determined by the school board protocols or the legislation in that province or state. The design of an Individualized Educational Plan (IEP) or Special Education Plan (SEP) is part of the school review process. Some systems institute a formal review of a child's progress at the end of each school year, others review the child's progress informally at a school case conference, and others request a review only when concerns arise. Parents can request a review at any time. When a child is enrolled in a new program, I recommend an initial review after 3 months and then at the end of the school year. *It is very difficult to predict academic prognosis despite the parent's desire to hear it; the audiologist should be cautious of offering such statements to the family. The clinical audiologist may wish to ask the family about the results of the most current academic review during the audiologic assessment.*

## Transitions through Elementary and Secondary School

Educational demands change as the child moves through the elementary and secondary years. The focus in early primary grades is the development of socialization, creativity, discovery, and problem-solving. As the child moves into the higher grades, there is a greater emphasis on assignments, group projects, and large group discussion, which are more verbally challenging and require a good general knowledge base and language skills. *It is not uncommon to see children who were relatively successful at the primary level begin to demonstrate some academic or social difficulties later.*

Although the upper grades in elementary school include limited rotary (moving from class to class for different subjects), students in high school must adjust to different teachers for every subject and to a wide variety of teaching styles and expectations. Long gone is the one classroom teacher who understood the needs of the child with hearing loss. Now the students with hearing loss must educate each of eight teachers per year about their academic needs. At the same time, the importance of socialization and acceptance into peer groups increases. Many students with hearing loss struggle emotionally through this time, wanting to appear the same as other students, yet having to advocate for needs that emphasize their differences. The students in the mainstream may reject FM amplification at this point because use of the FM system highlights their differences from others. *As discussed in Chapter 10, clinical audiologists need to be sensitive to social and emotional issues that can arise at the high school level.*

The transition to college or university is outside the scope of this chapter. Suffice to say that students once again face tremendous communication challenges in large college lecture halls and benefit from strong support systems within their college or university to supplement their advocacy efforts. For extensive information about the college years, refer to the text by Flexer, Wray, and Leavitt (1990).

In-servicing of school staff at the beginning of the school year, selection of a case manager, and routine meetings with school staff are critical to meeting the needs of students with hearing loss in all school settings.

# ROLE OF THE CLINICAL AUDIOLOGIST IN EDUCATIONAL MANAGEMENT

## Interpretation of Audiologic Findings for the School

The purpose of the initial audiologic assessment is diagnostic in nature. Unfortunately, the information in the resulting report is often written for the medical profession rather than the educational staff at the child's school. The following suggestions are offered to the clinical audiologist to enhance the usefulness of the audiologic report for school staff. Additional report suggestions for educational and rehabilitation personnel may be found in Appendix 5.

### Unaided and Aided Audiogram

• The shape of the hearing loss can give the teacher of the hearing impaired and the speech-language pathologist information about the vowels and consonants that the child may detect and potentially identify. Describe the speech sounds that are easiest for the child to hear and those sounds that will be difficult to detect.

• The aided thresholds and/or insertion gain measures will give the teacher of the hearing impaired and the speech language pathologist specific information about the child's auditory potential to detect and identify suprasegmental and segmental features of speech, which will be useful in speech training. Describe the conditions under which various speech sounds will be audible to the child, any particular amplification strategies that might increase audibility, and the child's predicted potential to identify various vowel and consonant contrasts.

### Speech Audiometry

The pure-tone audiogram is the best understood piece of information by most educational personnel and unfortunately, may be the only audiologic data reported at school reviews. Therefore, it is important to emphasize the richness of the information provided by speech audiometry in the body of the audiologic report.

• The aided Speech Awareness Threshold (SAT) or Spondee Threshold (ST) will provide the classroom teacher with expectations for the child's minimum level of audibility of speech, from which the audiologist can extrapolate expected levels of response in the classroom. Describe the softest level of speech that the child detects/identifies under ideal conditions and suggest the minimum level of loudness necessary to obtain the child's attention in a noisy classroom.

• The aided Word Recognition Score (WRS) provides the speech-language pathologist, the teacher of the hearing impaired, and the educational audiologist with information for planning auditory programming and provides the teacher with expectations for speech recognition in the classroom. Describe the child's capability to identify single words with or without contextual clues. If you record the child's responses, note any consistent errors in back, mid, or front vowel recognition, and/or voicing, manner, or place contrasts for consonant recognition. Note any differences among scores by listening only, speech reading only, and combined listening and speech reading, or between scores in quiet and in noise. (The WRS is similar to a spelling test given without contextual clues.)

### Middle Ear Function

• Impedance or immittance testing provides the teacher, the teacher of the hearing impaired, the speech language pathologist, and/or the educational audiologist with information about temporary changes in hearing levels due to middle ear dysfunction. The child may be more fatigued in the classroom as a result of middle ear dysfunction. Based on your information, those providing specific auditory programming may choose to decrease the auditory demands until middle ear function returns to normal. Describe the effects of the middle ear dysfunction on unaided and aided hearing levels, and the audibility of the speech spectra for the child, relative to previous results.

### *Sample Comments from an Audiologic Report*

Johnny has a bilateral high-frequency precipitous sensorineural hearing loss, with poor speech recognition scores for single words presented at normal conversational level within close distance.

These results suggest the following:

- His hearing loss is permanent in both ears.
- He has normal hearing for the lower pitches of speech, meaning that his vowel perception will be quite accurate and that he should alert to his name being called at close distance.
- He has difficulty detecting and identifying the voiceless consonants such as s, f, voiceless th, t, k.
- He will have more difficulty understanding speech in noise than other students and will need to be alerted to listen before giving instructions.
- He will need context to understand what you or other children have said, due to the omission or reduced intensity of the voiceless consonants.

The above information refers to completion of the standard audiologic test battery. To provide additional information on the development of children's listening skills over time, there are a wide variety of auditory assessment tools available (see Edwards, 1991; Moeller, 1982). *Clinical audiologists who wish to offer comprehensive assessments of children's listening skills are encouraged to evaluate many of these tests.*

### *Requests for Information*

There are times when the clinical audiologist may request some information about a child's overall functioning at school to determine if amplification is warranted. Given the amount of paperwork required of teachers, it is not reasonable to request a narrative report of a child's performance. Instead, it will prove helpful if the school staff is provided with an outline of the specific information desired (see Anderson, 1989 and Appendices 10 and 11).

### Liaison with Educational Audiologist

*The educational audiologist is a bridge between the clinical audiologist and the school staff and is a valuable resource to the clinical audiologist.* The exchange of information between the clinical audiologist and the educational audiologist can enhance the auditory management of children with hearing loss by tracking changes in hearing levels, middle ear function, and/or auditory responsiveness, and through improved dialogue when selecting and managing personal and classroom amplification systems. The clinical audiologist should also check with the educational audiologist before making recommendations for a specific make and model of FM equipment for a child to ensure compatibility with the equipment carried by the school district.

### Parent Support Groups

As discussed in Chapters 9 and 10, it is important that the clinical audiologist and other support personnel provide parents of children with hearing loss with information about individuals or groups who may provide support to the parents and family. At various times in the child's life, the parents may wish to meet other parents of children with hearing loss, adults who are hard-of-hearing, adults who are deaf, or other parents of children with special needs. The degree to which the parents seek out other groups beyond their neighborhood community is dependent on the child's needs. Parents of children who are mainstreamed and require little formal assistance often leave support groups after the preschool years. Those parents whose children continue to require specialized services may continue with a group of parents with similar concerns. *The clinical audiologist must be aware of various parent support groups and contacts within the adult hard-of-hearing and deaf communities in his or her region.*

## In-service in the Clinic

The clinical audiologist can provide considerable in-service to parents, children, and school staff within the context of clinic assessment. The following ideas can easily be incorporated into clinic routines.

- Invite the parents to observe the assessment. This will give them more familiarity with audiologic terminology and procedures and give you an opportunity to find out if there are any discrepancies between the child's auditory performance in the home and in the clinic.
- Invite the classroom teacher, teacher of the hearing impaired, and/or speech language pathologist to observe the session. Do they see the child's performance in the clinic as consistent with what they observe in the classroom?
- Occasionally children ask if some of their hearing friends would be able to observe one of their audiologic assessments. By scheduling ahead of time, some clinics are able to offer the interested friends this opportunity to share an experience together.
- Parents of children with minimal or mild sensorineural hearing loss, or fluctuating conductive hearing loss often have difficulty understanding the auditory difficulties of their children. Give them a pair of disposable earplugs and ask them to wear them for a day on the weekend to experience more clearly the type of hearing loss their children have. Often the parents return with a new appreciation of the effects of hearing loss. As discussed in Chapter 3, audiologists' efforts may be better served if the term *mild hearing loss* were replaced with *educationally significant hearing loss* in discussion with parents.
- There are many videotapes available on various aspects of hearing loss. Parents and children often spend time in the audiology clinic waiting room prior to the appointment. Arrange to have a VCR in the waiting room and run instructional videotapes continuously throughout the day.

- Brochures about many aspects of hearing loss are available from any of the professional associations in the fields of speech, language, and/or hearing disorders and can be displayed in the waiting room.
- There are a variety of books available from consumers about their experiences (Appendix 6). Have a lending library for children and adults. Young children with hearing loss can enjoy reading story books about other children wearing hearing aids.
- To provide some consumer training for adolescents with hearing loss, have the students record vital information about their hearing aids and earmolds (such as make, model, internal settings, earmold material, type, tubing, and other modifications) prior to the electroacoustic check of their hearing aids. At the conclusion of the assessment, explain the audiologic results to the students privately, and then ask them to explain the results to their parents in your presence. This allows you to check on how well the student understood the information and initiates them in their first steps as an educated consumer.

## SUMMARY

Parents and children with hearing loss have many decisions to make over many years about educational placement, support services, and technological support. The clinical audiologist has a number of roles to play in those decisions—as provider of information about the receptive communication skills of the child, as a source of information about hearing loss in general, as a professional fostering the growth of the child, as a consumer of services, and as a liaison to student and parent support groups. Watching the child and family grow through their experiences over the years can be highly gratifying. Over time, we as professionals may see that there is no single decision that can ever be a mistake. The only mistake we make is the inability to change paths when children are conveying to us that they need something different than what they are currently receiving, whether it be in the context of academics, speech, and language skills, communication methodology, social circles, or emotional support.

# REFERENCES

Anderson, K. (1989). *Screening Instrument for Targeting Educational Risk (SIFTER)*. Austin: Pro-Ed.

Brackett, D., and Maxon, A. (1986). Service delivery alternatives for the mainstreamed hearing-impaired child. *Language, Speech and Hearing Services in the Schools, 17*, 115–125.

Brill, R., Merrill, E., and Frisina, D. (1973). *Recommended Organizational Policies in the Education of the Deaf*. Paper presented at the Conference of Executives of American Schools for the Deaf, Washington, DC.

Davis, J., Shepard, N., Stelmachowicz, P. and Gorga, M. (1981). Characteristics of hearing impaired children in the public schools: Part II. Psychoducational Data. *Journal of Speech and Hearing Disorders, 46*, 130–137.

Edwards, C. (1991). Assessment and Management of Listening Skills in School-Aged Children. In C. Flexer (ed.), *Seminars in Hearing 12*(4), 389–401.

Flexer, C., Wray, D., and Leavitt, R. (1990). *How the Student with Hearing Loss Can Succeed in College: A Handbook for Students, Families and Professionals*. Washington, DC: Alexander Graham Bell Association for the Deaf.

Gibson, C., and Edwards, C. (eds.), (1994). *Children and Youth with a Hearing Loss: Promoting Mental Health*. Ottawa, Ontario: Health Canada.

Karchmer, M., and Kirwin, L. (1977). *The Use of Hearing Aids by Hearing Impaired Students in the United States*. Washington, DC: Office of Demographics Studies, Gallaudet College.

Maxon, A., and Brackett, D. (1987). The hearing impaired child in regular schools. *Seminars in Speech and Language, 8*, 393–413.

Moeller, M. P. (1982). Hearing and speechreading assessment with the severely hearing-impaired child. In D. Sims, G. Walter, and R. Whitehead (eds.), *Deafness and Communication: Assessment and Training*. Baltimore: Williams & Wilkins.

Montgomery, P., and Matkin, N. (1992). Hearing-impaired children in the schools: Integrated or isolated? In F. Bess and J. Hall (eds.), *Screening Children for Auditory Function* (pp. 477–495). Nashville: Bill Wilkerson Center Press.

Ross, M., Brackett, D., and Maxon, A. (1991). *Assessment and Management of Mainstreamed Hearing-impaired Children*. Austin: Pro-Ed.

# CHAPTER 17

---

# EDUCATIONAL AUDIOLOGY

*JAMES C. BLAIR*

## INTRODUCTION

While the previous chapter provided an overview of the educational management options for children with hearing loss, this final chapter discusses the professional area of educational audiology. This chapter presents a general overview of the children audiologists work with, and of the full range of services provided by educational audiologists on behalf of these children. As will be seen in this chapter, the direct impact educational audiologists have on the educational services provided to children with hearing loss makes this segment of our profession both challenging and rewarding.

## HISTORY AND DEVELOPMENT OF EDUCATIONAL AUDIOLOGY

The concept of educational audiology is of recent origin. It roots are found in the advent of the hearing aid in the early 1900s, which for all practical purposes defined individuals who were hard-of-hearing rather than deaf. As hearing aids became available for common use by children, the problems associated with children who were hard of hearing began to be researched. According to Berg (personal communication, 1991), the first person to use the term *educational audiology* was Ann Mulholland in 1965. She was referring to those audiologists who tested children with hearing losses in the public schools.

## Early Awareness

One of the earliest reports on hard-of-hearing children (Davis, 1967) pointed out some of the significant learning problems that children who are hard-of-hearing experience in the schools. A year earlier Berg (Blair and Von Almen, 1991) developed a training program for educational audiologists to begin to address the issues of school children who are hard-of-hearing. His conceptualization of the educational audiologist was a combination of a teacher of the deaf and an audiologist. The work done by Berg and Fletcher at Utah State University lead to a text, *The Hard of Hearing Child* (1970). The text outlined the plight of the hard of hearing child and helped other researchers begin to focus their interests on this heterogeneous population. The recognition for the need for services began to be documented (Alpiner, 1978; Northcott, 1973; O'Neil, 1964; Ross and Giolas, 1978; Yater, 1978). By the end of the seventies the need for services for the child who is hard of hearing had become well documented.

## The Development of Educational Audiology

### The Impact of Public Law 94-142

The major impetus toward establishing educational audiology as a specialty came in 1975 with the enactment of Public Law 94-142, the Education for All Handicapped Children Act. Audiology was identified as an area of need to be met by the new law. This law indicated that the school audiologist was to be involved with the following: (1) the identification of children with hearing loss, (2) the determination of the range, nature, and degree of hearing loss, including referral for medical and other professional attention for the rehabilitation of hearing, (3) the provision of rehabilitative activities, such as language habilitation, auditory training, speech reading, hearing evaluation, and speech conservation, (4) the creation and administration of programs for prevention of hearing loss,

(5) the provision of counseling and guidance of pupils, parents, and teachers about hearing loss, (6) the determination of the child's need for group and individual amplification, and (7) the selection and evaluation of the effectiveness of amplification.

### Barriers to Implementation of Services

Even as services for children who are hard of hearing began to be identified through the establishment of the law, barriers began to emerge that blocked the way for implementation of this law. Sarnecky (1981) identified three barriers to effective program implementation: (1) Audiologists are unfamiliar with the administration of the public school, (2) school personnel are unfamiliar with the role and responsibilities of the audiologist in the schools, and (3) school personnel do not understand the characteristics and needs of children with hearing losses. Later, Wilson-Vlotman (1984) added a fourth barrier, stating that educational audiologists are inadequately trained in organizational theory. This lack of training deters them from effectively and efficiently managing the residual hearing of the child with a hearing loss.

### Model for the Delivery of Services

Blair and Berg (1982) suggested a model of delivery that would allow the educational audiologist to overcome the barriers that had been identified. In this model it was suggested that the educational audiologist needs to be involved in the management of the child with a hearing loss from identification through management of direct services provided to the youngster. In 1983 the American Speech-Language-Hearing Association (ASHA) published a position statement for audiology services in the schools. This document suggested that audiologists can make significant contributions to meeting the needs of school children with hearing losses and provided several models for implementing audiology services in the schools. Despite the various models for services that had been proposed, there was no information available about the actual practice of audiology in the schools.

### The Practice of Educational Audiology

In an attempt to determine the practices, attitudes, and organizational structures of educational audiology, Wilson-Vlotman and Blair (1984) sent a survey to all of the known educational audiologists in the United States who were working full-time in the schools. Based on responses from 245 educational audiologists, it was determined that audiologists in the schools spent most of their time in audiological assessments (almost 40 percent of the time) and in hearing aid work (15 percent of the time).

In 1989 Blair, Wilson-Vlotman, and Von Almen partially replicated the earlier study and found a slight, but interesting shift in the way time is spent. Table 17.1 contrasts the findings of the two studies. On the average, in 1984 educational audiologists spent 48 percent of their time each month on diagnostic tasks, with the greatest amount of diagnostic time devoted to audiologic assessment (36.6 percent). In contrast, in 1989 only 35 percent of the total time per month was spent in diagnostic tasks. The area of audiologic assessment had decreased to 25 percent, yielding the largest average difference between the two surveys. In 1984, 2.4 percent of the time was reportedly spent in central auditory assessment, but in 1989 this percentage decreased to 1.7 percent of the time. Even though these percentages were small in both surveys, there may be a trend for educational audiologists to be less involved in these evaluations.

One of the most encouraging results of the survey was in the area of amplification management. In 1984 only a little more than 14 percent of the educational audiologists' time was spent working with amplification systems. In 1989 this time increased to almost 23 percent. These results suggested that the educational audiologist was beginning to spend more time providing services that are critical to the child with a hearing loss.

Time spent in consultation and counseling was also examined. Consultation related to select-

**TABLE 17.1**  Average Percentage of Time Spent per Month by Educational Audiologists on Various Tasks (1984 compared to 1989) as Reported by Blair, Wilson-Vlotman, and Von Almen (1989)

| TASKS | TIME PER MONTH 1984 | TIME PER MONTH 1989 |
|---|---|---|
| *Diagnostic* | | |
| Screening | 9.3 | 7.5 |
| Audiologic assessment | 36.6 | 25.5 |
| Central auditory assessment | 2.4 | 1.7 |
| *Amplification Management* | | |
| Hearing aids/equipment | 11.7 | 18.4 |
| Earmolds | 2.7 | 4.3 |
| *Indirect Service* | | |
| Consultation | 8.8 | 10.3 |
| Counseling | 5.6 | 2.8 |
| *Direct Service* | | |
| Tutoring | 7.0 | 4.8 |
| Educational assessment | 1.5 | 3.7 |
| *Leadership* | | |
| Administration | 9.0 | 9.5 |
| Supervision | 4.2 | 3.5 |
| Research | 0.8 | 0.8 |
| Professional growth | NR | 3.2 |
| *Other* | 0.5 | 3.8 |

NR = no response.

ing appropriate classrooms in terms of noise and reverberation, recommending classroom seating, working with teachers and administrators, and attending case management meetings with staff and parents. Counseling provided parents and children with information and support in regards to hearing loss, academic concerns, or other issues. The amount of time spent in these activities in 1989 was somewhat variable, but, on the average, it was not too different from that reported in 1984.

The percentage of time spent each month on consultation and counseling was 14 percent in 1984 and 13 percent in 1989.

The total amount of time spent providing direct services to children with hearing loss was no different in 1984 than in 1989 (8.5 percent of the time), but it was noted that the distribution of the time was a little different. In 1984 the audiologists indicated that they spent 7 percent of their time in tutoring activities, in 1989 this dropped to 4.8 percent of the time. In the 1984 survey, the audiologists reported 1.5 percent of their time was spent in educational assessment, and in 1989 this activity was reported to take 3.7 percent of the time.

There was very little difference on the two surveys in the time spent in leadership activities. Of the total available time each month, the audiologists only used 14 percent of their time in 1984 and 17 percent of their time in 1989 in this area. The 1989 survey included one additional category, professional growth. Without this area, the time spent in leadership activities was the same in 1989 as in 1984.

When asked to express their views of the distinction between their own role and that of a clinical audiologist, 32 percent of the educational audiologists indicated that there was a very clear distinction between the two roles—60 percent indicated that there was a moderately clear distinction, and 7 percent indicated that there was no distinction. The role distinctions seem to be clearer in 1989 than they were in 1984. Thus, it is clear that the practice of educational audiology is in the process of evolving.

## The Growth of Educational Audiology

### The Educational Audiology Association

Part of the evolution of educational audiology was the formation of the Educational Audiology Association in 1983. The association started with 8 members, and currently has a membership of more than 600. The focus of the association has been to promote the comprehensive delivery of services to children with hearing loss in the public schools. The main activities of the association have been the publication of a quarterly newsletter, and a biennial monograph, a biennial summer conference, and yearly meetings held in conjunction with the ASHA convention.

The Educational Audiology Association defined the role of the educational audiologist in the following way: "An educational audiologist is a specialist who ensures that all aspects of a child's hearing and learning are maximized in order for their educational and real life capabilities to be met."

Along with the development of the Educational Audiology Association has been an increased level of awareness of educational audiology and what educational audiologists do in the schools. One of the *Seminars in Hearing* journals (Flexer, 1991) was entirely devoted to educational audiology issues and highlighted the advances that have been made in this area over the past 10 years.

### The 1993 ASHA Guidelines

In 1993 ASHA updated its guidelines for audiology services in the schools. Members of the Educational Audiology Association were invited to be on the committee who developed the guidelines. These new guidelines described the roles and responsibilities of the audiologist in the schools in a more comprehensive and expanded fashion than those developed in 1983. The new guidelines indicate that the educational audiologist's role is as follows:

1. Provide community leadership to ensure that all infants, toddlers, and youth with impaired hearing are promptly identified, evaluated, and provided with appropriate intervention services.
2. Collaborate with community resources to develop a high-risk registry and follow-up.
3. Develop and supervise a hearing screening program for preschool and school-aged children.

4. Train audiometric technicians or other appropriate personnel to screen for hearing loss.
5. Perform follow-up comprehensive audiologic evaluations.
6. Assess central auditory function.
7. Make appropriate referrals for further audiologic, communication, educational, psychosocial, or medical assessment.
8. Interpret audiologic assessment results to other school personnel.
9. Serve as a member of the educational team in the evaluation, planning, and placement process to make recommendations regarding placement, related service needs, communication needs, and modification of classroom environments for students with hearing impairments or other auditory problems.
10. Provide in-service training on hearing and hearing impairments and their implication to school personnel, children, and parents.
11. Educate parents, children, and school personnel about hearing loss prevention.
12. Make recommendations about use of hearing aids, cochlear implants, group and classroom amplification, and assistive listening devices.
13. Ensure the proper fit and functioning of hearing aids, cochlear implants, group and classroom amplification, and assistive listening devices.
14. Analyze classroom noise and acoustics and make recommendations for improving the listening environment.
15. Manage the use and calibration of audiometric equipment.
16. Collaborate with the school, parents, teachers, special support personnel, and relevant community agencies and professionals to ensure delivery of appropriate services.
17. Make recommendations for assistive devices (radio/television, telephone, alerting, convenience) for students with hearing impairment.
18. Provide services, including home programming if appropriate, in the areas of speech reading, listening, communication strategies,

use and care of amplification, including co-chlear implants, and self-management of hearing needs (pp. 28–29).

### The Future of the Educational Audiology Association

Recently the Educational Audiological Associa-tion (EAA) has proposed some long-range plans to support the expanded role of educational audi-ologists. Some of the areas that were targeted for development were a speakers' network to provide presentations at professional meetings; the devel-opment of information packets to be used in the schools as a means for educating parents, teach-ers, and administrators; the development of a graduate level course outline with support mate-rial to improve preprofessional training in educa-tional audiology; and expanded publications and continuing education offerings for the members of EAA and other audiologists.

The current mission statement of the Educa-tional Audiology Association is:

> The Educational Audiology Association (EAA) is an international organization of audiologists and related professionals whose primary interest is the comprehensive management of individuals from birth through graduation from school in all educa-tional environments who have listening and/or hearing difficulties. The EAA advocates for the ac-cessibility of educational audiology services for all individuals and provides opportunities for the continuing education of its members. (Educational Audiology Monograph, 1989, p. 14)

## CHILDREN WITH HEARING LOSSES

It is not always easy to interpret prevalence of hearing loss in children from birth through 18 years of age. However, there are some estimates of prevalence. Berg (1986) and Lundeen (1991) have estimated that within a population of 1000 school-age students, 7 have bilateral and 16 to 19 have unilateral hearing losses. Included in this number are children with sensorineural hearing losses as well as children with middle ear infec-tions resulting in conductive hearing losses

greater than 25 dB. It has been suggested by Bess (1985) that the incidence of children with minimal or fluctuating hearing losses due to otitis media may be as high as 30 percent at some ages. In ad-dition, there are a significant number of children who have central auditory processing problems. The prevalence of children who are deaf is about 1 percent of the population.

The general effects of hearing loss are also dif-ficult to clearly articulate, since there is such great variability in the way children respond to their hearing losses. It is known that the earlier the hear-ing loss occurs in life, the more serious the effects upon the child's development. However, it is also true that the earlier the loss is identified and habili-tation begins, the less serious the ultimate impact.

The Guidelines for Audiology Services in the Schools (ASHA, 1993) suggest that hearing loss affects children in four major ways, causing: (1) a delay in the development of receptive and expres-sive communication skills (speech and language); (2) a language deficit that causes learning prob-lems that result in reduced academic achievement; (3) communication difficulties that often lead to social isolation and poor self-concept; (4) an in-fluence on vocational choices. These four prob-lems interact to create several "common characteristics," that impact on the vocabulary, sentence structure, academic achievement, and psychosocial functioning of the child.

### Slight and Mild Hearing Loss

Anderson and Matkin (1991) published a chart that describes the relationship between varying degrees of long-term hearing loss and the psycho-social impact of the loss and educational needs of the child. In this display children with hearing losses in the 16 to 25 dB HL range are described as having difficulty hearing faint or distant speech. With 15-dB loss the student can miss up to 10 percent of the the speech signal when the teacher is at a distance greater than 3 feet or when the classroom is noisy. (see Table 17.2.) This is especially true in kindergarten through third grade where verbal instruction predominates. Since the

TABLE 17.2 Summary of What Children Can Hear without Amplification by Degree of Hearing Loss

| DEGREE OF LOSS | DESIGNATOR | CONVERSATION MISSED WITHOUT AMPLIFICATION |
|---|---|---|
| 15 dB | Slight | 10 percent |
| 30 dB | Mild | 25 to 40 percent |
| 35 dB | Mild | 50 percent |
| 40 dB | Moderate | 50 to 75 percent |
| 50 dB | Moderate | 80 to 100 percent |
| 56–70 dB | Moderately severe | 100 percent |
| 71–90 dB | Severe | Loud voices only (1 foot from ear) |
| 91+ dB | Profound | Vibrations (not any tonal patterns) |

average distance between the student and a teacher is 12 feet and the signal-to-noise (S/N) ratio of a classroom is generally about +3 dB, it is likely that these children will experience some difficulty in the classroom. Anderson and Matkin (1991) suggest that children with minimal losses may be unaware of subtle conversational cues, causing the child to be viewed as inappropriate or awkward. The child may miss portions of fast-paced peer interactions that could begin to have an impact on socialization and self-concept. These children may also exhibit immature behavior and may show signs of inattention due to the strain of listening so hard all the time. It is unlikely that these children will actually fail a grade or qualify for special services. Their problems are more subtle, and their performance is at the low end of normal. The impact is therefore more likely to be poor self-image or self-esteem.

The child with the mild hearing loss (26–40 dB HL) experiences even greater problems. Anderson and Matkin (1991) suggest that with a 30-dB hearing loss the child may miss 25 to 40 percent of the speech signal. The degree of difficulty experienced in school will depend upon the noise level in the classroom, the distance from the teacher, and the configuration of the hearing loss. Without amplification the child with a 35- to 40-dB loss may miss at least 50 percent of class discussions, especially when voices are faint or the speaker is not in the line of vision. These children will not hear many of the consonants of speech, particularly when there is a high-frequency hearing loss present. Unfortunately, research suggests that children with hearing losses of 30 dB or less are unlikely to wear hearing aids, even though they can benefit from them (Davis, Shepard, Stelmachowicz, and Gorga, 1981). Those with losses of 35 to 40 dB will use amplification when they are fitted, but these children are usually identified late and miss a great deal of information during the early language-development years. Anderson and Matkin (1991) suggest that for these children barriers begin to build between the child with hearing loss and the peer group. Often these children are accused of hearing when they want to or of not paying attention. The child with a mild hearing loss begins to lose the ability for selective hearing and has increasing difficulty suppressing background noise, which makes the learning environment stressful. These children generally suffer a significant delay in vocabulary and the use of abstract concepts. They frequently experience a sense that they are less capable than their hearing peers and feel a sense of worthlessness. As suggested earlier, this group of youngsters is at high risk for social and emotional difficulty. Again, like those with slight hearing losses, these children rarely fail at school-related activities; they just score low on all the tests and are often viewed as being among the "slower" children.

## Moderate Hearing Loss

The child with a moderate hearing loss (41–55 dB HL) will understand conversational speech at a distance of 3 to 5 feet only if structure and vocabulary are controlled. If the child does not wear amplification, the amount of speech signal missed can be 50 percent to 75 percent with a 40-dB loss and 80 to 100 percent with a 50-dB loss. These children are likely to have delayed or defective syntax, limited vocabulary, imperfect speech production, and frequently an atonal voice quality. Often the impact on academics is significant with a 2- to 3-year delay in academic achievement common. These students generally present a "spotty" profile in that they will perform similarly to their peer group in some areas, such as math computation, but they will have significant delays in language-based areas, notably reading. Often they will develop good word-attack skills and, when asked to read aloud, will do so surprisingly well. Despite this their reading comprehension is very poor. The student with a moderate hearing loss will have difficulty following directions and participating in group discussions. Often these children associate well with their peer group until adolescence, and then there is generally a severe impact on self-esteem and peer interactions. Frequently there is a denial of hearing loss during this period and a rejection of hearing aids and/or hearing assistance technologies. Although these children seem to hear everything when amplified, it is apparent that they miss a tremendous amount of information and tend to misunderstand what is meant in a communicative exchange. One area in which their difficulties becomes very apparent is written language, which is generally full of significant syntactical and morphological errors. They also have considerable difficulty in clarity of expression.

## Moderately Severe Hearing Loss

The child with a moderately severe hearing loss (56–70 dB HL) will not hear conversational speech and will miss 100 percent of speech information without amplification. These youngsters experience marked difficulty in school situations that require verbal communication, both in one-to-one and group situations. The student with a moderately severe loss will usually demonstrate delayed language, delayed syntax, reduced speech intelligibility and atonal voice quality. In school settings these children will typically be significantly delayed, a 3-year academic delay is generally expected. However, there is great variability

within this population depending on the benefit derived from amplification. These children will often demonstrate poor comprehension of reading materials and yet will give the appearance that they are able to read. Even with full-time use of hearing aids or FM systems these students are often judged by both peers and teachers as less competent learners, resulting in poorer self-concept, a high degree of dependence on others, and frequently a sense of rejection.

## Severe Hearing Loss

The child with a severe hearing loss (71–90 dB HL) will hear loud voices only when spoken 1 foot from the ear unless amplification is worn. When these children wear amplification devices, optimally, they should be able to identify environmental sounds and detect all the sounds of speech. If the hearing loss is of prelinguistic onset, oral language and speech may not develop spontaneously or will be severely delayed. If the hearing loss is of recent onset, speech is likely to deteriorate with the voice quality becoming atonal. Often these children prefer other children with hearing losses as friends and playmates. This may further serve to isolate the child from the mainstream; however, peer relationships may foster improved self-concept over those with less severe losses. These children may develop a cultural identity with the Deaf, but they are often in the area between the hearing and the Deaf and may not have a clear sense of an identity at all.

## Profound Hearing Loss

Children with profound hearing losses (91 dB HL or more) are generally aware of vibrations but not of any tonal patterns. The detection of speech sounds is dependent upon the configuration of the loss and the ability to use amplification. Most of the children in this group rely on vision, rather than hearing, as their primary avenue for communication and learning. Speech and language will not develop spontaneously and are likely to deteriorate rapidly if the hearing loss is of recent onset. Generally speaking, if this child is not placed into an appropriate educational environment providing a good language base, the child will be functionally illiterate, will probably develop no true reading or writing skills, and will generally be forced to work in a job that is below his or her true potential. On the other hand, if this child is placed in a language-rich environment with a visual input, the child has all the potential of a normal-hearing child. This child is not a good candidate for mainstreaming unless there is a large group of other children with profound hearing losses with whom this youngster can interact.

### Unilateral Hearing Loss

The child with a unilateral hearing loss may have difficulty with faint or distant speech. Usually these youngsters have difficulty localizing sounds and voices, and they experience considerable difficulty understanding speech when the environment is noisy and/or reverberant. They demonstrate difficulty understanding soft speech from the side of the bad ear, particularly during a group discussion. These children may be accused of selective hearing due to discrepancies in speech understanding in quiet versus noise. As a day progresses these children may become tired from the expenditure of energy in listening. This fatigue may cause them to be inattentive or to demonstrate frustration by exhibiting behavior problems.

### Other Auditory Problems

In addition to children with educationally significant sensorineural losses of hearing sensitivity, there are students with fluctuating conductive hearing losses and those with central auditory processing disorders. The literature is not always clear concerning the magnitude of the problems that these two groups exhibit, but it is clear that both groups experience language deficits that lead to concerns about both identification and treatment. Unfortunately, neither group is easily identified, and protocols for management are not well-defined. Although there are guidelines for acoustic immittance screening (ASHA, 1990), the implementation of these guidelines, and even the efficacy of these guidelines in the school setting, has not been clearly delineated. There is even less formalization of procedures for central auditory processing, and there is no clear set of guidelines to follow in habilitation of children with central auditory problems.

## SERVICES NEEDED AND A DESCRIPTION OF EDUCATIONAL AUDIOLOGY

Although the concept of educational audiology is well established in the literature, there is still a crying need for these professionals in public school systems. With the federal mandates for services dictated by Public Law 94-142 (Education of All Handicapped, 1975) and Public Law 99-457 (Education of the Handicapped Amendments, 1986), the call for audiologic services in schools is becoming apparent and will continue to become more apparent with implementation of the Americans with Disabilities Act (1990). However, there are still only a few training programs that offer a full range of coursework in the area of educational audiology. According to the ASHA guidelines (1993), there should be one audiologist for every 12,000 children. Since there are approximately 39.5 million children in the public schools in the United States, this would place the need for educational audiologists above 3000. Currently ASHA estimates that there are only about 1000 full-time educational audiologists in the United States. This huge discrepancy is present because most school districts do not see a need for audiologists in their schools. Obviously a great deal of work needs to be done to help training programs and school systems realize the scope of training required and the need for these services in the schools.

### Ideal Delivery of Services

When audiologists are employed in the schools, what do they do under ideal circumstances? If there were an audiologist for every 12,000 children, it would be quite feasible to meet the guidelines suggested by ASHA (1993) and described by the model proposed by Blair and Berg (1982). This model was developed to demonstrate how audiologists could meet the identified needs of children with hearing losses in the public schools. Basically the model proposes that there are five essential competencies for a professional attempting to provide appropriate services to children with hearing losses. These competencies are to be able to: (1) obtain, integrate, and synthesize diagnostic information; (2) obtain additional educational and audiologic test results; (3) evaluate the available environmental and educational resources; (4) plan appropriate programs; and (5) implement these programs.

The proposed model is illustrated in Figure 17.1. Notice that the model is divided into nine components: the identification of children with hearing loss through effective screening programs; the diagnostic evaluation through both audiologic and otologic procedures; the assessment of language, speech, listening, cognition, emotion, motor, and academic skills by careful coordination of professionals working together to assess these areas; the selection, care, and management of amplification systems; the systematic evaluation, selection, or modification of classrooms; the appropriate selection, training, and support of classroom teachers; the training and support of school administrators; parent training and support; and direct provision of listening training or other services to children with hearing losses.

There are at least two different models for delivery of audiology services in the schools, the school-based model and the contractual agreement (ASHA, 1993). Interestingly, a study com-

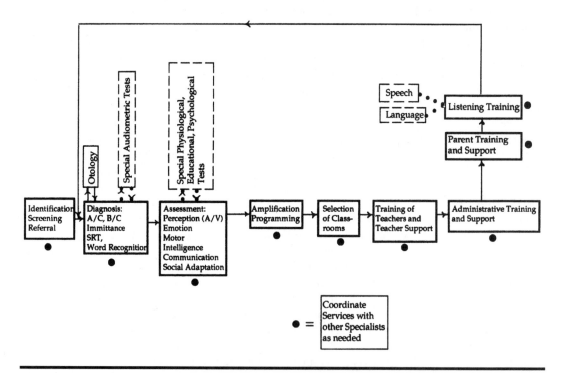

FIGURE 17.1   Delivery of services by the educational audiologist. The solid lines indicate that the educational audiologist will be directly involved with these activities. The dotted lines indicate that the educational audiologist may be involved with these activities.

pleted in Missouri (Allard and Golden, 1991) found that school-based models were superior to other forms of delivery, including some combinations of the two basic models. A major problem with the contractual arrangement is that schools will purchase only those services that they can afford from the contractor. In many instances this ends up being only part of the services that children with hearing losses really need in the schools. If the audiology contract would provide all of the services described in this chapter, then it might be just as effective as school-based models. This area needs to be explored more completely to determine what model or perhaps combination of models might be the best.

## THE IDEAL PRACTICE OF EDUCATIONAL AUDIOLOGY

### Screening

As can be seen in Figure 17.1, the first task of the educational audiologist is to establish an appropriate hearing screening program. Guidelines for screening are discussed in Chapter 5 and will not be the focus of this chapter. Instead, some frequently overlooked issues that need to be addressed in schools will be discussed. Although ASHA (1985) has published guidelines for puretone hearing screening, many school districts are at a loss as to what to do. As a director of special education said in a letter to me a few years ago: "Isn't there some rationale for increasing the levels at which we screen? We are finding too many children with mild hearing losses who are not having difficulty in school." It may be appropriate for audiologists to examine the levels at which they screen in light of the purpose of their screening programs and then communicate this information to the administrators. We need to do a better job of deciding what we are looking for in a screening program and what is going to be done about it once we have identified the children.

Immittance screening is even less clear, at least in terms of what we are looking for and why. If we are trying to find all children with middle ear problems, then screening once a year in the fall really makes no sense at all. We all know that middle ear problems for most children under 8 years of age are of a fluctuating nature. That means that at certain times of the year there will be a problem, and at other times there will be no problem. We need to screen more often. Also, once we have identified the children, if we are not completing follow-up studies over time, we are not providing the right kind of service to them. Too often it is the policy of a school program to identify children using immittance screening and then refer the child to a physician to determine if the child has a problem. The physician, in most instances, will use a nonpneumatic otoscope, which is less sensitive to changes in the middle ear than the immittance meter, and declare to the parent that there is no problem. The child goes back to school and may continue with an unresolved conductive hearing loss. If we are not following the child with tympanometry, there is no way to know if the child is better. We need to do a better job of screening, of working with local physicians to be certain that a child gets middle ear problems under control, and of monitoring the status of the child's middle ear system over time.

### Diagnosis of Hearing Loss— Audiometry in the Schools

While audiologists are generally well trained to work in a clinical setting, few have any training for working in a school setting. The needs of the consumer in schools are different from the needs in a clinical setting. Generally, for an adult client there is a need to have information that will lead to the appropriate fitting of a hearing aid or other rehabilitation. In the schools there is a need to fit the hearing aid and then to provide information to the classroom teachers that will allow them to teach that child in the most effective manner. This expanded need suggests that we should concentrate on speech testing in simulated or real classroom conditions. The classroom teacher needs to know what the child **can** hear, not what the child cannot hear. The teacher will benefit from knowing what modality works best for communication. Thus our speech recognition testing should be in a background of noise with the hearing aid on. The S/N ratio ought to be as close to the classroom environment as possible (+3 to +6 dB), and conditions that the child will likely encounter (auditory alone, auditory-visual together, visual alone) should be simulated. It might be useful to test at normal speech levels (50 dB HL) and at quiet speech levels (35 dB HL) to simulate the effects of distance on word recognition abilities. It would be helpful if the audiologist would use both single words and sentences to help the teacher understand what to expect from the child. These scores should then be reported to teachers in a document that is less than a page in length and simply states what the child can hear and what conditions must be met in order for this to happen.

## Assessment of Abilities

Unfortunately, we know that decisions about children with hearing loss are frequently made with little or no diagnostic information (Davis et al., 1981). The audiologist should be in a position to have expert information to provide about the child to establish the Individualized Education Plan (IEP). This suggests that the audiologist must be knowledgeable about hearing, but also about tests that can be used to assess children with hearing losses, or the audiologist should facilitate the completion of comprehensive testing before an IEP is written. The areas we need to make certain are covered are auditory and visual perception, psychosocial status, motor, intelligence, communication, and social maturity.

### Visual Problems

There is considerable evidence that children with hearing loss are at risk for other disabilities (Moores, 1982; Scheetz, 1993; Schildroth and Karchmer, 1986). It is also clear that visual problems among children with hearing losses are certainly as prevalent as among children with normal hearing and potentially occur more frequently. Yet there is little evidence to suggest that visual difficulties beyond those detected in a routine screening for nearsightedness, are ever considered when

evaluating children with hearing losses. It would be appropriate for the educational audiologist to suggest that a careful and complete visual evaluation of a child with a hearing loss be required before a new school year has begun, or at least that there be a record of such having been completed in the last 3 years.

### Emotional–Psychosocial Problems

In order for the child with the hearing loss to be educated properly, the child's psychosocial development and status need to be carefully considered. The literature extending back into the seventies (Nix, 1976) suggests that one of the best predictors of successful mainstreaming for children with hearing losses is their personality. Children who are well-adjusted, outgoing, and flexible have a far better chance of succeeding in the mainstream than do children who have a poor self-image, regardless of magnitude of hearing loss. Yet it seems that the whole area of psychosocial adjustment is often ignored (Davis et al., 1981).

### Motor Problems

The literature suggests (Mykelbust, 1960) that children with hearing losses are at risk for motor problems, particularly in gross motor balance. Yet there is no evidence to suggest that this area is even considered when discussing programs for the child who is deaf or hard-of-hearing. This certainly is worth examination before school placement is contemplated.

### Cognitive Abilities

Although the literature is not clear concerning the cognitive abilities of children who are deaf or hard of hearing, it is abundantly clear that most of these youngsters do not score as well on verbal tasks as do children with normal hearing. Certainly this is not a function of intelligence, but it does bear careful examination when considering the child's ability to compete with children who hear normally. It is also clear that there are those children who are deaf or hard of hearing who do not have the intellectual ability to successfully understand the information presented in typical fashion in the regular classroom even if their hearing had been normal. If a child has a cognitive deficit and a significant hearing loss, the effect is much greater than if the child possessed only one such deficit.

### Communication Abilities

There can be no attempt to make recommendations to a classroom teacher concerning a child's educational program without a complete assessment of the child's communication abilities. At a minimum the child with a hearing loss should be assessed following the schema suggested by Brackett (1982). Brackett divided the communication assessment into six areas: (1) the reception of spoken language, (2) the comprehension of spoken language, (3) the production of spoken language, (4) the production of speech, (5) the comprehension and production of written language, and (6) communicative competence. There is not space here to discuss this process in detail; however, it is critical that these areas be examined carefully before recommending classroom placement for a child with a hearing loss (see Blair, 1986, or Brackett, 1982, for a detailed discussion).

### Social Maturity

One of the primary functions in the assessment process is to determine how well an individual is able to function in society. Education is designed to help individuals obtain a level of independence such that they can work, live, and enjoy a happy, independent, and productive life. Too often the assessment of children leaves out the area of adaptation and only assesses academic achievement. Some measure of the child's adaptive skills needs to be in the child's folder in order to determine if more efforts in this area should be expended to enhance the child's independence. Too often children with hearing losses are trained to be too dependent on others (McCrone, 1979). For further information on assessment, the reader is referred to Salvia and Ysseldyke (1991) and Blair (1986).

## Amplification Management

It is obvious that the audiologist is the one professional who needs to be involved in the management of amplification systems in the schools. It is also clear that hearing aids and FM systems continue to malfunction at an alarming rate in the schools (Lipscomb, Von Almen, and Blair, 1990). If one area could be chosen that would have the potential for making the largest impact on children with hearing losses, wearing a functional hearing aid all day would be the area. Yet there is much evidence to suggest that the daily monitoring of hearing aids in the public schools is essentially nonexistent. Every teacher that has a child with a hearing loss needs to have instruction on troubleshooting hearing aids and have the materials to do the minor repairs that are necessary to keep them functional. Lipscomb and colleagues (1990) explain this process in detail.

A study currently underway suggests that FM systems need to be monitored just as much as hearing aids. Again, there is little evidence in the literature to suggest that an appropriate level of monitoring is ongoing in the schools. There is much work that needs to be done to provide the minimum amount of service in the area of amplification that children with hearing losses deserve.

Current emphasis on cochlear implants and the continuing need for auditory stimulation and training make it more critical that audiologists work with children in the schools. Too many children with cochlear implants are sent into the school systems with no one present to provide the guidance, stimulation, and monitoring necessary to ensure maximum use of these highly sophisticated and very expensive instruments. The need to follow children with cochlear implants is ever increasing, but the issue seems to be ignored by most school programs.

Finally, it is clear that there is a large body of children who, as they move into adolescence, modify their amplification systems by trying to make their amplification devices invisible. There are also a large number who refuse to wear any amplification. Unfortunately, creative, yet effective, methods for helping these youngsters continue to use amplification have not been developed. With appropriate intervention strategies, many of these youngsters could be helped to keep their amplification systems on and working through the crucial adolescent period. Without appropriate support and flexibility, too many spend 3 to 5 years without appropriate, and in many instances, no, amplification.

## Classroom Selection

Berg (1994) indicates that the area of classroom acoustics has been largely ignored by professionals in audiology. Yet research indicates that this area of study is critical if children with hearing losses are going to be able to reach their potential in school. We have known since 1975 (Finitzo-Hieber and Tillman, 1978) that noise and reverberation can make a significant difference in the word recognition ability of all children, but especially children with hearing losses. Yet there are few audiologists who actually select the classroom in which a child with a hearing loss needs to be placed. Barton (1989) found that the average S/N ratio in elementary schools was +3 to +6 dB. The literature suggests that an optimal classroom for children with hearing losses needs to have a S/N ratio of at least +12 dB, and preferably +20 dB, but there is often no attempt to even measure noise in the schools.

Research dating back to 1967 (Moncur and Dirks) suggests that reverberation is also a problem in classrooms. Finitzo (1988) reports that reverberation times in classrooms range from greater than 1 second down to .6 second. We have known for at least 20 years that reverberation times above .6 seconds are detrimental to children with hearing losses. Yet there is no protocol developed for the measurement of reverberation times in the schools.

In the schools a typical scenario is that we fit hearing aids on children and demonstrate in quiet that their scores are good enough that they should be able to do well in the mainstream. Then we place these children into acoustical conditions that make it impossible for them to use their hearing aids effectively. We essentially cause the child who is hard of hearing to function more like a deaf child. It is very important that audiologists begin to address the need for an environment in which noise and reverberation are at a minimum, or at least insist that children with hearing losses be fitted with FM systems to overcome the effects of noise and reverberation.

There is some compelling evidence to suggest that regular classrooms need to be fitted with appropriate sound-field amplification as discussed further in Chapter 14 (Berg, 1994). This will effectively improve the S/N ratio in the classroom, but if we are unwilling to deal with issues of reverberation the sound-field systems will still be less than adequate.

## Teacher Considerations

There is a thrust in special education for the inclusion of all children with disabilities into a regular public school classroom. While this movement may help many children to make better adjustments to society, it certainly places a large burden on the classroom teacher. Placing a child who is hard of hearing into the regular classroom without any support help makes no sense at all. There is ample evidence that hearing aids and FM systems must be monitored and maintained on a daily basis (Lipscomb et al., 1990; Thibodeau and Saucedo, 1990). Yet there is no provision for the classroom teacher to know the slightest thing about amplification. It is clear that many children who are hard of hearing require some extra help, yet often the help that is given is in the form of letters, checklists, or suggestions for the teachers to follow (EuDaly, 1993). Children with hearing losses are expected to get the same chance at an education as do children with normal hearing, yet the teacher, who is responsible for the educational growth of the child, is frequently uninformed about the needs of the child (EuDaly, 1993).

In order to provide meaningful support to classroom teachers, the following goals should be met: (1) Children need to be adequately assessed both audiologically and educationally before they are placed in a classroom; (2) Information from the tests must be communicated to the classroom teacher in a manner that is clear and understandable; (3) The teacher must be provided with appropriate training and given ongoing support; and (4) There must be some kind of amplification trouble-shooting program in the classroom.

### Direct Contact with the Classroom Teacher

Perhaps one of the best ways available to meet these objectives is through the implementation of a program similar to the one presented by Dodge and Mallard (1992), who describe a communication lab that is implemented once a week, for 30 minutes each time for a period of 9 weeks, in a regular classroom. The lab is designed to teach all children about good communication. Some of the topics suggested for this lab are observation, body language, listening, turn-taking, inflection, criticism and praise, and success and failure. If an educational audiologist or other related professional were to use this approach and add to it information on hearing loss and troubleshooting hearing aids, the children in the classroom and the teacher would learn how best to work with the child with a hearing loss as well as how to improve their communication with each other.

EuDaly (1993) recommends that audiologists who work in the schools have more direct contact with the classroom teacher. At the present time the only method that has been demonstrated to be effective with the classroom teacher is direct teacher contact on a fairly routine basis. This does not mean that a tremendous amount of time must be spent with the classroom teacher, but periodic, warm, accepting contact with the teacher with information or questions about the child should be initiated.

Experience has shown that the classroom teacher is only able to handle three recommendations for the child. If there are more than this, it is almost impossible to get them implemented into the class without extra help from the outside. Frequently the audiologist's recommendations may

not get to the classroom teacher, but instead are filed in the central or teacher's folder for the child without having been read, or at least not remembered (EuDaly, 1993).

## Parent Considerations

One of the most neglected areas in working with children with hearing losses is parents. While it is true that there have been tremendous strides made in early intervention and intensive parent programs for newly identified children with hearing losses (see Chapter 15), there has been little attempt made to continue to provide support to parents as their children enter school. It may be that we have assumed that parents have accepted their child and that there are no issues that need to be addressed as the children enter school and complete the educational cycle. Some literature (Luterman, 1991; Worden, 1982) indicates that there are predictable times when parents actively grieve the fact that their children have a hearing loss—at the time of identification of the loss, at the entrance to school, as the child enters into adolescence, and as the child nears the end of high school. Yet there is no attempt to help parents go through these periods in any systematic way. Perhaps there is no one way this can be done, but certainly the profession needs to have increased sensitivity to parents as they enter into these critical periods.

### Providing Support to Parents

There is also some evidence to suggest that many parents maintain a hope that their child will have normal hearing at some point in time. There is little attempt to continue to educate parents and to help them deal with their feelings after the diagnosis of the hearing loss. Clark (1994) indicates that, while audiologists often lack training in counseling, they have the responsibility to provide more than hearing management of clients. When dealing with children, it is evident that one must also deal with families; they are unavoidably connected.

There are some things we can do with parents to help make their educational involvement with their children successful. Probably the biggest single area of concern is helping the parents accept their child. The issue is one of understanding that parents all have a dream child whom they dream about doing all of the things that they themselves were not able to do or be. When a child fails to meet the dream, there is a tendency to deny the reality of the child and to continue to believe in the dream child. This tendency is true for all parents, but it is frequently more evident when children have disabilities. If the parent can deny the reality of the disability, then they are able to maintain hope in the dream child emerging over time. Unfortunately, children who are hard of hearing are similar enough to children who hear that it is easy to deny the reality of the hearing loss. It may be that their child is able to do very well, but the fact is that all children with hearing losses will experience some of the effects of the hearing loss. The problems are compounded when the parents deny the effects of the hearing loss and insist that their child perform as though the hearing loss were not present. Our responsibility is to help the parents see, as much as we can, the reality of the loss and its effect on the child.

In addition to providing parent counseling, we can also help to sponsor parent groups that meet together on a monthly or bimonthly basis to talk about the things that are going on in the lives of their children. Hopefully, the parent group will have parents of different aged children, so that perspective can be provided. Of course there is tremendous variability across children, but what is usually discovered is that the feelings parents have about their children are very similar. The parents' interaction with each other often provides insights about their own acceptance that cannot be provided by the professional. For more information on parent groups and how they can be formed, see Atkins (1994).

### *Guiding Parents*

Another important role audiologists can play in working with parents is providing guidance. Parents often do not know where financial assistance can be found, what equipment to purchase, or where to get the best education for their child. The audiologist is in the best position to provide this information to the parents. If a trusting relationship is developed, the parents will seek out the audiologist for information, counseling, and guidance. If the audiologist is open, honest, caring and genuine, the parents will, in most instances, be able to grow through their periods of grief and confusion and be better able to parent their child.

## School Administration Considerations

Schools are bureaucracies, and administrators, for better or for worse, are the individuals in the bureaucracy who make the major decisions about how schools will be run and the personnel that are needed to run those schools. We have the laws that have been written to help make certain that persons with disabilities are educated appropriately. However, the laws are subject to many interpretations, and ignorance does not help translate laws into a meaningful reality. The vast majority of school administrators do not have a clear understanding of all the issues that are involved in the schools. Generally, most school administrators have been teachers for a number of years and then have gone back to school to get a certificate in school administration. Their training is usually focused on issues of school law, supervision, educational evaluation, child learning, discipline, and what it means to be a building principal. Most have little or no background on children with disabilities. Thus they are generally not aware of the problems children with hearing loss experience, and their primary concern is meeting the requirements of the law as they understand it.

### *Administrators Initiate Change*

In spite of their lack of knowledge, administrators are the primary facilitators for initiating change or beginning programs in the schools. Without the school administration's support, it is difficult to provide effective programming for students with hearing losses. Issues such as the selection of teachers and personnel who work with children who have hearing losses, provision of appropriate classrooms, and procurement of suitable equipment and instructional materials, are generally under the direct supervision of the building administrative staff. It is therefore important for the educational audiologist to help the administration to understand what children with hearing losses need, what the law is, and how the law ought to be interpreted. It is also important that the administration be able to visualize how programs can be easily implemented and the benefits these programs will provide to the school, the district, and the children themselves. It is therefore essential that the educational audiologist understand the programs in the school and what needs to be in place. The following are some ways to help administrators visualize what needs to happen.

**1.** The educational audiologist must maintain high visibility in the schools. One of the biggest problems we have in schools is that no one knows who the audiologist is, what he or she does, and where to find him or her. Audiologists need to make the administrator aware of their presence and what they are doing in the schools. Both formal and informal contacts with the administrators need to occur on a regular basis.

**2.** About once a month the administration needs to get a letter of acknowledgment from the audiologist with copies to their supervisors, expressing appreciation for the administrators' support. The letter should explain some of the important accomplishments that have happened because of the ability to serve the children.

**3.** The administrator in charge of a given school needs to be educated on a regular basis on what the children with hearing losses are able to do, the growth that is being made, and the great service that is being rendered. The idea is to help the administrator understand that the program is one that is going to make the school a better school

and some important advantages to the school exist because of this program.

## Direct Services to Children
### *Communication Issues*
The educational audiologist in most states functions more as a case manager than as a clinician. However, there are some places where the audiologist provides direct services to children with hearing losses. The services most frequently provided are auditory training and communication training. According to the limited research in this area (Wilson-Vlotman, 1984) direct training frequently focuses around the use of the *Auditory Skills Curriculum* (Audiologic Services & Southwest School for the Hearing Impaired, 1976a) in conjunction with the use of *The Test of Auditory Comprehension* (Audiologic Services & Southwest School for the Hearing Impaired, 1976b), and the *Developmental Approach to Successful Listening* (Stout and Van Ert Windle, 1986).

As noted earlier, about 5 percent of the audiologist's time in the school is spent in some kind of tutoring activity. The most frequently reported activities are helping the students complete homework assignments that were not understood or helping the students understand some of the reading from their coursework. Additionally, some audiologists have developed techniques to help the students learn how to study, answer questions, and ask questions that will help them in class. The audiologists have also done some work in the area of pragmatics, helping students learn how to do some of the things described earlier in the discussion in the communication lab.

### *Language Issues*
Recently, more attention is being paid to American Sign Language in the deaf community, and many children who are hard of hearing are beginning to use this language more frequently. In the survey discussed previously (Blair et al., 1989) over 80 percent of the audiologists who work in the schools reported a need to have at least a

working knowledge of sign language. Most audiologists work in settings in which total communication is used, but there is a growing focus on a bilingual–bicultural approach across the United States. Based on the information available, audiologists working in the schools need to have an ability to use sign language at a level where they can communicate with individuals with hearing loss who use this language.

Audiologists are also in the position to influence decisions about children and the kinds of language to which they will be exposed. It is clear that a number of children are being placed in a regular classroom with an interpreter; however, many of the interpreters are poorly trained and do little to help the child with the hearing loss understand what is being said in the classroom. Audiologists need to understand the issues, techniques, and approaches that are being used to educate the child with a hearing loss so that they can give meaningful input to the IEP process in the schools. Too often audiologists present information on hearing, but have no input on the educational programming of the child. This is not an appropriate stance for audiologists to take; they need to be active in helping to manage the education of the child with a hearing loss.

## WORKING IN SCHOOLS

### School Organization

The need to work effectively in the schools means that audiologists must be able to understand the operation and structure of the school system. It also means that they must be able to work cooperatively with others in the system to see that the needs of children are met. It is not enough to perform routine audiologic assessments and then send a report with recommendations that the teacher may not receive, or, if the recommendations are read by the teacher, may not be understood.

Schools are organized to run from the top down. The building principal, either alone or in conjunction with other staff, place children into a particular teacher's classroom. The teacher then takes the children who are assigned. Based on information received through a survey (Blair, Wilson-Vlotman, and Von Almen, 1989) audiologists feel they have influence over the placement of children. If the ideas suggested in this chapter are implemented, then the audiologist's impact can be expanded to benefit the child with a hearing loss.

### Other Professionals

It is becoming clear that if we are going to provide maximum assistance to a child with a hearing loss the work in the schools must be a collaborative venture. It is critical that educational audiologists learn how to work with other professionals in the school system. If we fail to work with others, we cannot succeed in helping the children, as discussed in Chapter 16. The educational audiologist needs to be knowledgeable about all the other professionals who work in the schools and be able to work with these people effectively.

### In-service Training

Finally, it is important that the educational audiologist know how to present in-service training sessions that are effective, interesting, useful, and memorable. I have found that too often in-service training is given at the worst time of day, by audiologists who may be more concerned with their professional status, rather than with providing information that is interesting, relevant, and appropriate to the classroom teacher. If the teacher cannot go back to the room and use the information that was presented, it is probably not remembered at all. My colleagues and I have found that in over half of the instances in which an in-service has been delivered, the classroom teacher does not remember ever attending an in-service meeting where the audiologist presented any information.

## SUMMARY

Educational audiology is a growing and necessary area of focus in the schools. The role of this professional is extensive, and the services rendered are critical for the benefit of children with hearing losses. Unfortunately, the number of educational audiologists is not nearly sufficient to meet the need. Part of the problem is that audiologists themselves do not have an understanding of the scope of practice in the school systems, and they frequently lack interest in working in the school setting. Perhaps, as the scope of practice is better understood, the challenges and opportunities that are present in the schools will serve as a motivator for more people to seek out this employment setting. Of course, much still needs to be done to convince the school systems that educational audiology is a critical service. However, as districts become more aware of the law and the rights that it provides to children who are deaf or hard of hearing, it will become more important for the schools to hire qualified professionals to help ensure that the children's needs are being met.

# REFERENCES

Allard, J. B., and Golden, D. C. (1991). Educational audiology: A comparison of service delivery systems utilized by Missouri schools. *Language, Speech, and Hearing Services in Schools, 22*(2), 5–11.

Alpiner, J. (ed.), (1978). *Handbook of Adult Rehabilitative Audiology.* Baltimore: Williams & Wilkins.

American Speech-Language-Hearing Association (ASHA). (1983). Audiology services in the schools position statement. *Asha, 25*(5), 53–60.

American Speech-Language-Hearing Association (ASHA). (1985). Guidelines for identification audiometry. *Asha, 27*(5), 49–52.

American Speech-Language-Hearing Association (1990). Guidelines for screening for hearing impairments and middle ear disorders. *Asha, 32* (Suppl. 2), 17–24.

American Speech-Language-Hearing Association (ASHA). (1993). Guidelines for audiology services in the schools. *Asha, 35*(3) (Suppl.), 24–32.

Anderson, K., and Matkin, N. (1991). Relationship of degree of longterm hearing loss to psychosocial impact and educational needs. In K. Anderson (ed.), Hearing conservation in the public schools revisited, *Seminars in Hearing, 12*(4), 340–364.

Atkins, D. V. (1994). Counseling children with hearing loss and their families. In J. G. Clark and F. N. Martin (eds.), *Effective Counseling in Audiology* (pp. 116–146) Englewood Cliffs, NJ: Prentice Hall.

Audiologic Services & Southwest School for the Hearing Impaired (1976a). *Auditory Skills Curriculum.* North Hollywood, California: Foreworks.

Audiologic Services & Southwest School for the Hearing Impaired (1976b). *The Test of Auditory Comprehension.* North Hollywood, California: Foreworks.

Barton, L. (1989). *Sound Levels in Elementary School Classrooms.* Unpublished master's thesis, Utah State University, Logan, Utah.

Berg, F. (1986). Characteristics of the target population. In F. Berg, J. Blair, S. Viehweg, A. Wilson-Vlotman. *Educational Audiology for the Hard of Hearing Child* (pp. 1–24). New York: Grune & Stratton.

Berg, F. (1994). *Acoustics & Sound Systems in Schools.* San Diego: Singular Publishing Group.

Berg, F., and Fletcher, S. (eds.), (1970). *The Hard of Hearing Child.* New York: Grune & Stratton.

Bess, F. (1985). The minimally hearing impaired child. *Ear and Hearing, 6,* 43–47.

Blair, J. (1986). Assessing the the hearing impaired. In F. Berg, J. Blair, S. Viehweg, and A. Wilson-Vlotman. *Educational Audiology for the Hard of Hearing Child* (pp. 37–80). New York: Grune & Stratton.

Blair, J., and Berg, F. (1982). Problems and needs of hard-of-hearing students and a model of delivery of services to schools. *Asha, 24*(8), 541–546.

Blair, J., and Von Almen, P. (1991). Historical growth of educational audiology and the educational audiology association. *Educational Audiology Monograph, 2*(1), ii–iii.

Blair, J., Wilson-Vlotman, A., and Von Almen, P. (1989). Educational audiologist: Practices, problems, directions, and recommendations. *Educational Audiology Monograph, 1*(1), 1–14.

Brackett, D. (1982). Language assessment protocols for hearing-impaired students. *Topics in Language Disorders,* June, 46–56.

Clark, J. G. (1994). Audiologists' counseling purview. In J. G. Clark and F. N. Martin (Eds.). *Effective Counseling in Audiology: Perspectives and Practice* (pp. 1–17). Englewood Cliffs, NJ: Prentice Hall.

Davis, J. (1967). *Our Forgotten Children: Hard-of-hearing Pupils in the Schools.* Minneapolis, MN: Audio Visual Library Service.

Davis, J., Shepard, N. Stelmachowicz, P., and Gorga, M. (1981) Characteristics of hearing-impaired children in the schools: Part I. Demographic data. *Journal of Speech and Hearing Disorders, 46,* 123–129.

Dodge, E. P., and Mallard, A. R. (1992). Social skills training using a collaborative service delivery model. *Language, Speech, and Hearing Services in Schools, 23*(2), 130–135.

Education for All Handicapped Children Act of 1975. Public Law 94-142. U.S. Congress, 94th Cong., 1st sess., U.S. Code, sec. 1041–1456.

EuDaly, M. (1993). The effectiveness of modes of communication used by audiologists with classroom teachers. Unpublished thesis, Utah State University, Logan, Utah.

Finitzo, T. (1988). Classroom acoustics. In R. Roeser and M. Downs, (eds.), *Auditory Disorders in School Children* (2nd ed., pp. 221–233). New York: Thieme Medical.

Finitzo-Hieber, T., and Tillman, T. (1978). Room acoustics effects on monosyllabic word discrimination ability for normal and hearing-impaired children. *Journal of Speech and Hearing Research, 21,* 440–458.

Flexer, C. (ed.). (1991). Current audiologic issues in the educational management of children with hearing loss. *Seminars in Hearing 12*(4). New York: Thieme Medical Publishers.

Lipscomb, M., Von Almen, P., and Blair, J. (1990). Students as active participants in hearing aid management. *Language, Speech, and Hearing Services in the Schools, 23*(3), 208–213.

Lundeen, C. (1991). Prevalence of hearing impairment among children. *Language Speech and Hearing Services in Schools, 22,* 269–271.

Luterman, D. (1991). *Counseling the Communicatively Disordered and Their Families* (2nd ed.). Austin: Pro Ed.

McCrone, W. (1979). Learned helplessness and level of underachievement among deaf adolescents. *Psychology in the Schools, 16,* 430; 434.

Moncur, J. P., and Dirks, D. (1967). Binaural and monaural speech intelligibility in reverberation. *Journal of Speech and Hearing Research, 10,* 186–195.

Moores, D. (1982). *Educating the Deaf* (2nd ed.). Boston: Houghton Mifflin Company.

Mykelbust, H. (1960). *Psychology of Deafness.* New York: Grune & Stratton.

Nix, G. (ed.), (1976). *Mainstream Education for Hearing Impaired Children and Youth.* New York: Grune & Stratton.

Northern, J., and Downs, M. (1991). *Hearing in Children* (4th ed.). Baltimore: Williams & Wilkins.

Northcott, W. (ed.). (1973). *The Hearing Impaired Child in the Regular Classroom.* Washington DC: The Alexander Graham Bell Association for the Deaf.

O'Neil, J. J. (1964). *The Hard of Hearing.* Englewood Cliffs, NJ: Prentice Hall.

Ross, M., and Giolas, T. G. (1978). *Auditory Management of Hearing-impaired Children.* Baltimore: University Press.

Salvia, J. and Ysseldyke, J. E. (1991). *Assessment* (5th ed.). Boston: Houghton Mifflin Company.

Sarnecky, E. A. (1981). Eliminating barriers to successful implementation of audiology programs in schools. *Hearing Aid Journal. 7,* 4; 36–38.

Scheetz, N. A. (1993). *Orientation to Deafness.* Boston: Allyn and Bacon.

Schildroth, A. N. and Karchmer, M. A. (1986). *Deaf Children in America.* San Diego: College-Hill Press.

Stout, G., and Van Ert Windle, J. (1986). *The Developmental Approach to Successful Listening.* Houston: DASL.

Thibodeau, L., and Saucedo, K. A. (1990). Consistency of electroacoustic characteristics across components of FM systems. *Journal of Speech and Hearing Research, 34,* 628–635.

Wilson-Vlotman, A. (1984). Educational audiology: Practices, attitudes and organizational structures. Unpublished doctoral dissertation, Utah State University.

Wilson-Vlotman, A., and Blair, J. (1984). A survey of audiologists working full-time in school systems. *Asha, 28*(11), 33–38.

Worden, J. W. (1982). *Grief Counseling and Grief Therapy.* New York: Springer Publishing Co.

Yater, V. (1978). Educational audiology. In J. Katz (ed.), *Handbook of Clinical Audiology* (2nd ed., pp. 589–595). Baltimore: Williams & Wilkins.

# CHILDHOOD COMMUNICATION DEVELOPMENT CHECKLIST

| AGE | HEARING AND UNDERSTANDING | TALKING |
|---|---|---|
| Birth | Does your child listen to speech? Does your child startle or cry at noises? Does your child awaken at loud sounds? | Does your child make pleasure sounds? When you play with your child, does he or she look at you, look away, and then look again? |
| 0–3 Months | Does your child turn to you when you speak? Does your child smile when spoken to? Does your child seem to recognize your voice and quiet down if crying? | Does your child repeat the same sounds a lot (cooing, gooing)? Does your child cry differently for different needs? Does your child smile when he or she sees you? |
| 4–6 Months | Does your child respond to "no"? Changes in your tone of voice? Does your child look around for the source of new sounds, e.g., the doorbell, vacuum, dog barking? Does your child notice toys that make sound? | Does your child's babbling sound more speech-like with lots of different sounds, including p, b, and m? Does your child tell you (by sound or gesture) when he wants you to do something again? Does your child make gurgling sounds when left alone? When playing with you? |
| 7 Months– 1 Year | Does your child recognize words for common items like "cup," "shoe," "juice"? Has your child begun to respond to requests ("Come here," "Want more?")? Does your child enjoy games like peek-a-boo and pat-a-cake? Does your child turn or look up when you call his name? Does your child listen when spoken to? | Does your child have one or two words (bye-bye, dada, mama, no) although they may not be clear? Does your child's babbling have both long and short groups of sounds such as "tata upup bibibibi"? Does your child imitate different speech sounds? Does your child use speech or noncrying sounds to get and keep your attention? |

| AGE | HEARING AND UNDERSTANDING | TALKING |
|---|---|---|
| 1–2 Years | Can your child point to pictures in a book when they are named?<br><br>Does your child point to a few body parts when asked?<br><br>Can your child follow simple commands and understand simple questions ("Roll the ball," "Kiss the baby," "Where's your shoe?")?<br><br>Does your child listen to simple stories, songs, and rhymes? | Is your child saying more and more words every month?<br><br>Does your child use some one to two word questions ("Where kitty?" "Go bye-bye?" "What's that?")?<br><br>Does your child put two words together ("More cookie," "No juice," "Mommy block")?<br><br>Does your child use many different consonant sounds at the beginning of words? |
| 2–3 Years | Does your child understand differences in meaning ("go-stop," "in-on," "big-little," "up-down")?<br><br>Does your child continue to notice sounds (telephone ringing, television sound, knocking at the door)?<br><br>Can your child follow two requests ("Get the ball and put it on the table")? | Does your child have a word for almost everything?<br><br>Does your child use two to three word "sentences" to talk about and ask for things?<br><br>Do you understand your child's speech most of the time?<br><br>Does your child often ask for or direct your attention to objects by naming them? |
| 3–4 Years | Does your child hear you when you call from another room?<br><br>Does your child hear television or radio at the same loudness level as other members of the family?<br><br>Does your child answer simple "who," "what," "where," "why" questions? | Does your child talk about what he does at school or at a friend's home?<br><br>Does your child say most sounds correctly except a few, like r, l, th, and s?<br><br>Does your child usually talk easily without repeating syllables or words?<br><br>Do people outside your family usually understand your child's speech?<br><br>Does your child use a lot of sentences that have four or more words? |
| 4–4½ Years | | Does your child's voice sound clear like other children's?<br><br>Does your child use sentences that give lots of details (e.g., "I have two red balls at home")?<br><br>Can your child tell you a story and stick pretty much to the topic? |

| AGE | HEARING AND UNDERSTANDING | TALKING |
|-----|---------------------------|---------|
| 4½–5 Years | Does your child hear and understand most of what is said at home and in school? Does everyone who knows your child think he hears well (teacher, baby sitter, grandparent, etc.)? Does your child pay attention to a story and answer simple questions about it? | Does your child communicate easily with other children and adults? Does your child say all sounds correctly except maybe one or two? Does your child use the same grammar as the rest of the family? |

Used with permission from "Your Child's Speech and Hearing" developed by the Psi Iota Xi Sorority and the American Speech-Language-Hearing Foundation. Revised by the ASHA Consumer Division.

A wide range of developmental variability exists among children. However, substantial deviation from these guidelines may indicate a developmental lag signaling the need for more in-depth evaluation.

# APPENDIX 2

# CHILDHOOD MOTOR
# DEVELOPMENT CHECKLIST

| | |
|---|---|
| 0–3 Months | Can your child raise her head from a supine position? |
| | Does your child look at your face when you are directly before him? |
| | Do your child's eyes follow a moving object? |
| 4–6 Months | Can your child hold onto a rattle? |
| | Does your child reach for and grasp objects? |
| | Can your child turn over? |
| | Does your child turn in response to sound? |
| | Can your child sit with minimal support? |
| 7 Months–1 Year | Can your child move an object from hand to hand? |
| | Can your child sit alone momentarily? |
| | Can your child sit for several minutes without support? |
| | Can your child pull himself up by holding onto things? |
| | Can your child move around her playpen or crib, or walk while holding onto supports? |
| 1–2 Years | Does your child wave good-bye or wave in response to others? |
| | Can your child walk with only one hand held? |
| | Can your child walk alone? |
| | Can your child balance three blocks together? |
| 2–3 Years | Does your child run? |
| | Does your child go up and down stairs? |
| | Can your child jump with both feet? |
| | Can your child stack six or more blocks together? |
| 3–4 Years | Can your child build a nine-block tower? |
| | Can your child copy a circle? |
| 4–5 Years | Can your child stand on one foot? |
| | Can your child draw a cross from a picture? |
| | Can your child copy a square? |
| | Can your child skip? |

Modified from the "Rapid Developmental Screening Checklist" developed by the Committee on Children with Handicaps, American Academy of Pediatrics, New York Chapter 3, District II. Significant deviation from the normative values above may warrant further evaluation. Prior to 2 years of age, the checklist should be adjusted for premature birth by subtracting the number of weeks of prematurity from the child's age.

# APPENDIX 3

# PEDIATRIC CASE HISTORY

### IDENTIFYING INFORMATION

Person completing this form:_____ Date:_____

Relationship to child:_____ Phone:_____

Address:_____
         No./Street                   City/State                  Zip

Child's name:_____ Birthdate:_____
          First        Middle        Last

Age:_____ Sex:_____ Social Security Number (or guardian's):_____

Address:_____
         No./Street                   City/State                  Zip

Phone: _____

Referred by:_____

Address:_____
         No./Street                   City/State                  Zip

Reason for referral: _____

_____

Insurance provider_____

Mother's name: _____ Birthdate:_____

Address:_____
         No./Street                   City/State                  Zip

Home phone: _____ Business phone: _____Occupation:_____

Place of employment: _____

Education: _____ Social Security Number:_____

Father's name: _____ Birthdate:_____

Address:_____
         No./Street                   City/State                  Zip

Home phone: _____ Business phone: _____Occupation:_____

Place of employment: _____

Education: _____ Social Security Number:_____

### HEARING

Do you think the child hears adequately? _____ Is her/his hearing constant or does it vary depending on the situation?_____

Has the child's hearing been tested? _____

    By whom? _____

    When? _____

    Results:_____

Does the child wear a hearing aid? _____

    Type of aid: _____

    Model and number: _____

    Ear(s) fitted: _____

    Daily wearing time: _____

Does the child do the following?

| Yes | No | | Explain |
|-----|-----|-----|---------|
| ____ | ____ | localize (find) the source of a sound | _____ |
| ____ | ____ | listen selectively in the presence of noise | _____ |
| ____ | ____ | ignore environmental sounds | _____ |
| ____ | ____ | respond consistently to sound | _____ |
| ____ | ____ | need to have spoken information repeated | _____ |
| ____ | ____ | follow verbal instructions | _____ |

Has the child had?

| Yes | No | | Explain |
|-----|-----|-----|---------|
| ____ | ____ | frequent ear infections | _____ |
| ____ | ____ | drainage of pus from the ear(s) | _____ |
| ____ | ____ | drainage of blood from the ear(s) | _____ |
| ____ | ____ | too much wax in the ear(s) | _____ |
| ____ | ____ | dizziness or balance problems | _____ |
| ____ | ____ | ear deformity | _____ |
| ____ | ____ | tubes placed in the ear drums | _____ |
| ____ | ____ | ears lanced | _____ |

## SPEECH OR LANGUAGE CONCERNS

What concerns you about the child's communication? _____

_____

Who first noticed the problem? _____ When?_____

Did speech or language development ever seem to stop? _____

    When? _____

Does the child seem embarrassed or frustrated about her/his speech or language? _____

Has there been any change in the child's speech/language in the past 6 months? _____

    Describe: _____

_____

What efforts have been made to help the child with speech/language at home?_____

_____

How is the child at:

    following directions _____

    carrying on a conversation _____

    being understood by parents _____ siblings_____

    playmates _____ other adults_____

Has the child had speech or language therapy?_____

    Where?_____

    When? _____

    Results: _____

What problems other than speech or hearing does the child have that worry you? _____

_____

_____

_____

What specific questions about the child do you want answered? _____

_____

_____

_____

_____

## FAMILY HISTORY

| Brothers/sisters | Date of birth _ | Sex | Speech/hearing/medical problems |
|---|---|---|---|
| _____ | _____ | ___ | _____ |
| _____ | _____ | ___ | _____ |
| _____ | _____ | ___ | _____ |
| _____ | _____ | ___ | _____ |

| Other household members | Relationship to child |
|---|---|
| _____ | _____ |
| _____ | _____ |
| _____ | _____ |

Has any member of child's family had:

| Yes | No | | Relationship to child |
|---|---|---|---|
| ____ | ____ | speech or language problems | _____ |
| ____ | ____ | hearing problems in childhood | _____ |

| Yes | No | | Relationship to child |
|-----|-----|-----|-----|
| ____ | ____ | hearing problems acquired as adult | _____ |
| ____ | ____ | learning disability | _____ |
| ____ | ____ | cleft lip or palate | _____ |
| ____ | ____ | mental retardation | _____ |
| ____ | ____ | other (please specify) | _____ |

Languages Spoken in the Home (including ASL and Signed English)

What languages are spoken in the home? _____

What language is most commonly used by the parents at home? _____

What language is most commonly used by the child when conversing with parents? _____

 with siblings? _____ with other children in the neighborhood? _____

What language is predominantly used with the child at school?_____

## MATERNAL HEALTH DURING PREGNANCY

How was the mother's physical health during pregnancy? (good, fair, poor)_____

 Explain_____

How was the mother's emotional health during pregnancy? (good, fair, poor) _____

What medications did the mother take during pregnancy? _____

 For what? _____ Which month(s)? _____

Did any of the following occur during pregnancy?

| Yes | No | | Explain |
|-----|-----|-----|-----|
| ____ | ____ | Bleeding | _____ |
| ____ | ____ | Rh incompatibility of parents | _____ |
| ____ | ____ | Measles (which months?) | _____ |
| ____ | ____ | Accidents | _____ |
| ____ | ____ | Illnesses/Infections | _____ |
| ____ | ____ | Rashes (which month?) | _____ |

## BIRTH HISTORY

How long was the mother's pregnancy? _____

What was the child's birth weight? _____

What type of delivery (normal, breech, Caesarean)? _____

Was labor induced? _____

What medications were given to the mother? _____ to child? _____

Were forceps used? _____ How long was labor? _____

What was the child's apgar score?_____

Were any of the following present at the child's birth?

| Yes | No | | Explain |
|-----|-----|-----|-----|
| ____ | ____ | Cord wrapped around neck | _____ |
| ____ | ____ | Jaundice | _____ |

| Yes | No | | Explain |
|---|---|---|---|
| ___ | ___ | Rh incompatibility | _____ |
| ___ | ___ | Convulsions | _____ |
| ___ | ___ | Blood transfusions | _____ |
| ___ | ___ | Respiratory distress | _____ |
| ___ | ___ | Heart problems | _____ |
| ___ | ___ | Hemorrhage | _____ |
| ___ | ___ | Cyanosis (bluish discoloration) | _____ |
| ___ | ___ | Oxygen administered (how long?) | _____ |
| ___ | ___ | Congenital malformations | _____ |
| ___ | ___ | Birth injuries | _____ |
| ___ | ___ | Incubator required (how long?) | _____ |
| ___ | ___ | Sucking or feeding problems | _____ |
| ___ | ___ | Other (specify) | _____ |

Name of hospital where the child was born: _____

Address: _____

## MEDICAL HISTORY

Who is the physician who has primary care of the child? _____

    Address: _____ Phone:_____

Does the physician know the child is being seen at this Center? _____

Has the child's general health been good, fair, or poor? _____

    Explain _____

Has the child ever had:

| Yes | Date | No | | Yes | Date | No | |
|---|---|---|---|---|---|---|---|
| ___ | _____ | ___ | Whooping cough | ___ | _____ | ___ | Rickets |
| ___ | _____ | ___ | Mumps | ___ | _____ | ___ | Rheumatic fever |
| ___ | _____ | ___ | Scarlet fever | ___ | _____ | ___ | Polio |
| ___ | _____ | ___ | Measles | ___ | _____ | ___ | Diabetes |
| ___ | _____ | ___ | Chicken pox | ___ | _____ | ___ | Nephritis |
| ___ | _____ | ___ | Pneumonia | ___ | _____ | ___ | Earaches |
| ___ | _____ | ___ | Diphtheria | ___ | _____ | ___ | Chronic colds |
| ___ | _____ | ___ | Frequent headaches | ___ | _____ | ___ | Head injury |
| ___ | _____ | ___ | Meningitis | ___ | _____ | ___ | Asthma |
| ___ | _____ | ___ | Sinus | ___ | _____ | ___ | Allergies |
| ___ | _____ | ___ | Epilepsy | ___ | _____ | ___ | Encephalitis |
| ___ | _____ | ___ | Typhoid | ___ | _____ | ___ | Tonsillitis |
| ___ | _____ | ___ | Tonsillectomy | ___ | _____ | ___ | Broken bones |
| ___ | _____ | ___ | Adenoidectomy | ___ | _____ | ___ | Cerebral palsy |
| ___ | _____ | ___ | Mastoidectomy | ___ | _____ | ___ | Anemia |
| ___ | _____ | ___ | Poor coordination | ___ | _____ | ___ | Mental retardation |

Allergies_____

Hospitalizations _____

Surgeries _____

Serious illnesses_____

Has the child had any high fevers (104° or more for longer than 24 hours)? _____

    When? _____

Has the child's vision been tested? _____

    By whom? _____

    When? _____

    Results:_____

What medications is the child presently taking? _____

Please list any food or physical restrictions that the child has. _____

_____

## DEVELOPMENTAL HISTORY

At what age did the child do the following?

    Sit unsupported _____

    Walk _____

    Begin saying words _____

    Put 2–3 words together _____

    Answer questions and relate facts verbally _____

    Bowel control_____

    Bladder control_____

Approximately how large is the child's vocabulary?_____

Compared to others in the family, was speech development fast, slow, or average? _____

_____

Compared to others in the family, was motor development fast, slow, or average? _____

_____

What is the child's present weight? _____ Height?_____

## PSYCHOSOCIAL HISTORY

For his age, do you consider the child to be socially mature, immature or average? _____

_____

Does the child have any of the following?

| Yes | No | | Explain |
|-----|-----|-----|---------|
| ____ | ____ | Nail biting | _____ |
| ____ | ____ | Thumb sucking | _____ |
| ____ | ____ | Bed wetting | _____ |
| ____ | ____ | Food fadisms | _____ |

| Yes | No | | Explain |
|-----|-----|-----|---------|
| ____ | ____ | Sleeping problems | _____ |
| ____ | ____ | Frequent crying | _____ |
| ____ | ____ | Frequent day dreaming | _____ |
| ____ | ____ | Frequent temper tantrums | _____ |
| ____ | ____ | Abnormal aggressiveness | _____ |
| ____ | ____ | Pronounced disobedience | _____ |
| ____ | ____ | Destructiveness | _____ |
| ____ | ____ | Mood swings | _____ |
| ____ | ____ | Hyperactivity | _____ |

How is the child disciplined?_____

Has the child been seen by a psychologist or psychiatrist?_____ At what age?_____

    Name _____

    Address _____

## EDUCATIONAL HISTORY

What school does the child presently attend? _____

    Grade _____ Teacher _____ Principal_____

    Address _____

How is the child's general school performance? (excellent, average, poor) _____

What subject(s) is the child best in? _____

What subject(s) is most difficult? _____

Has the child ever been in a special education classroom?_____ For what? _____

Has the child ever received resource teacher help?_____ For what? _____

Has the child ever been retained? _____ What grade?_____

Has the child been tested at school? _____

    By whom? _____

    When? _____

    Results: _____

Please check and sign below if you give the Center permission to contact the following agencies if further information is needed:

Physician _____ School_____

Signature _____ Relationship _____

## SPECIAL PRECAUTIONS

Person (friend or relative) to call in case of an emergency when parent or guardian is not available:

Name _____ Telephone number_____

Relationship to child _____

List foods that must <u>NOT</u> be given to your child:_____

_____

# APPENDIX 4

# SYNDROMES/CONDITIONS RESULTING IN HEARING LOSS IN CHILDREN

| SYNDROME/ CONDITION | CLINICAL CHARACTERISTICS | MODE OF INHERITANCE* | CHROMOSOMAL LOCATION | GENE MUTATION | REFERENCES† |
|---|---|---|---|---|---|
| Alport syndrome | Progressive SNHL<br>Nephritis<br>Ocular changes | XLR (some families AD) | Xq | COL4A5 collagen | Barker et al., 1990 |
| Aminoglycoside-induced SNHL | Nonsyndromic SNHL induced by amino-glycoside exposure | MT | MT | Ribosomal RNA gene | Prezant et al., 1993 |
| Biotinidase deficiency | Seizures<br>SNHL<br>Visual disorders<br>Skin rash<br>Hair loss<br>Mental retardation<br>Some reversal of symptoms possible with early treatment with biotin | AR | unknown | Unknown | Wolf et al., 1985 |
| Branchio-oto-renal syndrome | Mild–profound SN, conductive, or mixed hearing loss<br>Preauricular pits<br>Branchial cysts or fistulae<br>Altered ear shape<br>Structural kidney changes | AD | 8q | Unknown | Smith, Coppage et al., 1992<br>Kumar et al., 1992 |
| Congenital stapes fixation | Progressive mixed hearing loss<br>Perilymphatic gusher at surgery for stapes fixation | XLR | Xq | Unknown | Brunner et al., 1988 |
| **Craniosynostosis Syndromes** | | | | | |
| Apert syndrome | Premature closure of sutures<br>Skull malformations<br>Fusion of fingers and toes<br>High forehead<br>Hypertelorism (wide spaced eyes)<br>Downward sloping eyes<br>Small nose | Sporadic, some cases AD | Unknown | Unknown | Gorlin et al., 1990 |

| SYNDROME/ CONDITION | CLINICAL CHARACTERISTICS | MODE OF INHERITANCE* | CHROMOSOMAL LOCATION | GENE MUTATION | REFERENCES† |
|---|---|---|---|---|---|
| Apert syndrome *continued* | Narrow palate or cleft palate<br>Low-set ears<br>Congenital fixation of stapes, conductive hearing loss<br>Mental deficiency in some | | | | |
| Crouzon disease | Premature closure of sutures<br>Hypertelorism<br>Downward displacement of eyeballs due to shallow orbits<br>Mild to moderate conductive hearing loss<br>Closure of external auditory canal | AD | 10q | Unknown | Gorlin et al., 1990 |
| Pfeiffer syndrome | Premature closure of sutures—mild<br>Broad thumbs, broad great toes, short fingers and toes<br>Hypertelorism<br>High arched palate<br>Downward sloping eyes<br>Absent external auditory canals, conductive hearing loss | AD | Unknown | Unknown | Gorlin et al., 1990 |
| Saethre-Chotzen syndrome | Premature closure of sutures (variable)<br>Low-set frontal hairline<br>Facial asymmetry<br>Eyelids drooping<br>Webbing of fingers<br>Various skeletal anomalies<br>Mild conductive hearing loss | AD | 7p | Unknown | Gorlin et al., 1990 |
| Down syndrome | Developmental delay<br>Mental retardation<br>Cardiac malformations<br>Hypotonia<br>Epicanthal folds<br>Small, anomalous auricles<br>Conductive hearing loss common<br>SNHL in some | Chromosome 21 trisomy or translocation involving chromosome 21 | 21 | — | Jones, 1988 |

| SYNDROME/ CONDITION | CLINICAL CHARACTERISTICS | MODE OF INHERITANCE* | CHROMOSOMAL LOCATION | GENE MUTATION | REFERENCES† |
|---|---|---|---|---|---|
| Hunter syndrome | SN, conductive or mixed hearing loss<br>Growth deficiency<br>Mental and neurological deterioration<br>Coarse facial features | XLR | Xq | Iduronate-2-sulphatase gene | Hopwood et al., 1993 |
| Hurler syndrome | Conductive hearing loss<br>Growth deficiency<br>Mental and neurologic deterioration<br>Coarse facial features | AR | 4p | Alpha-L-iduronidase gene | Scott et al., 1990 |
| Jervell and Lange-Nielsen syndrome | Profound congenital SNHL<br>Ventricular tachycardia of the heart resulting in fainting episodes and sudden death in some | AR | Unknown | Unknown | Fraser et al., 1964 |
| Low frequency hearing loss 1 | Low frequency progressive SNHL<br>Onset in later childhood | AD | 5q | Unknown | Leon et al., 1992 |
| Neurofibromatosis, Type II | Bilateral acoustic neuroma | AD | 22q | Tumor suppressor gene | Narod et al., 1992 |
| Norrie's disease | Ocular defects<br>Mental deterioration<br>SNHL | XLR | Xp | Unknown | Berger et al., 1992 |
| Osteogenesis imperfecta, Type I | Connective tissue disorder with brittle bones<br>Conductive or mixed hearing loss<br>Blue sclerae | AD | 17p<br><br>7q | COL1A1 or COL1A2 genes | Sykes et al., 1990 |
| Pendred syndrome | Profound early-onset SNHL<br>Enlarged thyroid due to defect in organification of iodine | AR | 8q? | Unknown | van Wouwe et al., 1986 |
| Stickler syndrome | Severe myopia<br>Retinal detachment<br>Pierre Robin anomaly<br>Arthritis<br>SN, conductive or mixed hearing loss | AD | 12q | COL2A1 procollagen gene | Knowlton et al., 1989 |

| SYNDROME/ CONDITION | CLINICAL CHARACTERISTICS | MODE OF INHERITANCE* | CHROMOSOMAL LOCATION | GENE MUTATION | REFERENCES† |
|---|---|---|---|---|---|
| Treacher Collins syndrome | Pinnae malformations<br>Downslanting eyes<br>Small chin<br>Eyelid colobomas<br>Conductive hearing loss | AD | 5q | Unknown | Dixon et al., 1991 |
| Usher syndrome, Type I | Profound congenital SNHL<br>Retinitis pigmentosa<br>Vestibular dysfunction | AR | 11p,<br>11q,<br>14q | Unknown | Smith, Lee et al., 1992<br>Kaplan et al., 1992<br>Smith et al., 1994 |

*AD = autosomal dominant; AR = autosomal recessive; XLR = X-linked recessive; SNHL = sensorineural hearing loss; MT = mitochondrial

Compiled by Kathleen S. Arnos, Jamie Israel, Lisa Devlin, and Mary Pat Wilson.

†Full reference citations at the end of Chapter 2.

# INCREASING THE INTERVENTION UTILITY OF AUDIOLOGICAL REPORTS

Consider the effects of the identified hearing impairment for each of the following skills when describing the implications of the hearing status within audiological reports to school personnel:

- Consistency of speech or auditory signal (due to fluctuating hearing levels)
- Speech recognition
- Hearing and speech recognition in presence of background noise
- Distance hearing
- Locating sound source
- Detection versus comprehension
- Speech reading
- Fatigue due to concentration required for listening
- Attention
- Language command (receptive, expressive)
- Use of amplification (hearing aids, FM systems, etc.)
- Cognition (thinking, reasoning)
- Social/emotional state
- Suspected or diagnosed auditory processing complications
- Primary language mode
- Academic achievement and school performance

Consider the following needs relative to the identified hearing impairment when making recommendations for a child or student:

## Amplification Alternatives
- Personal (hearing aid, cochlear implant, tactile device)
- Personal FM system (hearing aid + FM)
- Auditory trainer (utilized without hearing aid)

- FM system only (Walkman-style)
- FM speaker system (sound field)

## Communication Modifications
- Seating to facilitate hearing and listening (e.g., front row, end seat with better—right or left—ear to class and away from noise sources) that is flexible for different situations
- Attention obtained prior to speaking with child/student
- Limited auditory distractions
- Ease with which to see face and lips for speechreading cues (avoid hands in front of face, mustaches well trimmed, no gum chewing)
- Information presented in simple, structured, sequential manner
- Teacher to check for understanding of information presented
- Clearly enunciated speech
- Extra time for processing information
- Limited visual distractions

## Physical Environment Modifications
- Noise reduction (carpet, room location, ventilation)
- Specialized lighting
- Room design specifications
- Flashing fire alarm
- Telecommunication device for the deaf (TDD) (more recently known as text telephone (TT))

## Instructional/Material Modifications
- Visual supplements (overhead, chalkboard, charts, vocabulary lists, lecture outlines)
- Captioning or scripts for television, movies, filmstrips

- Buddy system for notes, extra explanations/directions
- Checking for understanding of information
- Down time/break from listening
- Extra time to complete assignments
- Materials at appropriate reading levels

**Supplemental Services**

- Instruction in speech, language, pragmatic skill development
- Instruction in auditory skill development
- Instruction in speechreading skill development
- Interpreter (oral, manual)
- Note taker
- Instruction in hearing aid use, orientation, maintenance
- Instruction in social skills, responsibility, self-advocacy
- Instruction in sign language

**Personal and Family Services**

- Medical attention
- Financial assistance
- Counseling
- Community resources
- Vocational rehabilitation
- Ear protection
- Sign language instruction
- Family support
- Recreational opportunities
- Assistive devices
- Independent living skills
- Career/job exploration
- Deaf peer interaction opportunities

Adapted by Cheryl DeConde Johnson from Student Staffing Checklist for Hearing, *Effectiveness Indicators for Audiological Services.* Colorado Department of Education, 1992.

# APPENDIX 6

## BIBLIOTHERAPY: SUGGESTED READINGS FOR CHILD AND FAMILY

### Preschool and Elementary

*A Button in Her Ear* (1976) by Ada Litchfield
Albert Whitman & Company, Niles, IL

*Anna's Silent World* (1977) by Bernard Wolf
J. B. Lippincott Company, Philadelphia

*Claire and Emma* (1976) by Diana Peter
John Day Company, New York

*Ear Gear* (1986)by Carole B. Simko
Gallaudet University Press, Washington, DC

*Hearing Aids for You and the Zoo* (1984) by Richard Stoker and Janine Gaydos
Alexander Graham Bell Association
for the Deaf
3417 Volta Place, NW
Washington, DC 20007-2778
(202)337-5220 (TDD/Voice)

*Lisa and Her Soundless World* (1984) by Edna Levine
Human Sciences Press, New York

*My Friend Leslie: The Story of a Handicapped Child* (1983) by Maxine Rosenberg
Lothrop, Lee and Shepard Books, New York

*Now I Understand* (1986) by Gregory S. LaMore
Gallaudet University Press, Washington, DC

*Tim and His Hearing Aid* (1975) by Ronnie, Eleanor & Jean Porter
Alexander Graham Bell Association for the Deaf
3417 Volta Place, NW
Washington, DC 20007-2778
(202)337-5220 (TDD/Voice)

*We Can!* (1980) by Robin R. Star
Alexander Graham Bell Association for the Deaf
3417 Volta Place, NW
Washington, DC 20007-2778
(202)337-5220 (TDD/Voice)

### Adolescents

*Chelsea: The Story of a Signal Dog* (1992) by Paul Ogden
Time Warner Co., Boston

*How the Student with Hearing Loss Can Succeed in College: A Handbook for Students, Families and Professionals* (1990) by Carol Flexer, Denise Wray, and Ron Leavitt
Alexander Graham Bell Association for the Deaf
3417 Volta Place, NW
Washington, DC 20007-2778
(202)377-5220 (TDD/Voice)

*Silent Night* (1990) by Sue Thomas and S. Rickley Christian
Alexander Graham Bell Association for the Deaf
3417 Volta Place, NW
Washington, DC 20007-2778
(202)377-5220 (TDD/Voice)

*What's That Pig Outdoors? A Memoir of Deafness* (1991) by Henry Kisor
Alexander Graham Bell Association for the Deaf
3417 Volta Place, NW
Washington, DC 20007-2778
(202)377-5220 (TDD/Voice)

### Families

*The ABC's to Better Hearing* by John Greer Clark
HearCare, Inc., Cincinnati
(513)661-4327

*A Difference in the Family, Living with a Disabled Child* (1981) by Helen Featherstone
Penguin Books, New York

*A Hug Just Isn't Enough* (1980) by Caren Ferris
Gallaudet University Press, Washington, DC

*Amy: The Story of a Deaf Child* (1985) by Lou Ann Walker
Lodestar Books, E. P. Dutton, New York

*Broken Ears, Wounded Hearts* (1983) by George Harris
Gallaudet University Press, Washington, DC

*The Deaf Can Speak* (1985) by Pauline Shaw
Alexander Graham Bell Association for the Deaf
3417 Volta Place, NW
Washington, DC 20007-2778
(202)377-5220 (TDD/Voice)

*Deaf Like Me* (1978) by T. Spradley and J. Spradley
Random House, New York

*Deafness in the Family* (1987) by David Luterman
College Hill Press, Boston

*Family to Family* (1980) by Betty Griffin
Alexander Graham Bell Association for the Deaf
3417 Volta Place, NW
Washington, DC 20007-2778
(202)377-5220 (TDD/Voice)

*Growing Together* (1991) National Information Center on Deafness
Gallaudet University Press
800 Florida Avenue, NE
Washington, DC 20002

*Hearing Aids: A User's Guide* (1991) by Wayne Staab
512 East Canterbury Lane
Phoenix, AZ 85022

*Hearing Aids: Who Needs Them?* (1991) by David Pascoe
Big Bend Books, St. Louis, MO

*Hearing Impaired Children—A Guide for Concerned Parents and Professionals* (1988) by Richard C. Bevan
Charles C. Thomas, Springfield, IL

*How to Get the Most Out of Your Hearing Aid* (1981) by Joan Armbruster and Maurice Miller
Alexander Graham Bell Association for the Deaf
3417 Volta Place, NW
Washington, DC 20007-2778
(202)377-5220 (TDD/Voice)

*Language Says It All* (video) (1991)
Tripod Grapevine
2901 North Keystone Street
Burbank, CA 91504

*Learning to Listen: A Book by Mothers for Mothers of Hearing-Impaired Children* (1981) by Pat Vaughn
Alexander Graham Bell Association for the Deaf
3417 Volta Place, NW
Washington, DC 20007-2778
(202)377-5220 (TDD/Voice)

*Legal Rights of Persons with Disabilities: An Analysis of Federal Law* (1990) (Supplement, 1992) by Bonnie Tucker and Bruce Goldstein
Alexander Graham Bell Association for the Deaf
3417 Volta Place, NW
Washington, DC 20007-2778
(202)377-5220 (TDD/Voice)

*Once Upon a Time* (video) (1991)
Tripod Grapevine
2901 North Keystone Street
Burbank, CA 91504

*Negotiating the Special Education Maze: A Guide for Parents and Teachers* (1990) by Winifred Anderson, Stephen Chitwood, and Deidre Hayden
Alexander Graham Bell Association for the Deaf
3417 Volta Place,NW
Washington, DC 20007-2778
(202)377-5220 (TDD/Voice)

*94-142 and 504: Numbers That Add Up to Educational Rights for Handicapped Children: A Guide for Parents and Advocates* (1989) by Daniel Yohalem and Janet Dinsmore
Childrens Defense Fund
122 C Street, NW
Washington, DC 20001-2193

*Parents in Action: A Handbook for Experiences with Their Hearing-Impaired Children* (1978) by Grant B. Bitter
Alexander Graham Bell Association for the Deaf
3417 Volta Place, NW
Washington, DC 20007-2778
(202)377-5220 (TDD/Voice)

*Parents Guide to Speech and Deafness* (1984) by
Donald R. Calvert, Ph. D.
Alexander Graham Bell Association for the Deaf
3417 Volta Place, NW
Washington, DC 20007-2778
(202)377-5220 (TDD/Voice)

*Raising Your Hearing-Impaired Child: A Guideline for Parents* (1982) by Shirley McArthur
Alexander Graham Bell Association for the Deaf
3417 Volta Place, NW
Washington, DC 20007-2778
(202)377-5220 (TDD/Voice)

*Talk with Me* (1988) by Ellyn Altman
Alexander Graham Bell Association for the Deaf
3417 Volta Place, NW
Washington, DC 20007-2778
(202)377-5220 (TDD/Voice)

*When Your Child Is Deaf: A Guide for Parents* (1991) by David M. Luterman and Mark Ross
Alexander Graham Bell Association for the Deaf
3417 Volta Place, NW
Washington, DC 20007-2778
(202)377-5220 (TDD/Voice)

From Thibodeau, L. M. (1994). Counseling for pediatric amplification. In J. G. Clark and F. N. Martin (eds.), *Effective Counseling in Audiology: Perspectives and Practice*. Englewood Cliffs, NJ: Prentice Hall, 147–183.

# NATIONAL SUPPORT PROGRAMS AND ORGANIZATIONS FOR PROFESSIONALS AND FAMILIES

**Alexander Graham Bell Association for the Deaf**
3417 Volta Place NW
Washington, DC 20007
(202) 337-5220 (V/TDD)

**Alliance of Genetic Support Services**
35 Wisconsin Circle, Suite 440
Chevy Chase, MD 20815-7015
(301) 652-5553
(800) 336-GENE

**American Academy of Audiology (AAA)**
1735 North Lynn Street, Suite 950
Alexandria, VA 22209-2022
(800) AAA-2336 (V/TDD)
(703) 524-1923 (V/TDD)

**American Academy of Otolaryngology—Head and Neck Surgery**
1 Prince Street
Alexandria, VA 22314
(703) 836-4444 (V)
(703) 519-1585 (TDD)

**American Academy of Rehabilitative Audiology (ARA)**
P.O. Box 26532
Minneapolis, MN 55426
(612) 920-6098 (V)

**American Hearing Research Foundation**
55 East Washington Street
Suite 2022
Chicago, IL 60602
(312) 726-9670

**American Society for Deaf Children**
814 Thayer Avenue
Silver Spring, MD 20910
(800) 942-2732 (V/TDD)

**American Speech-Language-Hearing Association (ASHA)**
10801 Rockville Pike
Rockville, MD 20852
(800) 638-8255 (V/TDD)
(301) 897-5700 (V/TDD)

**Auditory-Verbal International (AVI)**
2121 Eisenhower, Suite 22314
Alexandria, VA 22314
(703) 739-1049 (V)
(703) 739-0874 (TDD)

**Beginnings for Parents of Hearing Impaired Children**
1504 Western Boulevard
Raleigh, NC 27606
(800) 541-4327 (V/TDD)
(919) 834-9100 (V/TDD)

**Captioned Films for the Deaf Modern Talking Pictures Services, Inc.**
5000 Park Street, North
St. Petersburg, FL 33709
(800) 237-6213 (V/TDD)

**Cochlear Implant Club International (CICI)**
P.O. Box 464
Buffalo, NY 14223-0464
(716) 838-4662 (V/TDD)

**Cochlear Implant Hotline/Cochlear Implant Information Center**
Cochlear Corporation
61 Inverness Drive East, Suite 200
Englewood, CO 80112
(800) 458-4999 (V/TDD)
(303) 790-9010

**Dogs for the Deaf, Inc.**
10175 Wheeler Road
Central Point, OR 97502
(503) 826-9220 (V/TDD)

**Family Services of America (FSA)**
44 East 23rd Street
New York, NY 10010
(800) 221-2681

**The Family Support Institute**
300-30 East 6th Avenue
Vancouver, BC V5T 4P4
(604) 875-1119

**Gallaudet University**
800 Florida Avenue NE
Washington, DC 20002
(800) 672-6720

**John Tracy Clinic, Correspondence Courses**
806 West Adams Boulevard
Los Angeles, CA 90007
(213) 748-5481

**National Association of Counsel for Children (NACC)**
1205 Oneida Street
Denver, CO 80220
(303) 321-3963

**National Association of the Deaf (NAD)**
814 Thayer Avenue
Silver Spring, MD 20910
(301) 587-1788 (V)
(301) 587-1789 (TDD)

**National Center for Law and Deafness**
Gallaudet University
800 Florida Avenue, NE
Washington, DC 20002-3695
(202) 651-5373 (V/TDD)

**National Cued Speech Association**
1615-B Oberlin Road
P.O. Box 31345
Raleigh, NC 27622-1345
(919) 828-1218 (V/TDD)

**National Information Center for Children and Youth with Disabilities**
P.O. Box 1492
Washington, DC 20013
(800) 695-0285 (V/TDD)
(202) 416-0300 (V/TDD)

**National Information Center on Deafness**
Gallaudet University
800 Florida Avenue NE
Washington, DC 20002
(202) 651-5051 (V)
(202) 651-5052 (TDD)

**National Institute on Deafness and Other Communication Disorders—Clearinghouse**
P.O. Box 37777
Washington, DC 20013-777
(800) 241-1044 (V)
(800) 241-1055 (TDD)

**Outreach Services Pre-College Program**
Gallaudet University
800 Florida Avenue NE
Washington, D.C. 20002
(800) 526-9105 (V/TDD)

**Parent to Parent/House Ear Institute**
2100 West Third Street
Los Angeles, CA 90057
(213) 483-4431 (V)
(213) 484-2642 (TDD)

**Red Acre Farm Hearing Dog Center**
109 Red Acre Road
Stow, MA 01775
(617) 897-8343 (V/TDD)
(617) 897-5370 (V)

**Registry of Interpreters for the Deaf, Inc.**
8719 Colesville Road, Suite 310
Silver Spring, MD 20910-3919
(301) 608-0050 (V/TDD)

**Resource Point, Cochlear Corporation**
Englewood, CO 80112
(800) 523-5798

**Self Help for Hard of Hearing People, Inc. (SHHH)**
7800 Wisconsin Avenue
Bethesda, MD 20814
(301) 657-2248 (V)
(301) 657-2249 (TDD)

**Sibling Information Network (Connecticut's University Affiliated Program)**
991 Main Street East
Hartford, CT 06108
(203) 282-7050

**Ski-Hi Institute**
Utah State University
Logan, UT 84322
(801) 752-4601

**Tripod**
2901 N. Keystone Street
Burbank, CA 91504
(800) 352-8888 (V/TDD)
(818) 972-2080 (V/TDD)

**Verbotonal Program for the Hearing Impaired**
Dr. Carl Asp
South Stadium Hall
University of Tennessee
Knoxville, TN 37996-0740
(615) 974-5019

Compiled by Donald M. Goldberg

APPENDIX 8

# PARENTAL SUGGESTIONS FOR SIBLINGS OF CHILDREN WITH HEARING LOSS

1. Let your children know you are available to talk and listen to them.
2. Be open and share your feelings with your children to help them feel safe in discussing their feelings with you.
3. Children need permission to express their feelings and thoughts without threat of feeling judged. You may need to be creative in eliciting these thoughts. By using puppets with young children you can discuss issues that may be difficult for the child to address directly.
4. Admit that you do not have all the answers.
5. Avoid making comparisons among siblings and praise them for helping one another and for helping in the family.
6. Demand the same behavior in the child who has a hearing impairment that you demand from your other children.
7. Responsibilities and chores should be equally divided according to ability and age.
8. Help siblings to develop their own identity and pursue their own interests.
9. Reassure all siblings of their importance in the family by asking for their input and advice in family discussions. Value them.
10. Emphasize the positive interactions that you observe among siblings.
11. Periodically provide your hearing child with correct and age-appropriate information about hearing loss, language, listening, and hearing aids so they will have the information when questioned by friends or strangers.
12. Role-play situations to provide siblings with specific responses they can give when they are asked questions.
13. Allow siblings to watch and to participate in activities designed to help the child with a hearing loss.
14. Reserve time in your schedule to spend with each child alone; let this be consistent and something the children and you can count on.
15. If a decision must be made that inconveniences the hearing siblings in favor of the child who has a hearing impairment, discuss it openly before it happens.
16. Make sure that your hearing children know that they are not responsible for their sibling's hearing loss.
17. Invite the siblings' friends to your home or on outings to see how the child with a hearing impairment functions within your family.
18. Notice if your hearing children are making up for what they perceive as your disappointment in having a child with a hearing impairment.
19. All brothers and sisters have difficulties relating to each other from time to time. Don't confuse normal sibling interaction with behavior related to the hearing impairment.
20. Attempt to keep the lives of all children somewhat separate with regard to toys, friends, special programs so that the individuality of each child can be ensured.

From: Atkins, D. (1994) Counseling children with hearing loss and their families. In J. G. Clark and F. N. Martin (eds.), *Effective Counseling in Audiology: Perspectives and Practice.* Englewood Cliffs, NJ: Prentice Hall, 116–146.

# GUIDELINES FOR THE CLASSROOM TEACHER

**Provide Preferential Seating:** The child with a hearing loss should be seated within 10 feet of the teacher and, if one ear has better hearing, slightly to one side so that the better hearing ear is toward the teacher and the class. Unless the child has a swivel seat it is difficult to visually follow a teacher around the room. If classroom activities necessitate the teacher be within a particular area of the room, the student with a hearing loss should be encouraged to move about the room to better see and hear the teacher. As a person's ability to recognize and meaningfully interpret speech sounds decreases in the presence of background noise, the child should be seated away from sources of auditory distraction such as open doors or windows, air conditioning vents, pencil sharpeners, etc.

**Always Remain Visible:** Clear visibility of a talker's facial expressions, gestures and body language can increase speech understanding by as much as 20 percent. As such, teaching position should remain as constant as possible during recitations. Light should be directed on the talker's face. Standing in front of a window, or other light source obscures facial movements and features. An exaggeration of lip and jaw movements in a conscious or unconscious attempt to make speech more clear will actually make speechreading more difficult. Speaking at a moderate speed with occasional pauses to facilitate comprehension is more appropriate.

**Do Not Assume Comprehension:** There is no particular lip or jaw movement that is specific to any single consonant of speech. While talker visibility is important, it does not ensure comprehension. We all have been guilty of feigning comprehension when we shied from asking for multiple repetitions. An affirmative nod when asked if understood can be misleading. It is often beneficial to ask the child to summarize what was said to determine if it was understood. If a repetition is needed, rephrasing the sentence can be beneficial as certain words may be more difficult to hear or visually discern than others or may not be within the child's vocabulary. When addressing the child individually, always begin with the child's name to ensure you have his attention. *Attention always precedes comprehension.*

**Watch for Fatigue:** The extra concentration required of the child with hearing loss just to keep up may result in exhaustion early in the day. To compensate, more difficult lessons should be scheduled for the early part of the day when the child is fresh, or alternated with activities that do not require greater concentration from the child with the hearing loss than from the others in the class.

**Use Visual Aids:** Visual perception will assist comprehension whenever noise or reverberation make auditory perception difficult; and a combined auditory/visual presentation will almost always yield higher comprehension. Key vocabulary words should be listed on the chalkboard or an overhead projector and defined prior to instruction. Summary statements may be similarly presented during lengthy classroom discussions. Movies, filmstrips, and taped materials should be accompanied by an outline summarizing the main points or preceded by a reading assignment on the same topic. The incorporation of visual aids into class presentations is beneficial to the normal-hearing student as well.

**Use the "Buddy System":** Even with instructional augmentation, teaching-style modifications, preferential seating, and appropriate amplification, the child with a hearing loss can miss key instructions and become frustrated with and lost within classroom instructions. A "buddy" can be extremely helpful even if the buddy's only job is to ensure the student with a hearing loss is on the correct page and that assignments are heard correctly. The teacher should also make arrangements with the school office so that the buddy's class notes may be photocopied for use by the student with hearing loss.

**Encourage Participation:** The child's presence in the regular classroom without participation in class activities is not indicative of educational or social progress. The child should be urged to participate in a variety of group activities including story telling, reading, drama, and conversation. If the child appears to be withdrawing from group activities, further counseling for the child and for the class may be in order.

**Use Outside Resources:** Parents and educational resource personnel such as the speech-language pathologist can help expose the child to vocabulary and language topics prior to the introduction of classroom instructional topics. Pre-instructional reading assignments on a subject area to be covered in the classroom can increase familiarity of vocabulary and concepts thereby facilitating classroom interaction. Keeping parents abreast of a child's performance and difficulties fosters their understanding of anticipated problem areas and helps to encourage their outside assistance.

**Monitor Performance of Hearing Aids and Assistive Listening Systems:** For more than a quarter of a century, research studies have revealed that children quite often attend school with malfunctioning amplification devices. Many young children do not recognize the difference between distortions from their hearing aids and distortions in their ears caused by the hearing loss. A day in school with malfunctioning hearing devices is a day lost to the child's education. Check with the school audiologist for guidance to ensure that all personal and classroom listening devices are functioning properly on a daily basis.

**Seek Assistance as Needed:** An open dialogue with other professionals enhances the educational success of the child with impaired hearing. If questions arise regarding the child's hearing status or performance in the classroom, the teacher should not hesitate to consult with the educational audiologist, the school speech-language pathologist, or the community audiologist who dispensed the child's hearing aids.

Revised from Clark, J. G. (1980). *Audiology for the School Speech-Language Clinician.* Springfield: Charles C. Thomas.

# OBSERVATIONS ON STUDENT PERFORMANCE IN THE CLASSROOM PRE–HEARING AID OR FM FITTING

Name: _____

Grade: _____

Age: _____

Teacher: _____

School: _____

Speech Language Pathologist: _____

Dates of Observation: _____

### Baseline Observations

Rate the student's performance relative to the average student in the classroom.

Attending in large group for teacher directed activity

Less _____     Same _____     More _____

Attending to classroom discussion

Less _____     Same _____     More _____

Participation in classroom discussion

Less _____     Same _____     More _____

Appropriateness of answers during classroom discussion

Less _____     Same _____     More _____

Ability to follow directions

Less _____     Same _____     More _____

Rate of response to questions posed during classroom discussion or when following directions

Less _____     Same _____     More _____

Watches speaker's face

Less _____     Same _____     More _____

Speaker repeats information at the child's request

Less _____     Same _____     More _____

Child moves closer to speaker where possible

Less _____     Same _____     More _____

Ease/comfort in listening situations

Less _____     Same _____     More _____

Overall listening skills

Poorer _____     Same _____     Better _____

Prepared by Carolyn Edwards.

# APPENDIX 11

# OBSERVATIONS OF STUDENT PERFORMANCE IN THE CLASSROOM POST–HEARING AID OR FM FITTING

Name:_____

Grade: _____

Age: _____

Teacher: _____

School:_____

Speech Language Pathologist:_____

Dates of Observation: _____

## I. Hearing Aid or FM Usage

Wears hearing aid or FM in school consistently
Yes _____ No _____

Positive attitude towards hearing aid or FM usage
by student     Yes _____ No _____

Positive acceptance of hearing aid or FM system
by classmates     Yes _____ No _____

## II. Observations during Trial Period

Attending in large group for teacher-directed activity
Improved _____ Same _____ Poorer _____

Attending to classroom discussion
Improved _____ Same _____ Poorer _____

Participation in classroom discussion
Improved _____ Same _____ Poorer _____

Ability to follow directions
Improved _____ Same _____ Poorer _____

Rate of response to questions posed during discussion or when following directions
Improved _____ Same _____ Poorer _____

Watches speaker's face
Improved _____ Same _____ Poorer _____

Speaker repeats information at the child's request
Less _____ Same _____ More _____

Child moves closer to speaker where possible
Less _____ Same _____ More _____

Ease/comfort in listening situations
Improved _____ Same _____ Poorer _____

Overall listening skills
Improved _____ Same _____ Poorer _____

Prepared by Carolyn Edwards.

# ASSISTIVE LISTENING AND ALERTING DEVICE MATERIALS

Compton, C. L. (1991). *Assistive Devices: Doorways to Independence.* Washington, DC: Gallaudet University. Available from Academy of Dispensing Audiologists, Columbia, SC, 1-800-445-8629.

This open-captioned videotape and book provide an overview of assistive devices and is designed to be used in waiting rooms, training centers, nursing homes, etc.

Interactive Product Locator
Support Syndicate for Audiology
1-800-869-0758

This software includes a needs assessment, catalogue of assistive devices and distributors, and a database of patient files. It may be used to determine which devices are needed, to preview the devices, and to identify appropriate distributors.

Knowledge Is Power
Mississippi Bend Area Education Agency
729-21st Street
Bettendorf, IA 52722-5096
319-359-1371

This is an educational program designed for audiologists, teachers of the hearing impaired, and speech-language pathologists to use with individual students or small groups of children with hearing loss. It is designed to teach children in preschool through high school basic information about hearing loss, coping skills, and communication strategies through learning activities, discussions, and handouts. Topics include anatomy of hearing, causes of hearing loss, hearing measurement, hearing aids, assistive listening devices, communication strategies, and resources.

Project PALS
Self Help for Hard of Hearing People, Inc.
7800 Wisconsin Avenue
Bethesda, MD 20814
301-647-2248 Voice
301-657-2249 TDD

PALS is a database of places with assistive listening systems. For a small fee, persons who travel may request a listing of churches, theaters, auditoriums, etc. in the area of interest in order to learn of available assistive devices.

SHHH Pamphlets
Self Help for Hard of Hearing People, Inc.
7800 Wisconsin Avenue
Bethesda, MD 20814
301-647-2248 Voice
301-657-2249 TDD

#251  Beyond the Hearing Aid with Assistive Listening Devices
#351  Travel for Hard of Hearing People
#451  Your Legal Rights as a Hearing Impaired Person
       Audio Induction Loops
       Budget Assistive Devices: The "Rube Goldberg" Approach
       A How-to-do-it . . . How-to-use-it Guide to a Personal Assistive Listening Device
       TV Listening: Some Do-it-Yourself Suggestions for Hard of Hearing People

Prepared by Linda M. Thibodeau

# EDITORS' NOTE

By virtue of the education and training received, audiologists will continue striving to ensure that, whenever possible, a child's residual hearing will be utilized to the fullest extent possible. For the vast majority of children with hearing loss, early identification and aggressive (re)habilitative intervention will provide a key to the entrance into and successful interaction within the society at large. However, as Ross (1992) discusses we cannot pursue our work without recognizing that the outcome of our endeavors will have some serious implications for some of the children we serve.

Despite our best efforts, audiologic successes with children who have profound hearing loss do not create "hearing" children. Significant barriers to aurally based communication will always remain, as will social barriers, as these children attempt to fully integrate within a hearing society. When these children become older and are aware of the presence of a separate Deaf community, they may reject contact with the Deaf culture that some would argue was their inherent destiny. Conversely, as Ross (1992) notes, some of these children may embrace this newfound culture with a bitterness toward the undue impositions placed upon them over the years by those striving for another audiologic success.

Despite the obvious caveat presented here, audiologists cannot presume to make decisions on Deaf culture. This decision can be made only by the child and family. Certainly, the more effectively the residual hearing has been developed, the wider will be the range of options these children and their parents will have as time goes on.

We hope that this book serves readers in their efforts on behalf of children living within a silenced world, so that through available technology they may begin to receive meaningful sound. With full recognition of the value and inherent integrity of members of the Deaf culture, audiologists must continue to strive toward "audiologic successes," which must always be measured in terms of the hearing world we hope to open for our young patients. To provide these children with less than our full knowledge and expertise as audiologists is not an option.

## REFERENCE

Ross, M. (1992). Implications of audiologic success. *Journal of the American Academy of Audiology 3:* 1–4.